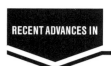

RECENT ADVANCES IN

KV-638-041

Surgery

Edited by

I. Taylor MD ChM FRCS
Professor of Surgery,
University of Southampton,
Southampton, UK

C. D. Johnson M Chir FRCS
Senior Lecturer in Surgery,
University of Southampton,
Southampton, UK

NUMBER FOURTEEN

CHURCHILL LIVINGSTONE
EDINBURGH LONDON MELBOURNE NEW YORK AND TOKYO 1991

CHURCHILL LIVINGSTONE
Medical Division of Longman Group UK Limited

Distributed in the United States of America by Churchill
Livingstone Inc., 1560 Broadway, New York, N.Y.
10036, and by associated companies, branches and
representatives throughout the world.

First published 1991

ISBN 0 443 044031
ISSN 0 143–8395

British Library Cataloguing in Publication Data
Recent advances in surgery. —No. 14
   1. Surgery—Periodicals
   617'.005   RD1

Library of Congress Catalog Card Number 79–41063

Printed in Great Britain at The Bath Press, Avon

Preface

Surgical practice continues to progress at a pleasingly rapid rate. Innovations, novel concepts, improvements in perioperative care and applications of the new biology to surgical practice all contribute to an exciting future for patients (and surgeons). Keeping up with these diverse advances becomes increasingly difficult. Nevertheless it is most important for individual surgeons to be aware of the possibilities that exist for their patients in the broad field of 'general surgery'. Not surprisingly the Royal Colleges have recognized the changing climate of surgical practice and the new regulations for the Fellowship examinations reflect this philosophy.

Recent Advances in Surgery is designed to reflect the rapid changes which are occurring in surgical practice and thought. It will now be published annually combining *Recent Advances in Surgery* (so expertly edited by Mr C. Russell) and *Progress in Surgery* (edited by Irving Taylor). The topics chosen are those in which surgeons would wish to familiarize themselves with the most up-to-date knowledge. Each author is an expert in the field and has been asked to provide a 'pithy', compact appraisal of the topic. The information should be valuable both to surgeons in training who are about to sit the Part II FRCS examinations, and to consultant surgeons wishing to keep abreast of the literature.

We would like to thank all the contributors for giving their time to write the reviews and the staff of Churchill Livingstone for their cooperation. We hope that readers enjoy the contributions as much as we have enjoyed assembling them.

Southampton 1991   I. Taylor
                                                                 C. D. Johnson

Contributors

John Bancewicz MB ChM FRCS
Reader in Surgery, University of Manchester; Consultant Surgeon, Hope
Hospital, Salford, UK

D. C. C. Bartolo MS FRCS
Consultant Surgeon, Royal Infirmary of Edinburgh, Edinburgh, UK

Irving S. Benjamin BSc MD FRCS
Professor and Director of Surgery, King's College School of Medicine and
Dentistry, King's College Hospital, London, UK

Jack Collin MA MD FRCS
Reader in Surgery, University of Oxford; Consultant Surgeon, John
Radcliffe Hospital, Oxford, UK

A. V. Darzi FRCSI
Registrar in General Surgery, Beaumont Hospital, Dublin, Republic of
Ireland

G. S. Duthie FRCS(Ed)
Department of Surgery, Royal Infirmary of Edinburgh, Edinburgh, UK

Colin D. Johnson MChir FRCS
Senior Lecturer in Surgery, University of Southampton; Honorary
Consultant Surgeon, Southampton General Hospital, Southampton, UK

Stephen J. Karran MChir (Cantab) FRCS FRCS (Ed)
Reader in Surgery, University of Southampton; Honorary Consultant
Surgeon, Southampton General Hospital, Southampton, UK

Francis B. V. Keane MD FRCS
Senior Lecturer, Trinity College, Dublin; Consultant Surgeon, Meath and
Adelaide Hospitals, Dublin, Republic of Ireland

Lt Colonel S. G. Mellor MB FRCS
Consultant Surgeon, Royal Army Medical College, London, UK

A. J. G. Miles FRCS
Surgical Registrar, Westminster Hospital, London, UK

M. Mughal MB ChB ChM FRCS
Senior Lecturer in Surgery, University of Manchester; Consultant
Surgeon, Hope Hospital, Salford, UK

R. David Rosin MS MB FRCS FRCS(Ed)
Consultant in General & Oncologic Surgery, St Mary's Hospital, London,
UK

L. F. A. Rossi MB FRCS
Consultant Surgeon, Wessex Regional Burns Plastic Surgery Unit,
Odstock Hospital, Salisbury, UK

Stuart D. Scott MS FRCS
Lecturer in Surgery, University of Southampton, Southampton, UK

P. G. Shakespeare BSc PhD
Director, Laing Laboratory for Burn Injury Investigation, Odstock
Hospital, Salisbury, UK

James A. Smallwood MS FRCS
Consultant General Surgeon, Southampton General Hospital,
Southampton, UK

W. A. Tanner MD FRCSI
Senior Lecturer, Trinity College, Dublin; Consultant Surgeon, Meath
Hospital, Dublin, Republic of Ireland

I. Taylor MD ChM FRCS
Professor of Surgery, University of Southampton, Southampton, UK

Christopher Wastell MS FRCS
Professor of Surgery, Westminster Hospital, London, UK

David Weeden MB BS FRCS FRCS(Ed)
Consultant Thoracic Surgeon, Wessex Regional Cardiothoracic Centre,
Southampton General Hospital, Southampton, UK

Contents

1

Alternatives to cholecystectomy for gallbladder stones

F. B. V. Keane   W. A. Tanner   A. Darzi

INTRODUCTION

Five years ago it would have been difficult to predict the changes and innovations that have occurred in the management of biliary lithiasis. One might wonder why these innovations did not occur earlier, but most of them are dependent on new technologies, which could only recently have been applied to gallstones. The rapidity of application of these new technologies has been fuelled by competition between the various proponents but most still require critical short-term and long-term evaluation.

Gallstones are common. The high prevalence of gallstones has become more apparent since the introduction of ultrasonography. An overall frequency of 8.2% was found amongst male civil servants in Rome, with an increase with age from 2.3% in the second decade to 14.4% in the seventh decade (GREPCO 1988). The incidence is thought to be higher in women in whom stones also occur at an earlier age.

As well as identifying the frequency of gallstones, ultrasonography has also helped to emphasize that gallstones are often harmless. Up to a few years ago prophylactic cholecystectomy for asymptomatic gallstones was performed routinely, especially for those under 50 years of age, in the expectation that they would soon develop symptoms, and that some might suffer serious or life threatening complications. William Mayo suggested that there was no such thing as an 'innocent' gallstone. However, recent data have shown that this practice and philosophy are incorrect. In 1983, Ransohoff et al summarized the outcome of 123 patients with asymptomatic gallstones with a follow-up ranging from 11–24 years. They found that only 13% developed biliary pain, while complications developed in 2%. By subjecting these and other data to decision analysis, they suggested that the burden of disease was insufficient to warrant surgical intervention in patients with silent gallstones (Ransohoff et al 1983).

Furthermore, the threat of developing gallbladder cancer does not alter the conclusion that prophylactic cholecystectomy should not be performed for silent gallstones. It has been calculated that cholecystectomy would have to be performed on 200 Caucasian women, with gallstones, to prevent

1

one gallbladder cancer (Weiss et al 1984). The risk is even less in black races, and only in American Indians is there a particular risk.

Until further data become available, conventional wisdom would dictate, therefore, that only symptomatic gallstones should be treated by whatever modality, be it surgery or otherwise. This review will concentrate on only that large group of patients who present electively with symptomatic gallstones, in other words, those with chronic cholecystitis or biliary colic, who require *elective* treatment. Little reference will be given to the complications of gallstones, especially acute cholecystitis, obstructive jaundice or acute pancreatitis, as these often require their own specific modes of therapy.

CHOLECYSTECTOMY—THE OPTIMUM TREATMENT?

Cholecystectomy has enjoyed a largely unchallenged supremacy as the treatment of choice in cholelithiasis since it was first performed by Carl Langenbusch in 1882. The risk of complications (7% or less) or death (0.5% or less) in the average case is low, and those deaths that do occur do so usually in those who display risk factors, particularly elderly patients with cardiopulmonary disease. Cholecystectomy, however, does inflict considerable discomfort on the patient, requires hospitalization for about one week, and loss of work for up to one month. This has considerable cost implications for both the patient and the health providing system. Moreover, up to 47% of patients continue to complain of some persistent symptoms and dyspepsia after cholecystectomy (Ros & Zambon 1987). Not surprisingly, therefore, both patients and their doctors are seeking gentler and more efficient forms of therapy for this essentially benign condition.

Nevertheless, not only does cholecystectomy eradicate the more specific symptoms of gallstones, but it also prevents their complications. When comparison is made to those techniques which are aimed at dealing with gallstones on their own, then cholecystectomy holds an obvious advantage in that, to all intents and purposes, gallstone recurrence is prevented. Nor does there seem to be a physiological price to be paid for removing the gallbladder. The so called post-cholecystectomy syndromes have been thought to be variously due to stones left behind within the bile duct, long cystic stump remnants, ampullary stenosis, or sphincter of Oddi dysfunction. Whilst these might have been corrected or prevented at surgery, they cannot be considered an outcome of cholecystectomy itself. An increased risk of developing large bowel cancer after cholecystectomy has been reported by some investigators but this has not been confirmed by others.

If cholecystectomy is to maintain its role as the main therapeutic option in the management of symptomatic stones then, clearly, its use should be confined to treating only those with the specific symptoms of gallstones.

Furthermore, the technical details of cholecystectomy are becoming more important, if comparisons are to be made with alternative techniques for dealing with gallstones. Surgeons should aim to cause less discomfort and to minimize hospital stay after cholecystectomy. There are already reports suggesting that hospital stay can be considerably reduced, even to as little as 24 hours (Moss 1986). The benefits of early ambulation after surgery are now well established. Nasogastric tubes can often be omitted or removed soon after surgery, and early post-operative feeding can usually be instituted safely. The necessity of draining the sub-hepatic space following cholecystectomy is no longer accepted as routine, and, indeed, may lead to more complications and prolonged hospital stay (Monson et al 1986).

Patient comfort and hospital stay can further be improved if the wound is less painful. Shorter incisions or mini-laparotomies cause less discomfort, and these can give adequate exposure for safe biliary surgery, particularly if the surgeon uses a modern fixed retraction system. This limited exposure will often prevent a full inspection of the abdominal contents, but the yield of laparotomy is small and indeed full abdominal exploration may lead to more post-operative discomfort, prolonged paralytic ileus, and a slower recovery. The use of long-acting local anaesthetics and subcutaneous wound closure, with or without sterile tapes, may also contribute to less wound discomfort. The benefit of many of these techniques is unproven, but may become more apparent after prospective assessment.

Laparoscopic cholecystectomy

The effort to reduce cholecystectomy to its least invasive form has led to the recent development of laparoscopic cholecystectomy (Reddick & Olsen 1989, Dubois et al 1990). This development has continued the widening spectrum of laparoscopic procedures that can now be performed, including many gynaecological operations, division of adhesions and appendicectomy. The rationale for laparoscopic cholecystectomy is based on the good cosmetic result, rapid resolution of post-operative pain, and a reduction of hospitalization with the ability to return to work soon after surgery.

Instruments for laparoscopic cholecystectomy are similar to those that are used in gynaecological surgery but a number of specific tools have been and are being evolved. A particular requirement at present is a video monitor attached to the laparoscope, such that both the surgeon and his assistants can interact during the surgical procedure.

After general anaesthesia and carbon dioxide insufflation of the patient's peritoneal cavity, a 10 mm port is inserted into the umbilicus for carrying the laparoscope. Subsequently, two 5 mm ports are inserted under laparoscopic vision into the right upper quadrant. These will be used to carry retracting forceps held by the assistant. A second 10 mm port is inserted below the xiphoid process in the midline, and to the right of the falciform ligament. This will carry the surgeon's dissecting forceps and clip applicator. After dividing adhesions to the gallbladder, the cystic duct and artery are freed by blunt dissection. The proximal and distal end of each are clipped, after which they can be divided. Before division of the cystic duct a cholangiogram can be performed by cannulating the cystic duct. Freeing of the gallbladder from the liver may then proceed using either an electro-cautery probe or laser dissection for haemostasis.

When the gallbladder is freed from the liver bed it can then be grasped by forceps inserted through the umbilical port. Meanwhile, the laparoscope is transferred to the upper 10 mm port and under direct vision the gall-bladder is then withdrawn with the port through the umbilical incision. When part of the gallbladder appears on the surface of the abdomen the gallbladder may be opened and its contents evacuated, prior to the delivery of the remainder of the gallbladder through the wound.

Laparoscopic cholecystectomy has developed in different centres with minor variations, and its advocates are excited by its early promise and suggest that over 90% of patients coming to cholecystectomy are suitable for this procedure. However, a unified approach has not yet been developed to cope with the 10–15% of patients coming to cholecystectomy who have stones in the common bile duct. One approach is to perform intravenous cholangiography, pre-operatively, in any patients coming to surgery and if choledocholithiasis is confirmed then a formal open operation is performed. Alternatively, if bile duct stones are found at a laparoscopic operation, on cholangiography, then either this procedure can be abandoned and an open operation with bile duct exploration can be performed, or an ERCP and stone removal can be carried out at a later date.

Because open operation might be required at any time during a laparo-scopic cholecystectomy, the procedure should always be performed by biliary surgeons. There are many potential hazards, particularly if there has been previous surgery with adhesion formation. Surgeons should learn and develop the necessary hand to eye coordination skills that are required in laparoscopic surgery carried out on a video screen.

ALTERNATIVES TO CHOLECYSTECTOMY

Dissatisfaction with some aspects of conventional cholecystectomy has led to a burgeoning of alternative techniques. The guiding concept behind many of these has been the idea that it is gallstones themselves that cause symptoms, and not the gallbladder, and if the gallstones are removed, then the symptoms will disappear. This approach seems logical if biliary colic is the primary symptom, but it pays scant attention to the entity of acalculus gallbladder disease, or, indeed, to the possibility of pain or symptoms coming from a diseased gallbladder in which gallstones may coexist incidentally.

The oldest of these cholecystectomy 'substitutes' was simple cholecyst-otomy, with stone removal (cholecystolithotomy). This has now been looked at with renewed interest using modern innovations. There are also the dissolution therapies to which extracorporeal shock wave lithotripsy has now been added. All of these procedures leave behind an intact gallbladder and it is therefore important that the possibility of recurrent stone formation and its prevention be considered subsequent to the successful application of these remedies.

Cholecystolithotomy

Although once popular, cholecystolithotomy has seldom been used in recent years except as an expeditious manoeuvre in gravely ill patients with acute cholecystitis or an empyaema. Its regular use fell into disfavour because of the reported high incidence of recurrent cholelithiasis of up to 80%. Many of these recurrences after cholecystolithotomy are likely to have resulted from stones being overlooked at operation. Indeed, it is suprisingly difficult to confirm gallbladder clearance when blind instrumentation is used to assess gallbladder contents through a small abdominal incision and a small opening in the gallbladder fundus.

Using contemporary endoscopic and radiological techniques, it is now easier to establish gallbladder clearance after simple cholecystotomy. Mini-cholecystotomy can be carried out under direct vision and local anaesthesia which may be particularly suitable in elderly high-risk patients (Leahy et al 1989). The correct site of the skin incision may at first be identified by ultrasound localization, and then at operation, when the fundus of the gallbladder is identified, it can be opened and the stones removed with forceps. Inspection of the gallbladder interior can then be carried out endoscopically, using a standard nephroscope, and residual stones may be removed or, if they are large, fragmented and then removed. Subsequent to gallbladder clearance, although it may be reasonable to close the gallbladder opening, it is more usual to intubate the gallbladder with a Foley catheter for up to 7–10 days. This permits contrast radiology prior to tube removal so that any residual fragments may be cleared. If bile duct stones are present then these may be dealt with by either instrumentation via the cystic duct or by ERCP.

Percutaneous direct cholecystotomy, with tract dilation, under ultrasound and radiological control and subsequent endoscopic stone removal further minimizes the surgical insult. Kellett and colleagues have adopted a one-stage procedure under general anaesthesia (Kellett et al 1988). The technique starts with a direct needle puncture of the gallbladder under ultrasound control. A catheter is then inserted into the gallbladder which is used to drain bile and subsequently to fill the gallbladder with a radiological contrast medium. A guide wire is then re-inserted into the gallbladder and along the guide wire the tract is dilated, using either balloon dilatation or telescoping metal dilators. When adequate dilatation has been achieved, an Amplatz sheath is inserted along the tract into the gallbladder through which a nephroscope can then be passed, allowing the inside of the gallbladder to be inspected and the stones to be removed. Any large fragments or stones can be fractured mechanically or by contact ultrasound, or electrohydraulic or laser lithotripsy, and can then be extracted. A Foley catheter is then placed through the sheath into the gallbladder and its balloon is inflated. Contrast can be injected through the Foley catheter to confirm gallbladder clearance and also to outline the biliary tree. Although hospital stay may be as short as 2–3 days, post-operative intubation with the Foley catheter is still required for 7–10 days and bile duct stones may also require treatment at a later date.

Unfortunately, as these techniques of cholecystolithotomy become less invasive, it then appears that more dependence is placed, not only on sophisticated radiology and instrumentation, but also on the specific skills of many personnel including surgeons, radiologists and anaesthetists. Also, not all patients coming to this form of elective treatment may be suitable, particularly those who are obese or those with shrunken contracted gall-bladders. There are also dangers associated with percutaneous puncture of the gallbladder, including severe hypotension and biliary peritonitis as well as haemorrhage and inadvertent intestinal puncture. These procedures should, therefore, be performed in an operating theatre setting so that surgical exploration can be resorted to, if required.

An alternative technique for gallbladder access has recently been described, using laparoscopic control (Jago 1990). This allows direct visualization of the gallbladder during puncture and cannulation, so avoiding some of the problems of ultrasound-guided puncture. Furthermore, obesity is thought not to be a problem with this technique.

Whilst in elderly high-risk patients it is unlikely that recurrent stone formation will be a significant clinical problem, it remains to be seen what the frequency of stone recurrence will be in younger patients coming to elective cholecystolithotomy. It may be contended that even if the incidence is high, then the procedure may be repeated, when required. Endoscopic access to the gallbladder does allow for the possibility of 'chemical' cholecystectomy, which might prevent gallstone recurrence. This will be discussed further when considering the prevention of gallstone recurrence.

Oral dissolution therapy for gallstones

In Western communities about 80% of gallstones are predominantly composed of cholesterol and are theoretically amenable to dissolution by drugs that increase cholesterol solubility in bile (Fromm 1986). Patients who form cholesterol gallstones are thought to do so because they secrete bile that is saturated with cholesterol and this may result from either increased secretion of cholesterol or reduced bile acids in bile. Bile acids given therapeutically not only increase the concentration of bile acids in bile but also inhibit cholesterol synthesis thus decreasing cholesterol saturation in bile. Chenodeoxycholic acid and ursodeoxycholic acid are two naturally occurring bile acids that may be given orally for gallstone dissolution. Both these bile acids reduce cholesterol saturation in bile and dissolve gallstones, but their effects are mediated by different mechanisms. Chenodeoxycholic acid by reducing HMG-CoA reductase activity reduces the synthesis and secretion of cholesterol but has no effect on cholesterol absorption while ursodeoxycholic acid reduces cholesterol secretion but has little effect on cholesterol synthesis. Bile acid synthesis from cholesterol in the liver may be increased by ursodeoxycholic acid but is reduced by chenodeoxycholic acid.

Both chenodeoxycholic acid and ursodeoxycholic acid have been widely used in clinical practice and appear to be safe. Chenodeoxycholic acid may cause diarrhoea and it also causes minor lipid alterations and thus carries a small theoretical risk of promoting atherosclerosis. Finally, it may also cause minor reversible elevations in serum liver enzymes. Ursodeoxycholic acid on the other hand causes no adverse effects and is therefore the preferred single agent in treating gallstones but it is more expensive.

Both these bile acids may be prescribed as a single preparation at a dose of approximately $15\,\mathrm{mg\,kg}^{-1}$ per 24 hours. However, they are often prescribed together at about $7\,\mathrm{mg\,kg}^{-1}$ per 24 hours each, because this not only reduces cost and side effects but also theoretically embraces their differing modes of action. Bile acids should not be given in pregnancy and caution should be exercised when there is associated hepatobiliary disease, inflammatory bowel disease or peptic ulceration.

Only one orally administered non-bile acid compound has been reported to dissolve gallstones in humans. Rowachol is an inexpensive preparation of six cyclic monoterpene oils, including menthol. It has been shown to depress HMG-CoA reductase and possibly to inhibit nucleation of crystals in bile. It also has choloretic and antispasmodic properties and is safe, with minimal side effects. In addition, it enhances the cholelitholytic effect of bile acids.

Patients suitable for treatment with these gallstone dissolving drugs should have a functioning gallbladder, as demonstrated either by opacification on oral cholecystography or by satisfactory contraction of the gallbladder after a fatty meal on ultrasonography. Stones should also be radiolucent and less than 15 mm in size. Small, floating, lucent stones on oral cholecystography are commonly rich in cholesterol and are particularly suitable for dissolution therapy. Such stones will be successfully dissolved in up to 90% of patients. However, dissolution therapy has no effect on calcified (radio-opaque) or pigment stones, nor on stones within a non-functioning gallbladder. Stones of 5–10 mm in diameter will dissolve within 1–2 years and smaller stones may take a shorter time. Patients require monitoring of the stone size during treatment which should be abandoned if there is no alteration after one year. Although gallstone symptoms may continue, the risk of complications does not appear to be increased during dissolution therapy.

Oral dissolution therapy for gallstones has not proved to be popular. Fewer than 20% of all patients with gallstones fulfil the requirements for dissolution therapy. Furthermore, dissolution therapy offers, at best, a 60% success rate in those patients who are suitable and who comply with the treatment for up to 18–24 months. Nevertheless, it remains a safe and convenient option for those who are unwilling or unfit to undergo cholecystectomy if that is the only alternative. It is perhaps the treatment of choice in patients with lucent, floating stones, who have only occasional symptoms. (The likelihood of recurrent stones after successful treatment will be discussed later.)

Extracorporeal shock wave lithotripsy

Extracorporeal shock wave lithotripsy (ESWL) has become the treatment of choice for renal calculi and its success in this setting has fostered the enthusiasm for biliary lithotripsy. Renal calculi pass spontaneously after fragmentation but the biliary tract does not offer such a simple passage for fragmented stones. Gallbladder stone fragments do not lie conveniently within an orthograde stream as do renal fragments, but usually lie inconveniently on the floor of the gallbladder. The gallbladder can contract, but the contraction is slow and incomplete, and often leaves a residual volume of 50% or more in patients with gallstones. Furthermore, the cystic duct is not an easy channel to navigate, as it comes from the posterior superior region of the gallbladder, is often only 1–3 mm in diameter, may be long and tortuous, and has a spiral valve. It is probably, therefore, as an adjunct to pharmacological dissolution therapy that ESWL has a role in the treatment of gallbladder stones. By fragmentation of stones to smaller particles or to a sand, lithotripsy should increase the surface area of the stones thus not only widening the spectrum of the stones that can be treated by dissolution therapy but also making that dissolution more rapid.

Table 1.1   Lithotripters for external biliary shock wave lithotripsy

Shock wave generation	Manufacturer	Lithotripters
Electrostatic	Direx	Direx X-1
Spark-Gap	Dornier	Dornier MPL
	Medstone	Medstone STS
	Northgate	Northgate SD-3
	Technomed	Sonolith 3000
Electromagnetic	K. Storz	Modulith SL 20
	Siemens	Lithostar
Piezoelectric	Diasonics	Therasonic
	EDAP	EDAP LT01
	R. Wolf	Piezolith 2300

This new technology has been greeted with perhaps exaggerated enthusiasm and a number of lithotripters have been developed (Table 1.1). All of these lithotripters fragment stones using shock waves that are generated under water and transmitted to the stones through a water bath or water-filled cushion and then through the soft tissues of the abdominal wall. Shock waves are generated in three ways. The spark-gap lithotripters create their shock waves using a high voltage spark between two electrodes. The resulting shock wave is then focussed by a semi-ellipsoid reflector so that the peak pressure is concentrated on a focal zone several centimetres in front of the generator. The piezoelectric lithotripters generate shock waves by applying an electrical current to many ceramic crystals set in a semi-ellipsoid fixed array. The crystals expand instantaneously, producing a shock wave that is tightly focussed on a small high pressure zone in front of the generator. Finally, electromagnetic lithotripters are constructed rather like a loudspeaker in which the shock wave is set up by rapidly repelling a metal plate. The resulting shock wave is then focussed by an acoustic lens.

Each of these devices produces a shock wave that differs in many respects and this makes their comparison difficult. Not only are there differences in the pressure produced but also in the configuration of the pressure wave, as well as in the size and shape of the peak pressure zone. All lithotripters can fragment stones and most now do not require the patient to have either anaesthesia, intravenous analgesia or sedation. However, the differences in the machines will probably influence the kind of stones that can be treated and the number of re-treatments that will be required. Targeting of the shock waves is done either by ultrasound or fluoroscopy. Ultrasound is the most satisfactory for gallbladder stones while fluoroscopy appears to be necessary for the treatment of bile duct stones.

Cavitation, induced by the negative rebound of the shock wave, is probably responsible for stone fragmentation during ESWL but this process may also cause tissue damage. The balance between efficacy and safety has, therefore, to be established for each kind of lithotripter. Indeed, the many variables in this form of treatment make its assessment very difficult at this stage. Investigators not only use different machines but often have very different approaches. Some require patients to stay in hospital while some invariably treat their patients as outpatients. Some try to treat their patients at a single session with perhaps the more powerful spark-gap machines, whilst others invariably re-treat their patients but the intervals between re-treatments may also vary between daily, weekly or even monthly. Most investigators treat their patients with concurrent oral dissolution therapy and this is based on both theoretical principles and accumulated evidence to date. Dissolution therapy varies from group to group but most commonly consists of bile acids, either singly or in combination, to which Rowachol may be added. A few patients have been shown to clear stone fragments a few days or weeks after lithotripsy and this has led to some investigators withholding dissolution therapy. It would seem unlikely, however, that this approach will work for many patients (Darzi et al 1990).

Complete stone clearance is the end-point of most published studies but so far there are few data on symptomatic relief after ESWL, with or without dissolution therapy. It may be that acalculous gallbladder pain may persist after stone clearance or, indeed, it may be that a small amount of tiny particulate matter detectable only by ultrasonography may be of no clinical relevance.

The initial published data relating to stone clearance after ESWL and dissolution therapy were obtained in highly selected patients. The Munich pioneers of ESWL require patients to have a functioning gallbladder in which the stones themselves should be solitary and radiolucent with a diameter of up to 30 mm, or up to three radiolucent stones, with a similar stone mass (Sackman et al 1988). They have also included some patients with a calcified rim on the gallstones. Using these criteria, they have achieved over 90% stone clearance for solitary stones, at between 12 and 18 months, whereas, the success rate for multiple stones at this time interval was about 60%. While these figures are very encouraging it is important to reflect that these selection criteria only included 28% of their gallstone population. Other investigators suggest that this figure may be closer to 15% in their own gallstone patient populations.

In an attempt to recruit more gallstone patients for this form of treatment, we and others have attempted to widen the selection criteria (Darzi et al 1989, Ponchon et al 1989). While it appears that more patients can achieve successful gallstone clearance than initially proposed by the

Table 1.2 Our selection and exclusion criteria for patients undergoing extracorporeal shock wave lithotripsy and dissolution therapy

Selection criteria
1. Symptomatic gallstones
2. Functioning gallbladder on oral cholecystogram
3. Lucent stones of any number, provided they fit into the size and calcification criteria
4. Size criteria—stones between 0.5 and 3 cm
5. Calcification criteria. Stones with a calcified rim 3 cm or less in size. Not stones with diffuse calcification or multiple calcified stones or stones with a calcified nucleus

Exclusion criteria
1. Pregnancy
2. Symptomatic and proven peptic ulceration—bile salts will aggravate symptoms
3. Elderly with severe cardiac or respiratory complaints or with back problems who are unable to lie prone for 30 minutes
4. Radiological evidence of common bile duct stones
5. Jaundice and/or hepatitis, and/or cirrhosis
6. Patients with acute cholecystitis
7. A recent attack of acute pancreatitis
8. Patients on anti-coagulants or cholesterol lowering drugs

Munich group, so too is it likely that by widening the selection criteria the failure rate may also increase. Clearly, more accurate definitions of patient suitability will have to be developed. Our own current criteria for ESWL and dissolution therapy are shown in Table 1.2.

The complications of combined ESWL and dissolution therapy may relate to either aspect of the treatment and those of dissolution therapy have already been discussed. Some lithotripters give more discomfort than others and require analgesia or sedation and there may be occasional mild post-treatment discomfort, some skin ecchymosis and haematuria. The incidence of acute pancreatitis is surprisingly low during follow-up, at 1–2%. However, the incidence of episodes of biliary colic occurring during post-lithotripsy dissolution therapy is high, often being greater than 30%. Our own experience has been lower than this, at around 13%, which we feel may be related to the spasmolytic properties of Rowachol which we include in our dissolution regime, together with bile acids.

Direct contact gallstone dissolution therapy

One of the major drawbacks of oral dissolution therapy, with or without ESWL, is the length of time required for complete gallstone clearance. Thistle and colleagues have adopted a more rapid approach to the dissolution therapy of gallstones. Pivotal to this concept has been the identification of an aliphatic ether liquid, methyl tert-butyl ether (MTBE) which rapidly dissolves cholesterol gallstones (Thistle et al 1989).

Their technique involves the insertion of a 5-French pigtail polyethylene catheter, transcutaneously and transhepatically into the gallbladder. This is carried out using local anaesthesia and under a combination of fluoroscopic and ultrasound control. Once the catheter is inserted, 5–10 ml of MTBE is repeatedly instilled and aspirated through the catheter thus constantly agitating the gallbladder contents. Suitable cholesterol stones can usually be cleared in a matter of hours although some take up to 3 days, especially if the stones are multiple. At the end of the procedure, the catheter may be removed, and during its removal, a Gelfoam plug can be injected into the tract to prevent bile leakage.

Whilst MTBE dissolution appears to be an attractive option for gallstone treatment, there are notable drawbacks. Firstly, the gallbladder itself has to be accessible. Next, the use of MTBE is limited to cholesterol gallstones and should the stones contain calcium then dissolution is ineffective. Calcium solvents, such as ethylene diamine tetra-acetic acid (EDTA) have, as yet, not been proven to be of clinical value.

The procedure itself is slow and painstaking if carried out by hand. The toxicity of MTBE is also a cause for anxiety, being both highly flammable and explosive. Side effects include nausea, vomiting, duodenal erosion, haemolysis and inadvertent anaesthesia. However, some of the tedium and side effects can be reduced using a microprocessor assisted pump, which prevents over-distension of the gallbladder and also achieves more efficient recovery of MTBE. Finally, non-dissolved fragments may remain in the gallbladder thus forming a potential nidus for future gallstone formation.

Contact gallstone dissolution therapy with MTBE is unlikely at present to have a wide role in clinical practice. Its use remains experimental and should be confined to those centres that have the special equipment and skills required. Perhaps the matter will not rest there and maybe new solvents will be developed. Alternatively, combined treatments using contact dissolution together with ESWL or trans-catheter fragmentation using tunable dye or neodymium-Yag laser pulses may find an application.

GALLSTONE RECURRENCE AND ITS PREVENTION

Prevention of gallstone formation has been considered under the headings of primary, secondary or tertiary prevention. Primary prevention would be the inhibition of the formation of stones in those who have not previously had gallstones. Secondary prevention might be considered as the successful management of silent gallstones by either clearing them or preventing them from becoming symptomatic. Tertiary prevention is the prevention of gallstone recurrence in those who have an intact gallbladder but have already had their gallstones cleared or dissolved either by cholecysto-lithotomy or by oral dissolution therapy with or without ESWL, or by contact dissolution therapy. It is tertiary prevention that we are most concerned with here.

Previously reported high recurrence rates after cholecystolithotomy are difficult to interpret because neither the tools nor the radiological skills were available to confirm absolutely complete gallbladder clearance. Most available information on gallstone recurrence comes, therefore, from studies carried out on patients after dissolution therapy. These suggest that the recurrence rate in patients followed for 2–12 years after confirmed complete gallstone dissolution is between 30 and 65%. However, few patients have been followed for more than 5 years, and so, the most reliable data are based on studies conducted over this period of time, and it is in these studies that recurrence rates range from 30–50%.

Early reports, and our own experience, suggest that the frequency of gallstone recurrence after successful lithotripsy and dissolution therapy is similar to the recurrence rate after dissolution therapy on its own. It is, however, too early to assess the frequency of recurrence after cholecysto-lithotomy using endoscopic procedures. Arguably, these procedures offer the most accurate means of confirmation of complete gallstone clearance and this in itself might lead to a lower incidence of recurrence. Never-theless, the incidence of gallstone recurrence appears to be high if the gallbladder is left in-situ. This raises a number of issues to which, so far, there are no clear answers. For example, do these recurrent stones, like their forbears, cause symptoms? Should patients be followed-up, and if so, for how long? Finally, can these recurrences be prevented, and if so, is prevention more cost effective than re-treating stones when they recur?

As in primary gallstone formation, the development of recurrent stones probably requires two, or maybe even three abnormalities. Predominantly, there is the development of supersaturated bile. When bile acid therapy is withdrawn there is a rapid and inevitable rebound of biliary cholesterol saturation, but as this does not always lead to gallstone recurrence, other factors may be involved. These could include nucleation defects and impaired gallbladder motor function.

To date, efforts to prevent cholesterol gallstone recurrence have largely been based on attempts to modify pharmacologically the rebound in biliary cholesterol saturation. However, few trials have been designed scientifically as prospective, random allocation studies, and most have only included small numbers of patients which make it difficult to identify sub-groups at-risk. Despite this, there is evidence to suggest that ursodeoxycholic acid probably reduces the incidence of gallstone recurrence when taken at a dose of about 300 mg per day, particularly in young patients (Villanova et al 1989).

An alternative pharmacological approach to the prevention of gallstone recurrence may be by the manipulation of nucleation factors. Patients with solitary primary stones are less likely to develop recurrences than those who initially had multiple stones, perhaps because of differences in the propensity to induce 'seeding' of stones from supersaturated bile. Non-steroidal anti-inflammatory drugs (NSAID) are thought to inhibit prostaglandin-mediated stimulation of mucin secretion by the gallbladder, and mucin may in turn act as a nucleating agent. In one study, which looked at patients' drug history whilst assessing recurrence rates after gallstone dissolution, it was found that those taking NSAID had significantly reduced incidence of recurrence (Hood et al 1987). Further evidence supporting NSAID as candidates for preventative therapy comes from animal studies in which aspirin has been shown to prevent primary cholesterol gallstone formation in prairie dogs fed a lithogenic diet (Lee et al 1981).

Cholecystolithotomy, by allowing access to the gallbladder, offers an alternative method for preventing stone recurrence. So-called, 'chemical' cholecystectomy requires two components; gallbladder mucosal ablation and cystic duct obstruction (Becker & Kopecky 1988). A number of chemicals have been shown to destroy gallbladder mucosa in the experimental animal over short periods. However, in many instances re-epithelialization takes place from the cystic duct. Cystic duct occlusion, using a bipolar electrocoagulation catheter has overcome this and has been successfully described in experimental animals. Thus, chemical cholecystectomy, in combination with stone removal, offers a theoretical option for managing gallbladder stones and preventing their recurrence using a minimalist one-stage technique. But this procedure is still experimental

Table 1.3 Cost implications when considering therapies for elective treatment of patients with symptomatic gallstones

	New equipment	Cost of one treatment	Hospitalization	Pre- or re-treatments required?
Oral dissolution therapy	Nil	Small	None	Always
ESWL and oral dissolution	High (Lithotripter)	Moderate	None	—Always dissolution —Usually ESWL
MTBE contact dissolution	Moderate	High	2–3 days	Unusual
Percutaneous cholecystolithotomy	Moderate	High	2–3 days	Unusual
Laparoscopic cholecystectomy	Moderate	High	2–3 days	Never
Conventional cholecystectomy	Nil (Already present)	High	7 days	Never

and anxiety must remain that such an ablative iatrogenic process may possibly increase the likelihood of gallbladder cancer.

CONCLUSION AND KEY POINTS FOR CLINICAL PRACTICE

These new techniques for dealing with gallbladder stones and the rapidity of their development and introduction has led to some confusion for the surgeon working at the coal face of clinical practice. Added to this, many of the newer treatments, although attaining wide publicity and often requested by patients themselves, have never been subjected to controlled

Table 1.4 Patient related factors when considering therapies for symptomatic gallstones

	Percentage of gallstone population suitable (%)	Pain or discomfort	Cosmesis	Potential complications	Work disability	Chance of recurrence
Oral dissolution therapy	10	Minimal (30% colic)	No scar	Minimal	Nil	High
ESWL and oral dissolution	30	Minimal (30% colic)	No scar	Minimal	Nil	High
MTBE contact dissolution	40	Moderate	Minor scar	Moderate	1 week	? High
Percutaneous cholecysto-lithotomy	70	Moderate	Minor scar	Moderate	1 week	? High
Laparoscopic cholecystectomy	80	Moderate	Minor scar	Moderate	1 week	Nil
Conventional cholecystectomy	98	Most	Scar	Moderate	1 month	Nil

clinical studies and analysis. In the light of this, cholecystectomy must still remain the acceptable treatment for the large majority of patients with symptomatic gallstones.

Concern must be expressed about the new profusion of players in the field of gallstones and their management. Therapies are now being instituted by primary care doctors and a variety of hospital specialists, perhaps inappropriately. This may lead to surgeons having to deal with a later and more complicated form of gallstone disease, and may be in older patients, with the inevitable consequence of increased morbidity and mortality. Surgical trainees, whilst getting less exposure to straightforward biliary surgery may also have to deal with more complicated and difficult cases.

Nevertheless, progress is inevitable and the concept of minimally invasive treatment is an aspiration that surgeons must espouse. We have attempted to summarize the methodologies that have been discussed. Table 1.3 reviews the cost implications that have to be considered with each of the modalities, while Table 1.4 looks at patient related factors. Clearly there are factors that have implications in both tables. Take, for example, the 'chance of stone recurrence'. Whilst this will probably have implications for the patient, it may also have important cost implications. The tabulated summaries, although crude and approximate, are aimed at providing surgeons with a global view of the important points that should be considered before adopting any of the techniques that have been discussed. Two other factors, not included in this tabulated assessment, include post-treatment symptomatology, which requires assessment for each modality and then comparison made with cholecystectomy. Finally, it must be remembered that approximately 15% of patients with symptomatic gallstones have associated stones within their bile ducts. Only conventional cholecystectomy allows concurrent removal of these stones, whilst the alternative techniques will always require some supplementary approach, mainly based on endoscopic retrograde cholangiography and sphincterotomy with stone removal.

REFERENCES

Becker G J, Kopecky K K 1988 Can the newer interventional procedures replace cholecystectomy for cholelithiasis?—The potential role of cystic duct ablation. Radiology 167: 275–279

Darzi A, Monson J R T, O'Morain C et al 1989 The selection criteria for gallstone extracorporeal shock wave lithotripsy can be widened. Br Med J 299: 302–303

Darzi A, Leahy A, O'Morain C et al 1990 Does gallstone clearance require both extracorporeal shock wave lithotripsy and chemical dissolution? Br J Surg (in press)

Dubois F, Icard P, Berthelot G et al 1990 Coelioscopic cholecystectomy. Ann Surg 211: 60–62

Fromm H 1986 Gallstone dissolution therapy. Gastroenterology 91: 1560–1567

Hood K, Gleeson D, Ruppin D C et al 1987 The British/Belgian Gallstone Study Groups post dissolution trial. Gut 28: A1359

Jago R 1990 What are the limitations of percutaneous cholecystolithotomy? Gut 31: A590

Kellett M J, Wickham J E, Russell R C 1988 Percutaneous cholecystolithotomy. Br Med J i: 453–455

Leahy A L, Darzi A W, O'Gorman S et al 1989 Minimal surgery for symptomatic gallstones: A safe new procedure in high-risk patients. Br J Surg 6: 1343

Lee S P, Carey M C, Lamont J T 1981 Aspirin prevention of cholesterol gallstone formation in prairie dogs. Science 211: 1429–1430

Monson J R, MacFie J, Irving H et al 1986 Does drainage increase the risk of sub-hepatic collections following cholecystectomy? Br J Surg 73: 993–994

Moss G 1986 Discharge within 24 hours of elective cholecystectomy. Arch Surg 121: 1159–1161

Ponchon T, Barkur A N, Pujol B et al 1989 Gallstone disappearance after extracorporeal lithotripsy and oral bile acid dissolution. Gastroenterology 97: 457–463

Ransohoff D F, Gracie W A, Wolfenson L B et al 1983 Prophylactic cholecystectomy or expectant management for patients with silent gallstones. Ann Intern Med 99: 199–204

Reddick E J, Olsen D O 1989 Laparoscopic laser cholecystectomy. Surg Endoscopy 3: 131–133

Ros E, Zambon D 1987 Post-cholecystectomy symptoms. A prospective study of gallstone patients before and two years after surgery. Gut 28: 1500–1504

Sackman M, Delius M, Sauerbruch T et al 1988 Shock-wave lithotripsy of gallstones. The first 175 patients. New Engl J Med 318: 393–397

The Rome Group for Epidemiology and Prevention of Cholelithiasis (GREPCO) 1988 The epidemiology of gallstone disease in Rome, Italy Part 1 and Part 2. Hepatology 8: 904–913

Thistle J L, May G R, Burder C E et al 1989 Dissolution of cholesterol gallbladder stones by methyl tert-butyl ether administered by percutaneous transhepatic catheter. New Engl J Med 320: 633–639

Villanova N, Bazzoli F, Taroni F et al 1989 Gallstone recurrence after successful oral bile acid treatment. Gastroenterology 87: 726–731

Weiss K M, Ferrell R E, Harris C L et al 1984 Genetics and epidemiology of gallbladder disease in new world native peoples. Am J Hum Genet 36: 1259–1278

2

Gastro-oesophageal reflux— pathophysiology and treatment

M. Mughal   J. Bancewicz

INTRODUCTION

Gastro-oesophageal reflux is a common condition. A recent study has shown that over 60% of the population suffer or have suffered from dyspepsia of whom 69% give a history of heartburn (Jones & Lydeard 1989). Only about a quarter of them seek medical advice. Measurement of oesophageal pH has shown that gastro-oesophageal reflux is physiological; it only becomes pathological when it is excessive, resulting in symptoms or complications and is then called gastro-oesophageal reflux disease (GORD). Oesophagitis is often, but not invariably associated with GORD and similarly, hiatus hernia may or may not be relevant. Clearly, therefore, GORD, oesophagitis and hiatus hernia are not synonymous.

PATHOPHYSIOLOGY

Before tests of oesophageal function became available, knowledge of the oesophagus was mainly anatomical, from dissection and barium studies. Not surprisingly, therefore, competence of the cardia was perceived in purely physical terms. Although physical factors are important, studies of oesophageal function by manometry and prolonged pH monitoring indicate that other, more important factors are involved and have clarified our understanding of gastro-oesophageal reflux.

Lower oesophageal sphincter

Although an anatomical sphincter at the cardio-oesophageal junction is difficult to show, a high pressure zone can be demonstrated by manometry in the most distal 1 to 4 cm of the oesophagus (Fyke et al 1956). The resting pressure in this zone is between 20 and 40 mmHg in normal subjects. This falls to equal gastric pressure on swallowing, in anticipation of a primary peristaltic wave propelling a bolus into the stomach. The pressure in this zone is responsive to many endogenous and exogenous stimuli. It rises on administration of cholinergic and alpha-adrenergic agents, and is decreased by secretin, cholecystokinin and glucagon. Certain drugs, for example, theophylline, and foodstuffs such as coffee and fatty foods also decrease this

17

pressure. This behaviour, together with the high density of VIP-containing nerve fibres in the region (as in other gastrointestinal sphincters) indicates the existence of a functional lower oesophageal sphincter (LOS).

Although most individuals with very low LOS pressure have GORD, the basal pressure in many sufferers of GORD is within normal limits. The basal LOS pressure does not therefore clearly separate normal subjects from those with GORD. Recently, Bombeck et al (1987) have described a computer generated analysis of the length and pressure of the LOS, the vector volume, which identifies more clearly those with reflux. Prolonged studies of the LOS pressure by Dent et al (1980), using a special manometry sleeve, have shown that episodes of inappropriate LOS relaxation, i.e. unrelated to swallowing, commonly occur after meals, allowing reflux to occur in both normal subjects and in those with GORD. But whereas this transient LOS relaxation is the mechanism for 97% of reflux episodes in normal subjects, it accounts for only 65% of the episodes in those with oesophagitis. The remainder of the reflux episodes occur either during transient increases in intra-abdominal pressure which overcome a hypotensive sphincter, or are free reflux across an atonic sphincter.

Pathological reflux therefore results from an interplay of a number of different factors. A vagal mechanism has been proposed to explain transient relaxation of the LOS (Jamieson 1987). It is postulated that stretch receptors in the fundus are activated by distension of the stomach and transmit impulses via afferent fibres to the dorsal nucleus of the vagus. This leads to the discharge of impulses down the efferent fibres of the vagus to the non-adrenergic, non-cholinergic inhibitory fibres in the region of the LOS, which then opens. The concept of 'inappropriate' LOS relaxation has been disputed by a recent study that found electromyographic and manometric evidence of pharyngeal contraction and peristaltic activity in the upper oesophagus associated with LOS relaxation. Transient relaxation of the LOS rarely occurs during sleep, and interestingly, both the fundal stretch theory, and the latter study indicating that the phenomenon is not strictly 'inappropriate' are consistent with this observation.

Oesophageal acid clearance

Swallow-induced primary peristalsis is the main mechanism for oesophageal clearance, aided by secondary peristalsis in response to oesophageal distension. It has been shown that, on average, we swallow saliva once every minute while awake. This, combined with the acid neutralizing effect of saliva, which is rich in bicarbonate, makes a very effective oesophageal clearance mechanism (Helm et al 1983).

A deficiency of oesophageal clearance is found in many patients with GORD and there is some evidence in favour of this being a primary and not a secondary abnormality. Clearance depends on the volume of refluxed material, salivary secretion, oesophageal motility and gravity. Minor motility abnormalities such as damped peristalsis and increased tertiary activity are often associated with GORD and do not, in our experience, significantly influence oesophageal clearance. Propagation of the peristaltic contraction is the main factor which determines clearance. Propagation is diminished or absent in conditions such as achalasia, scleroderma and diffuse oesophageal spasm. This explains why oesophagitis complicating scleroderma and that resulting from achalasia, treated by an over-enthusiastic myotomy is often very severe.

Gravity is an important factor in oesophageal emptying and may be employed with benefit to minimize nocturnal reflux by elevation of the head end of the bed. It is notable that patients with GORD who are found to reflux in both the erect and supine positions on 24-hr pH monitoring (the so-called 'combined' refluxers), who by implication lack an adequate oesophageal clearance mechanism, develop more severe oesophagitis with an increased risk of oesophageal strictures (Little et al 1980).

Physical factors

A number of anatomical factors are thought to play a role in the maintenance of the competence of the LOS. These are the right crus of the diaphragm which forms the oesophageal hiatus, the 'mucosal rosette', the length of the oesophagus within the abdomen, and the angle between the oesophagus and the fundus of the stomach.

The right crus of the diaphragm, a muscular structure, forms the oesophageal hiatus and exerts a 'pinchcock' action on the oesophagus. For many years this belief was based on purely anatomical findings, but has now been confirmed by manometric studies which show a rise in the LOS pressure in deep inspiration. The 'mucosal rosette' is used to describe the cross-sectional profile of the mucosa in the region of the LOS, which appears to 'plug' the lumen. This appearance results from the fact that the oesophagus, being a distensible muscular tube, appears to have mucosal redundancy in the contracted state. The 'mucosal rosette' may play a part in the production of a water-tight seal, but it has no fundamental role in the maintenance of LOS competence.

The length of the intra-abdominal oesophagus is believed by some to be of fundamental importance in preventing gastro-oesophageal reflux, as it is subject to any rises in intra-abdominal pressure which supplement LOS pressure (Joelsson et al 1982). It has been shown, however, that when there is no intra-abdominal oesophagus, as in a sliding hiatus hernia, that the portion of the oesophagus which lies below the insertion of the phreno-oesophageal ligament is still subject to intra-abdominal pressure, despite being anatomically within the thorax. Furthermore, LOS pressure is known to rise in response to an increase in intra-abdominal pressure, irrespective of the situation of the cardia, a response which is mediated through the vagus.

The theory that the acute angle of His forms a flap valve, thereby preventing reflux has been laid to rest by the failure to demonstrate an increase in reflux in monkeys subjected to excision of the fundus. However, the acute angle of entry of the oesophagus into the stomach and the local arrangement of mucosa at the cardia may form a flap valve of a different sort. Hill (1977) has shown that it is possible to reconstruct this valve with a novel operation.

Although many patients with hiatus hernia have GORD, most of those with GORD do not have a hernia. It is not altogether true that the presence or absence of a hiatus hernia is irrelevant to GORD, since careful barium studies have shown that as a bolus is stripped down the oesophagus into the stomach, some is sequestered in the hiatus hernia, only to reflux back into the oesophagus when the LOS next opens either in response to a swallow or 'inappropriately'. It is also true that patients with the more severe forms of reflux are more likely to have a hiatus hernia.

Gastric factors and bile reflux

Both the nature of gastric contents and the rate of gastric emptying have some bearing on gastro-oesophageal reflux. Although the maximal acid output in those with GORD does not differ significantly from asymptomatic controls, patients with duodenal ulcer disease have a propensity to develop oesophagitis and tend to have abnormal gastro-oesophageal reflux on 24-h oesophageal pH monitoring.

The role of delayed gastric emptying in either causing or exacerbating GORD is controversial, with as many studies showing that it is an important factor as those which fail to establish its relevance. On the other hand, there is both clinical and experimental evidence to show that gastric distension has a distracting effect on the cardia, and will eventually overcome the tone of the LOS and force it open. Indeed, it is postulated that the anti-reflux action of both a fundoplication and the Angelchik prosthesis is at least partly through the prevention of distraction of the LOS secondary to gastric distension.

If bile refluxes into the stomach, it will reach the oesophagus if the patient is susceptible to gastro-oesophageal reflux. Minor duodeno-gastric reflux is undoubtedly a common phenomenon in normal individuals but bile reflux is only important in the context of gastro-oesophageal reflux when the quantity of bile in the stomach in excessive, as after certain gastric operations. Normally, however, only minute quantities of bile are found in the oesophageal refluxate of those with GORD, and such amounts are unlikely to be significant in causing either symptoms or oesophagitis. It will be appreciated that whatever the quantity of bile in the stomach, it will not be able to produce any deleterious effects on the oesophagus unless there is significant gastro-oesophageal reflux.

In summary, although the aetiology of GORD is not entirely clear, the role of the vagus appears to be of central importance. It may be the mediator of transient relaxation of the LOS and it undoubtedly has an important function in the facilitation of oesophageal peristalsis and therefore oesophageal clearance. Abnormalities in the function of both afferent and efferent vagal fibres have been demonstrated in many patients with GORD, with strong evidence to show that these abnormalities are primary (Ogilvie et al 1985).

DIAGNOSIS

Symptoms

No pain receptors have been identified in the oesophagus. Pain due to exposure of the oesophageal mucosa to extremes of temperature is indistinguishable from that produced by oesophageal distension, and although acids and alkalis are sensed by chemoreceptors, the resulting symptoms are similar to those due to other stimuli (Jones & Chapman 1942). Oesophageal histology in patients with GORD shows that the rete pegs are more prominent and there is attenuation of the stratus corneum (Ismail-Beigi et al 1970). The nerve endings are thus closer to the oesophageal lumen and this explains why the infusion of acid into the lower oesophagus produces heartburn in those with oesophagitis but not in normal subjects (Bernstein & Baker 1958).

Whether symptoms are due to hypersensitivity of the oesophagus or motility abnormalities resulting from exposure to acid was elegantly investigated by Atkinson & Bennett (1968). They showed that the infusion of acid into the lower oesophagus of those with GORD produced pain with or without an associated abnormality of oesophageal motility. When the two occurred together, the pain could be relieved by the infusion of bicarbonate without any effect on motility and conversely, abnormal motility could be abolished without relief of pain. Hence in most cases the motility abnormality resulting from acid infusion is merely an association and not the cause of the pain.

The most common symptom of GORD is heartburn, usually after meals and often relieved by drinking milk or taking antacids. Regurgitation of gastric contents is another common symptom, also precipitated by heavy meals, recumbency or bending down. Dysphagia is usually a sign of severe GORD but is not always due to a stricture. It may be the result of oedema associated with severe oesophagitis or, more commonly, an associated motility disorder. Although dysphagia is usually felt in the lower sternal region, in some cases there is a clear history of high dysphagia without a demonstrable mechanical problem at this level. This is thought to arise from cricopharyngeal spasm, which can be produced experimentally by infusion of acid into the lower oesophagus.

Some patients present to cardiologists because their predominant symptom is chest pain, often radiating into the jaw and the arm and clinically indistinguishable from cardiac angina. With the widespread use of coronary angiography to investigate angina, it has become clear that in many patients no cardiac cause for the angina can be found. A number of studies have shown that a proportion of such patients have oesophageal disease. The issue of whether such symptoms arise from the heart or the oesophagus is often difficult to resolve, since some patients with normal coronary angiography will be found to have microvascular angina, and some patients whose symptoms are provoked by infusion of acid into the oesophagus or by the administration of edrophonium (to induce oesophageal spasm) will show electrocardiographic evidence of cardiac ischaemia with classical symptoms of cardiac angina.

Two other symptoms of GORD not often enquired about are odynophagia, or painful swallowing, and pulmonary symptoms. Odyno-phagia on swallowing hot or cold liquids, acidic drinks and spirits is an early, and in our experience a reliable symptom of GORD. Pulmonary complications are not uncommonly associated with GORD, but this association is not widely appreciated. Such complications may be gross, resulting in aspiration pneumonitis, or subtle, such as the exacerbation of asthma. Bronchospasm may be triggered by microaspiration of gastric contents or may result from a vagally mediated reflex initiated by gastro-oesophageal reflux. This phenomenon has been clearly demonstrated in animal experiments.

Bleeding may occur as a result of severe oesophagitis, but it is important to exclude other causes, in particular gastrointestinal malignancy, before ascribing anaemia to oesophagitis.

Unfortunately, the history is not very reliable in the diagnosis of GORD, as some patients with seemingly classical symptoms turn out not to have the disease, while others with quite severe oesophagitis, and perhaps even stricture formation, have minimal symptoms. Although a careful history is important, appropriate investigations are essential in establishing a diagnosis of GORD.

Investigations

Endoscopy

Careful endoscopy should be the first investigation in the diagnosis of GORD. The diagnosis of oesophagitis depends on the diligence of the endoscopist and whether mucosal histology is considered. Histological evidence of oesophagitis is often found in mucosa which looks normal but this depends very much on the number of biopsies taken and their depth.

Table 2.1 Severity of oesophagitis according to Savary & Miller modified by Little et al (1980)

Grade I	Erythema and/or friable mucosa
Grade II	Superficial non-confluent linear ulceration
Grade III	Confluent or circumferential areas of deeper ulceration or 'cobblestone' mucosa
Grade IV	Extensive mucosal ulceration or complication e.g. stricture, shortening or Barrett's oesophagus

Suction biopsy instruments obtain better material than pinch biopsy forceps, but histological changes are often patchy, and therefore may be completely missed unless multiple biopsies are taken. Furthermore, biopsies from the lowest 2 cm of the oesophagus in normal subjects may show histological changes consistent with a diagnosis of GORD. Histology is therefore potentially confusing, but is obviously useful for distinguishing oesophagitis from cancer.

Careful macroscopic inspection of the oesophagus is quite reliable. It is also possible to grade the severity of oesophagitis using objective criteria and those developed by Savary and Miller and modified by Little and colleagues (1980) are both simple and reliable (Table 2.1). In this way changes in severity, particularly in response to treatment can be objectively recorded.

Subtle degrees of sliding hiatus hernia and Barrett's oesophagus can be missed easily on endoscopy. Endoscopic diagnosis of a hiatus hernia is made when the squamo-columnar junction lies 2 cm above the diaphragmatic hiatus, the level of which may be difficult to determine, but is indicated by the pinchcock action of the right crus of the diaphragm when the cooperative patient is asked to sniff. A Barrett's oesophagus is diagnosed by the presence of columnar epithelium extending into the oesophagus at least 3 cm beyond the anatomical gastro-oesophageal junction, which can be identified by the transition from the rugose gastric mucosa to the smooth oesophageal mucosa. The healthy squamo-columnar junction is normally irregular, hence the term 'Z-line', with projections of the columnar epithelium up to 1.5 cm above the gastro-oesophageal junction. Islets of columnar mucosa in the lower oesophagus are also considered to represent a Barrett's oesophagus.

Barium studies

Although severe oesophagitis may be apparent on a carefully performed barium swallow, barium studies are more useful in delineating anatomical details such as the presence and severity of a stricture—the length and calibre of which is much better gauged by this test than by endoscopy. A hiatus hernia is easier to diagnose on barium swallow than endoscopy, but

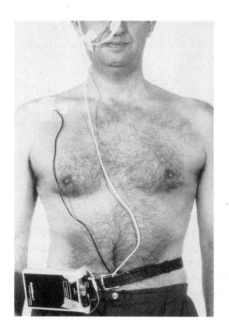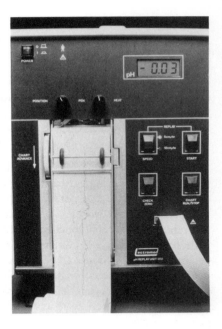

Fig. 2.1 Ambulatory oesophageal pH monitoring. **A** Patient connected up for monitoring, **B** pH trace being generated by the chart recorder connected to the 24-h pH recorder. (Reproduced by kind permission of the Department of Medical Illustration, Salford Health Authority.)

its presence has little bearing on management unless surgical treatment is considered. A barium swallow and meal is therefore an adjunct to endoscopy in the diagnosis of GORD.

Oesophageal pH monitoring

After endoscopy, oesophageal pH monitoring is the single most useful test for assessing GORD and has revolutionized the management of this condition. Reasonably inexpensive and reliable equipment for performing 24-h ambulatory oesophageal monitoring is now commercially available. This technique is particularly useful when the symptoms suggest GORD but endoscopic evidence of oesophagitis is lacking.

Oesophageal pH is sensed by a pH electrode passed through the nose so that its tip is positioned 5 cm above the gastro-oesophageal junction. Changes in pH are stored on a digital recorder (Fig. 2.1) and analysed after 24 h of recording. A reflux episode is conventionally defined as a drop below pH 4 lasting at least 30 s. The individual is encouraged as far as possible to go about his normal activities during the recording period, and to record events such as meals, recumbency and most importantly the onset and severity of symptoms by pressing the appropriate buttons on the recorder.

The data obtained are used both to calculate the total amount of reflux and to study any relationship between symptoms and reflux episodes. A number of formulae are available to convert the data into clinically useful information, some of which are now available commercially on computer software. Most of these are variations of the original formula of Johnson & DeMeester (1974). Although many aspects of reflux are considered in this formula, the main determinants of abnormal reflux are the total amount of reflux, i.e. more than 5% of the time, and supine (usually nocturnal) reflux.

Oesophageal manometry

Oesophageal manometry is useful to complete the investigation of gastro-oesophageal reflux. For example, there may be an associated motility disorder such as scleroderma or the presentation may be with atypical symptoms such as angina-like pain, which may be due to either reflux or a motility disorder. Occasionally patients with achalasia have symptoms indistinguishable from reflux. Manometry also forms an important component of the assessment for re-operation after failed anti-reflux surgery. Some investigators have suggested that it is mandatory before anti-reflux surgery to exclude abnormalities of oesophageal motility and to determine the mechanical efficiency of the LOS. They define a mechanically deficient sphincter as that which has a resting pressure of less than 5 mmHg or an intra-abdominal length of less than 1 cm, and indicate that patients with these characteristics do best after surgery (Joelsson et al 1982). It is also suggested that there is a high likelihood of producing dysphagia if a fundoplication is performed around a mechanically competent LOS so rendering it supercompetent, or if there is an oesophageal motility disorder. Many patients coming to surgery in our practice have abnormalities of oesophageal motility and have a mechanically competent LOS but we have not observed a higher incidence of post-operative dysphagia provided that the operation has been well performed and does not produce oesophageal obstruction (Mughal et al 1990).

Acid perfusion test

Bernstein & Baker, in 1958, showed that classical heartburn could be reproduced in a large proportion of patients with oesophagitis by perfusion of the lower oesophagus with 0.1 M HCl via a nasogastric tube and that the symptom could be abolished by the perfusion of sodium bicarbonate. They found only a 15% false positive and false negative rate. However, the test has a much lower accuracy if used to distinguish those with reflux but no oesophagitis from normal subjects and has therefore largely been superseded by 24-h ambulatory oesophageal pH monitoring.

Radionuclide studies

Oesophageal scintigraphy has been extensively studied for detecting gastro-oesophageal reflux, particularly in children, because it is non-invasive. It also has the theoretical advantage that it detects the volume of reflux, irrespective of the pH of the refluxate. However, to date, the majority of studies have found that it is not sufficiently sensitive to be of clinical value, and it remains a research tool.

TREATMENT

Treatment depends on the severity of symptoms, the severity of reflux and the presence of complications. Most individuals with symptoms of gastro-oesophageal reflux treat themselves with simple antacids and only seek medical advice when symptoms worsen. In the latter case the patient's family doctor will usually prescribe effective treatment and only a small proportion will be referred for specialist opinion. Most of this selected group will be treated quite satisfactorily by conservative means, and only a tiny fraction of the original population of symptomatic individuals will be considered for surgery.

Medical

After establishing the diagnosis and explaining the nature of the disease the importance of general measures is emphasized. These include weight reduction if indicated, propping up the head end of the bed by 15 cm if nocturnal symptoms are particularly troublesome, and avoiding large meals, fatty foods, chocolate, coffee and smoking. In those without oesophagitis, these measures are supplemented with the use of antacids to be taken as and when necessary. This will alleviate symptoms in a large proportion of patients.

Those with oesophagitis are best treated with a combination of an H_2 receptor antagonist such as cimetidine and an antacid–alginate mixture in addition to the measures outlined above. The dose of H_2 receptor antagonist required is usually higher than that used for the treatment of peptic ulcer disease, and we usually commence with cimetidine at a dose of 400 mg four times daily or an equivalent dose of ranitidine. If symptoms are unchanged at review six weeks later, changes are made in the therapy, depending on the dominant symptom. If heartburn has been relieved but regurgitation remains a problem, the addition of a drug to enhance the LOS pressure and oesophageal clearance may be helpful. Metoclopramide, bethanecol and domperidone are largely ineffective, but the new prokinetic drug cisapride has been shown to heal oesophagitis as effectively as an H_2 receptor antagonist. If heartburn remains unchanged, the endoscopy may be repeated and treatment with omeprazole is started. This is highly effective and some have suggested that it is the treatment of choice for oesophagitis.

Once an effective combination of drugs has been found, treatment usually needs to be prolonged for at least three months to allow sufficient healing of the oesophagitis to occur. Long-term follow-up studies have shown that the maximum benefits of H_2 receptor antagonists occur within the first two to three months, and once healing has been confirmed the dose can often be reduced. Some patients can be weaned off H_2 receptor antagonists completely but those referred to hospital are a more resistant group and may require continuous treatment at full dosage.

Peptic strictures

The majority of peptic strictures can be dilated, and are successfully managed by periodic dilatations and medical treatment of GORD. In most cases the frequency of dilatation decreases with time (Patterson et al 1983). Dilatation is safely performed with sedation and analgesia, by the passage of dilators over a guidewire placed through the stricture at endoscopy. A variety of dilators are available ranging from the Eder–Puestow metal olives to the more recently developed KAD dilators (Keymed Advanced Dilator, Keymed, Southend on Sea). We currently use the Celestin dilators which allow dilatation to 18 mm in only two passages provided that the size of the stomach has not been reduced significantly by previous surgery.

We perform oesophageal dilatation as a day-case procedure, and a chest X-ray is only performed after the procedure if it has been difficult or the operator suspects a perforation. A luminal calibre of 12 mm is required to alleviate dysphagia and 16 to 18 mm to restore normal swallowing. The aim is to dilate safely and full dilatation may be easily achieved in most cases at the initial session. Some tight strictures are best dilated gradually, over a period of weeks until a calibre of 12 to 15 mm has been achieved.

The principle of balloon dilatation, producing a radial as opposed to an axial dilating force, is attractive, but in practice this method of dilatation is less effective than conventional dilatation. Dilatable strictures in young people with severe reflux are best treated by dilatation and anti-reflux surgery. Only fibrotic strictures resistant to dilatation require resection, but these are rare.

Barrett's oesophagus

Barrett's oesophagus is a condition in which the mucosa of the lower oesophagus becomes replaced by columnar epithelium. Clinical and experimental evidence indicates that the aetiological factor is gastro-oesophageal reflux damaging the squamous mucosa which is replaced by columnar mucosa (Gillen et al 1988). Because columnar mucosa is more resistant and less sensitive to acid than squamous mucosa, patients with this condition may have no symptoms and the diagnosis is sometimes made during endoscopy for some other purpose. The condition has a malignant potential, with a 44-fold risk of developing adenocarcinoma (Spechler et al 1984). Adenocarcinoma complicating Barrett's oesophagus tends to occur in the sixth and seventh decades and is usually aggressive with a poor prognosis.

The management of Barrett's oesophagus is to treat symptomatic reflux. There is considerable controversy about the usefulness of endoscopic surveillance. Annual review is probably prudent for younger patients with the condition, but many are elderly and poor candidates for any form of surgical treatment. The role of anti-reflux surgery is similarly controversial. Two well conducted studies have shown regression of

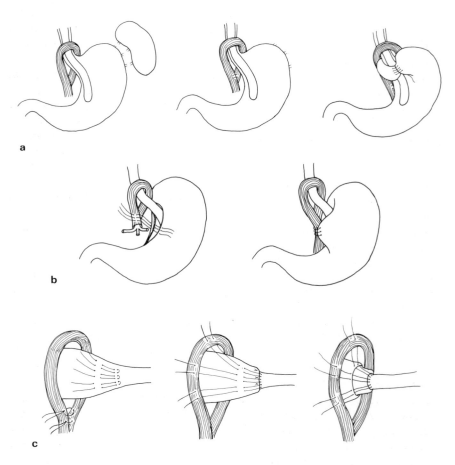

Fig. 2.2 Illustration of the principles of **A** the Nissen fundoplication, **B** the Hill operation and **C** the Belsey Mk IV operation. (Reproduced by kind permission of the Department of Medical Illustration, Salford Health Authority.)

Barrett's mucosa in a proportion of cases following surgery. Interpretation of post-operative endoscopic findings can be difficult because of anatomical changes caused by the surgery. Prophylactic oesophagectomy is difficult to justify in this condition. It is reserved for cases presenting with frank carcinoma or when severe dysplasia or in situ carcinoma is detected by endoscopic surveillance. In such cases it is essential that oesophageal resection is performed by specialist surgeons to minimize post-operative mortality.

Surgery

About 5 to 10% of patients referred to hospital are resistant to medical treatment and this is the most common indication for surgery. In general, heartburn responds rather better to medication than the symptom of reflux itself. Surgery is also indicated for the complications of GORD such as stricture in young patients, penetrating ulcers which fail to heal and respiratory problems.

Since oesophagitis was believed to be a consequence of a hiatus hernia, the earliest operations were designed to correct this anatomical abnormality. The best known of these, the Allison repair, consisted of reducing the hiatus hernia and narrowing the oesophageal hiatus by suturing the crura. Others, such as the Boerema operation concentrated on 'restoring' the acute angle of His, by pulling the lesser curve of the stomach down and suturing it to the linea alba. Long-term results from such operations were poor, and they have largely been superseded by those designed to stop reflux rather than correct anatomical abnormalities. The most commonly performed are the Nissen fundoplication, the Belsey Mk IV repair, and the Hill operation. The salient principles of these operations are illustrated in Figure 2.2.

The complete fundoplication was first described by Nissen in 1936 but until recently its mode of action has been unclear. Nissen performed his original fundoplication after resecting the cardia, and he found no evidence of oesophagitis on reviewing the patient 16 years later. Thus a fundoplication works without a LOS, and it has also been shown to work in the chest. It is unlikely, therefore, that its mode of action depends on 'bolstering' the LOS or increasing the intra-abdominal length of the LOS. There is some experimental evidence that the fundoplication works by protecting the cardia from the distracting force exerted by a distended stomach, a mechanism of action also attributed to the Angelchik prosthesis.

The Nissen fundoplication is very effective in controlling reflux and has very good long-term results. Its main disadvantages were the high incidence of gas-bloat and dysphagia associated with the original operation. However, by making the wrap loose and short (the 'floppy Nissen'), the incidence of these complications is markedly reduced without adverse effects on reflux control (Donahue et al 1985). The great advantage of the operation is that it is simple in its concept, simple to teach and perform, and has very good long-term results.

The Belsey Mk IV operation is a 270° fundoplication together with a reduction of a hiatus hernia performed through the chest. It too has very good long-term results without significant complications, but is a more difficult operation to learn and perform well. The principle of the Hill operation is to create a good length of intra-abdominal oesophagus by securing the lesser curve to the median arcuate ligament which is a condensation of the pre-aortic fascia above the coeliac axis. The sutures are placed in such a way as to also plicate the cardia and produce a pressure of 40 to 50 mmHg in the LOS when tied. This requires intra-operative manometry and it is technically a difficult operation to perform to a high standard.

The Angelchik prosthesis is a C-shaped, silicone filled ring with a silicone tie-strap. Placement is very easy and requires minimal mobilization of the lower oesophagus. The device is slipped round the oesophagus and the tapes are tied to produce a loose collar. There is no doubt that it prevents reflux and probably works in the same way as a fundoplication. However, there have been numerous reports of disruption and migration of the prosthesis and one recent prospective study comparing it with the Nissen fundoplication has shown it to be less effective than the Nissen in controlling reflux with 10% of the prostheses having to be removed because of sepsis or dysphagia (Stuart et al 1989). Whatever its efficacy, its long-term safety remains to be proven.

An operation based on an altogether different rationale for controlling reflux is the Roux-en-Y gastrectomy. The aim is to reduce the volume and acidity of gastric secretions and prevent bile reflux into the stomach remnant. Although it has been used successfully in the primary surgical treatment of GORD, we would regard it as too radical an operation in this context. We reserve this procedure for certain situations during re-operation after failed primary surgery as described later.

All the operations described above have been found to have a low morbidity and good results in the hands of enthusiasts. However, the Nissen fundoplication alone has been assessed most rigorously and has been found to have the best long-term results. It is our choice for primary reflux surgery and the technique is briefly described below.

Floppy Nissen fundoplication—surgical technique

The operation can be performed through the chest or the abdomen. We prefer the latter route unless a thoracic approach is deemed more desirable, as for instance with a shortened oesophagus. A laparotomy is performed through an upper midline incision and the decision is made whether to proceed with the fundoplication. A 50 Fr gauge Maloney bougie is passed into the stomach alongside a 16 Fr gauge nasogastric tube, after oesophageal dilatation if a stricture is present. It is essential to obtain good access to the oesophageal hiatus by the use of fixed retractors such as the Polytract (Pilling Ltd, UK) which pull the rib cage and sternum upwards. The gastro-oesophageal junction is mobilized after dividing the phreno-oesophageal ligament, taking care to avoid damaging the vagus nerves, and about 5 cm of distal oesophagus is mobilized. The short gastric vessels are ligated and divided to mobilize the fundus. The flimsy lesser omentum is divided from the oesophageal hiatus to a point just short of the hepatic branches of the vagus. The remainder of the lesser omentum is left intact and it is essential not to divide the left gastric artery which is a convenient support for the fundoplication.

The oesophageal hiatus can be clearly inspected. If it is wide it is narrowed with interrupted silk or Goretex (Gore Ltd, UK) sutures. The fat pad at the cardia is carefully removed, again taking care not to damage the vagus nerves. Removal of this pad produces a denuded area which encourages proper adherence of the fundal wrap to the lower oesophagus. The fundus is passed round the back of the oesophagus to emerge on the medial side of the cardia. A fundoplication is created with six to eight interrupted silk or Goretex sutures centred on the cardia. The

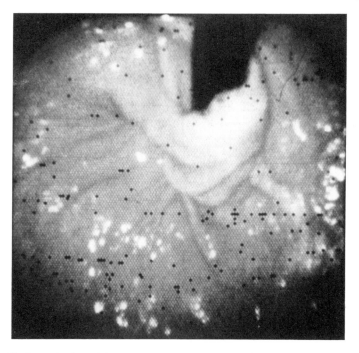

Fig. 2.3 Endoscopic view of the 'nipple' of a properly constructed floppy Nissen fundoplication. (Reproduced by kind permission of Mr T O'Hanrahan.)

bottom suture may include the cardia, but the others are not inserted into the oesophagus. The length of the fundoplication is 2 to 3 cm and it should be loose enough to permit a 36 Fr gauge dilator to be passed easily between the fundoplication and the oesophagus with the bougie within it. There must be no tension on the fundoplication when it is complete. The bougie is removed leaving the nasogastric tube in place and the abdomen is closed. The nasogastric tube is left in place for 48 h to prevent gastric dilatation which can lead to the disruption of the fundoplication, but fluids are allowed from the day after the operation. Figure 2.3 shows an endoscopic view of the 'nipple effect' achieved by a properly constructed fundoplication.

Most patients lose their symptoms very quickly but mild dysphagia and gaseous distension are common in the first few weeks after operation. With

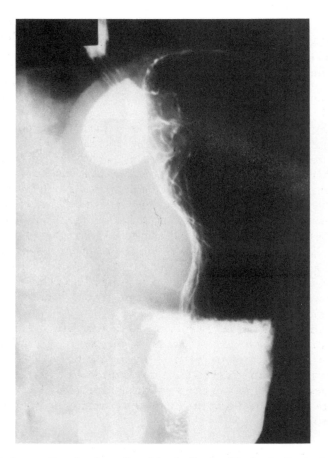

Fig. 2.4   Barium swallow showing a slipped fundoplication. The fundoplication is seen as a waist round the upper part of the stomach.

a properly constructed fundoplication these symptoms settle completely. Systematic audit of our practice has confirmed that excellent results are obtained in most cases. Reflux is controlled in 96% of cases as judged by pH recording and endoscopy. Overall patient satisfaction is 86%—a higher proportion than that obtained following most other forms of gastro-intestinal surgery.

Re-operation for failure or complications of anti-reflux surgery

Re-operative surgery has a higher morbidity and mortality and lower success rate than primary surgery, emphasizing the need for careful assessment and technique for the initial operation. Re-operations on the cardia, which require dismantling of some previous procedure, carry a risk of damage to the stomach and the oesophagus, and are best undertaken by surgeons experienced in oesophageal surgery with the ability to perform oesophageal replacement should this be necessary. Before any re-operation, details of the previous surgery should be studied and a thorough assessment should be performed including barium studies, endoscopy, manometry and 24-h ambulatory oesophageal monitoring.

The procedure selected will depend on the reasons for re-operation and the nature of the previous surgery. Complications of a previous fundoplication such as disruption, slippage (Fig. 2.4) or over-tightening, can usually be corrected by re-doing the procedure, although this can sometimes be extremely difficult. If pre-operative studies indicate that there is significant oesophageal shortening, a common cause of a slipped fundoplication performed through the abdomen, it may be prudent to plan for a thoraco-abdominal approach. This allows safe and full mobilization of the cardia and the lower oesophagus which is essential if the complication is not to be repeated. When the oesophagus is significantly shortened, a Collis gastroplasty combined with a fundoplication is a very effective procedure. In this operation the oesophagus is lengthened by cutting down from the angle of His for the required length parallel to the lesser curvature of the stomach. This is very simply achieved by using a linear stapler with a 50 Fr gauge bougie in the oesophagus and using the new fundus for a Nissen fundoplication round the neo-oesophagus.

If the cardia and the lower oesophagus become severely damaged during mobilization, it may be necessary to excise the damaged portion and replace it with a jejunal or colonic graft. A useful alternative to a tedious and hazardous dissection of the cardia is to perform a Roux-en-Y gastrectomy to decrease the volume and acidity of the gastric secretions. However, the results of this indirect approach seem less predictable than other, more direct methods.

KEY POINTS FOR CLINICAL PRACTICE

GORD is a very common chronic relapsing condition usually presenting with classical symptoms. Successful treatment is based on accurate diagnosis and endoscopy is the first investigation. If normal, 24-h ambulatory oesophageal pH monitoring should be undertaken. This often clinches the diagnosis. Manometry is only necessary when an associated motility disorder, such as scleroderma, is suspected and in those with atypical symptoms such as angina-like pain. The vast majority of patients can be managed quite satisfactorily with a combination of general measures and medical treatment. A highly successful first-line treatment is a combination of cimetidine 400 mg and an antacid–alginate mixture, both four times daily, reserving omeprazole for the very resistant cases. Surgery is indicated in about 10% of cases for failure of medical treatment and complications of GORD. Dilatable strictures can be managed very successfully with medical treatment and dilatation.

It is important to assess the patient carefully before operation and ensure that there is no doubt about the diagnosis. A floppy Nissen fundoplication is the operation of choice. It is easy to perform, has a low morbidity and excellent long-term results, and can be combined with a Collis gastroplasty if there is significant oesophageal shortening. Patients with failed anti-reflux surgery or complications are best managed by specialists in oesophageal surgery.

REFERENCES

Atkinson M, Bennett J R 1968 Relationship between motor changes and pain during esophageal acid perfusion. Am J Dig Dis 13: 346–350
Bernstein L M, Baker L A 1958 A clinical test for esophagitis. Gastroenterology 34: 760–781
Bombeck C T, Vaz O, DeSalvo J et al 1987 Computerised axial manometry of the esophagus. A new method for the assessment of antireflux operations. Ann Surg 206: 465–472
Dent J, Dodds W J, Friedman R H et al 1980 Mechanisms of gastroesophageal reflux in recumbent asymptomatic subjects. J Clin Invest 65: 256–267
Donahue P E, Samelson S, Nyhus L M et al 1985 The floppy Nissen fundoplication: effective long term control of pathological reflux. Arch Surg 120: 663–668
Fyke F E, Code C F, Schlegel J F 1956 The gastroesophageal sphincter in healthy human beings. Gastroenterologia 86: 135–150
Gillen P, Keeling P, Byrne P J et al 1988 Experimental columnar metaplasia in the canine oesophagus. Br J Surg 75: 113–115
Helm J F, Dodds W J, Riedel D R et al 1983 Determinants of esophageal acid clearance in normal subjects. Gastroenterology 85: 607–612
Hill L D 1977 An effective operation for hiatal hernia: an eight year appraisal. Ann Surg 166: 681–692
Ismail-Beigi F, Horton P F, Pope C E 1970 Histological consequences of gastroesophageal reflux in man. Gastroenterology 58: 163–174
Jamieson G G 1987 Anti-reflux operations: how do they work? Br J Surg 74: 155–156
Joelsson B E, DeMeester T R, Skinner D B et al 1982 The role of the esophageal body in the antireflux mechanism. Surgery 92: 417–423
Johnson L F, DeMeester T R 1974 Twenty-four-hour pH monitoring of the distal esophagus: A quantitative measure of gastroesophageal reflux. Am J Gastroenterol 62: 325–331
Jones C M, Chapman W P 1942 Studies on the mechanism of pain of angina pectoris with particular relationship to hiatus hernia. Trans Assoc Am Physicians 57: 139–151
Jones R, Lydeard S 1989 Prevalence of dyspepsia in the community. Br Med J 298: 30–32

Little A G, DeMeester T R, Kirschner P T et al 1980 Pathogenesis of esophagitis in patients with gastroesophageal reflux. Surgery 88: 101–107
Mughal M M, Bancewicz J, Marples M 1990 Oesophageal manometry and pH recording does not predict the bad results of Nissen fundoplication. Br J Surg 77: 43–45
Ogilvie A L, James P D, Atkinson M 1985 Impairment of vagal function in reflux oesophagitis. Q J Med 54: 61–74
Patterson D J, Graham D Y, Smith J L et al 1983 Natural history of benign esophageal stricture treated by dilatation. Gastroenterology 85: 336–350
Spechler S J, Robbins A H, Rubins H B et al 1984 Adenocarcinoma and Barrett's esophagus: an overrated risk? Gastroenterology 87: 927–933
Stuart R C, Dawson K, Keeling P et al 1989 A prospective randomized trial of the Angelchik anti-reflux prosthesis versus Nissen fundoplication. Br J Surg 76: 86–89

3

Aortic aneurysm—screening and management

J. Collin

One of the great joys of medical practice is daily contact with the endless diversity of human personalities, abilities and experience. Differing needs and expectations produce varying demands on a doctor's time and critical faculties. Requests for explanations, information and advice are influenced by the intelligence, educational background and anxiety of patients. At one extreme is the man who on being told that a surgeon is proposing to amputate his head and replace it with a cabbage replies 'very good doctor, you know best'. At the other is the 'North Oxford Don' who insists on an explanatory dissertation in reply to every question and believes nothing which cannot be proved. In the closing decade of the twentieth century the former type of patient is rapidly becoming extinct while the latter has spread far beyond his original breeding grounds and is now to be found in every city.

Any surgeon who wants to be well equipped to deal with the changing management of the consumer-orientated patient of the future will need to have detailed answers to their questions. Patients with aortic aneurysms ask a number of simple questions, but as any examination candidate can testify, the questions may be easy but the answers are difficult. Let us consider each in turn.

WHAT IS AN AORTIC ANEURYSM?

By definition an aneurysm is an abnormal dilatation of a blood vessel. But how much dilatation is abnormal, and in comparison with what? Before we can begin to answer these questions an even more fundamental problem arises.

What to measure and how?

There is no agreement as to which diameter of the aorta is more important, anteroposterior, transverse, a mean of anteroposterior and transverse or the maximum diameter in any plane. Transverse diameter is usually greater but anteroposterior diameter may be a better predictor of subsequent aneurysm rupture (Cronenwett et al 1985). The diameters of infrarenal aortas, like other biological measurements, when collected in sufficient numbers fit into a normal distribution curve (Collin et al 1988). It is likely that the shape of this curve depends on the age, sex and ethnic origin of the population studied but no data have been published.

Measurement of the external diameter of the abdominal aorta is now relatively easy using ultrasonography or computerized tomography and both techniques have excellent reproducibility with little inter-observer variation. Nuclear magnetic resonance imaging is becoming available in some centres and provides another non-invasive method of measurement which has yet to be evaluated in this application. Plain abdominal radiography is unsuitable for general application since only around 40% of aortic aneurysms have sufficient calcium in their walls to be visible. Aortography is invasive and generally useless for sizing an aneurysm since the amount of mural thrombus is variable while the contrast material is confined to the flowing column of blood. There are two direct measurements which can be performed for the intellectual edification of the surgeon but neither can easily be recommended to a patient. Per-operatively, after dissection of the aorta, the anteroposterior diameter may be measured by transfixion of the vessel with a needle or the transverse diameter may be read from callipers. At necropsy, although ample time is available for accurate measurement, aortic diameters will be reduced by tissue shrinkage and removal of the dilating effect of blood pressure.

The above considerations point to ultrasonography as the best current technique for general use. It is readily available, cheap, accurate, rapid, reproducible between observers and instruments to within 5 mm, absolutely safe and can be repeated as often as required with minimal inconvenience to the patient. The dilated aorta is generally tortuous in the transverse and rarely in an anteroposterior plane. For this reason the anteroposterior diameter is a more reliable measurement than either transverse or oblique diameters. To avoid confusion between false and true lumen of an aneurysm the external diameter of the aorta should be measured.

The detailed arguments involved in formulating a precise definition of an aortic aneurysm have been pursued in detail elsewhere (Collin 1990a) and my proposed definition is given below.

Definition of an aortic aneurysm

An aortic aneurysm is present when the maximum anteroposterior external diameter of the aorta is at least 4.0 cm. When dilatation is confined to the infrarenal aorta an aneurysm is also present when its diameter exceeds that of the suprarenal aorta by at least 0.5 cm.

The lack of an agreed definition of aortic aneurysm presents a problem for the numerous screening programmes which are currently being introduced. As can be seen in Table 3.1 the variability of definitions used is

Table 3.1 Screening studies for abdominal aortic aneurysm

	Author (reference)	Study group	Number screened	Aneurysm definition	AAA prevalence
Healthy subjects	Collin (1988)	Men 65–74 years	426	> 4.0 cm or 5 mm > suprarenal aorta	5.4%
	Scott et al (1988)	Men and Women 65–80 years	1312	⩾ 3.0 cm	5.8%
Hypertensives	Twomey et al (1986)	Men > 50 years	200	⩾ 3.0 cm	7.0%
	Allen et al (1987)	Men 65–85 years	94	5 mm > suprarenal aorta	7.4%
		Women 65–85 years	71		2.8%
Atherosclerosis/ hypertension/ obesity	Allardice et al (1988)	Consecutive patients attending Vascular Clinic	90	Localized dilatation	11.1%
	Thurmond & Semler (1986)	Men and women > 50 years attending Cardiology Clinic	120	⩾ 4.0 cm	5.0%
	Graham & Chan (1988)	Men > 55 years waist measure > 101 cm hypertensive or atherosclerotic	45	⩾ 3.0 cm	13.3%
	Lederle et al (1988)	Men 60–75 years with hypertension and or coronary heart disease	201	> 1.5 times suprarenal aortic diameter	9.0%
	Berridge et al (1989)	Men and women attending Vascular Clinic	104	> 3.5 cm or 5 mm > suprarenal aorta	7.7%

one of the important factors which hinders comparisons of data obtained from these studies.

HOW COMMON IS AORTIC ANEURYSM?

In the last 30 years there has been a linear increase in the number of recorded deaths from aortic aneurysm in England and Wales. This can be explained in part by the progressive growth in the number of elderly people in the population but age specific death rates for aortic aneurysm have also increased over the age of 60 (Collin 1988). Some of the increase may be real but much of the apparent change may be due to enhanced awareness of the disease, improved diagnosis and altered referral patterns associated with the establishment of specialist vascular units. This issue is difficult to resolve because of the unreliability of national records of cause of death which ultimately depend on the diagnostic acumen of the reporting doctor and are seldom supported by autopsy evidence. In the United States a similar but more rapid increase in age adjusted mortality for aortic aneurysm occurred between 1951 and 1968 but recorded deaths then reached a plateau and in white males have declined at 2% per annum since 1976 (Lilienfeld et al 1987). These differences between England and the Unites States are best explained by dissimilar health care provision in the two countries. The seminal world event was the first successful resection of an abdominal aortic aneurysm by Dubost in 1951. It is likely that in the United States the operation rate for aortic aneurysm has been high enough

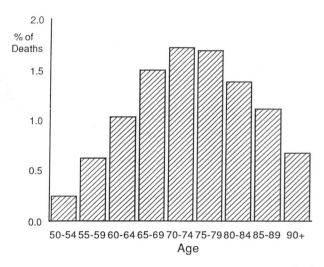

Fig. 3.1   Deaths from ruptured abdominal aortic aneurysm as a percentage of all deaths for men in England and Wales, 1986.

since the mid-1970s, at least in the white population, to produce a measurable impact on total mortality from the disease. In England, elective aneurysm operation rates are less than one-third of the transatlantic figure due to a combination of chronic underfunding of health care and the slower growth of vascular surgery as a speciality.

Incidence

In much of the United Kingdom the commonest presentation of aortic aneurysm is death. The disease predominantly affects men past middle age and is uncommon in women except for the very elderly. The chances of dying from ruptured abdominal aortic aneurysm increase relentlessly with age and reach an apparent peak only in the 85 + age group (Mortality Statistics Cause 1986). The absolute number of deaths from abdominal aortic aneurysm reaches a peak at age 75–79 in men and 80–84 in women. The greatest relative importance of the disease is in men aged 70–74 in whom it accounts for 1.72% of all deaths (Fig. 3.1). The disease is particularly common as a cause of unexpected death and in one study of 322 sudden deaths between 18 and 69 years of age, ruptured aortic aneurysm was the cause in 4.2% of men and 1.2% of women (Thomas et al 1988). If only deaths over 50 years had been considered the incidence would undoubtedly have been substantially higher.

The total annual incidence of the disease is the sum of deaths and diagnoses made without patients having to experience the inconvenience of dying first. It is known that fewer than half of all patients with a ruptured abdominal aortic aneurysm reach hospital alive (Ingoldby et al 1986, Budd et al 1989). Subsequent survival rates among those who do reach hospital vary considerably but for the country as a whole the figure is unlikely to be more than one-third. Combining this information with our own recent experience (Collin et al 1989a) we can calculate approximate total annual incidence rates. In men aged 65–74 the current total annual incidence of abdominal aortic aneurysm is around 0.13%. This almost certainly is a substantial underestimate due to misdiagnosis of the cause of death. It is a sad fact that the number of deaths investigated by autopsy has been declining steadily and is now under 15% of all deaths. In the elderly the number of necropsy examinations is even smaller and many deaths allegedly from myocardial infarction are likely to be due to aneurysm rupture.

Prevalence

The majority of aortic aneurysms are asymptomatic and impalpable, consequently their prevalence in the community can be determined only by ultrasound screening. Although the results of many screening studies have been published, most are fundamentally flawed as measures of prevalence.

The incidence of aortic aneurysm increases rapidly with age and is much higher in men than women. Prevalence studies must therefore differentiate each 5- or 10-year age group and men from women. Studies in patients with hypertension, atherosclerosis or other diseases cannot produce prevalence data relevant to the whole population. Examination of all the data (see Table 3.1) does, however, allow a number of conclusions to be drawn. In men aged 65–74 the prevalence of abdominal aortic aneurysm of all sizes is 5.4% and of aneurysms of at least 4.0 cm is 2.3%. In patients with hypertension or atherosclerotic occlusive disease of the coronary, carotid or limb arteries the prevalence of abdominal aortic aneurysm is around 50% higher than in the general population.

IS IT SERIOUS DOCTOR?

The only substantial danger posed by an aortic aneurysm is that of death from aneurysm rupture. As deaths go it tends to be pleasanter than most, often being almost immediate and never taking longer than three days. Many men would rank it close to the ideal exit from this vale of tears, which must be to be shot to death by a jealous husband at the age of 85. But both exits are unnecessary and with a little forethought and prophylactic measures both can be avoided.

Rarely morbidity may occur from distal arterial embolization and ureteric or renal artery occlusion. Occasionally an aortic aneurysm may thrombose and sometimes this will cause critical ischaemia of one or both lower limbs. These morbidity risks are small, however. They are often curable if they do occur and are too infrequent to justify undergoing prophylactic surgery.

The risks of premature death from aortic rupture increase proportionately with the diameter of the aneurysm and how dangerous an aneurysm is, therefore, depends largely on how big it is.

Large aneurysms > 6.0 cm diameter

Patients with aneurysms of more than 6.0 cm diameter are nowadays invariably advised to have elective surgery. What we know of the natural history of large aneurysms comes from studies before 1951 or contemporary studies in patients too ill to undergo a major elective operation.

The only substantial study before 1951 was that of Estes (1950) who reviewed 97 patients with non-syphilitic aneurysms diagnosed at the Mayo Clinic up to 1947. Fewer than half survived for 3 years and 63% of all deaths were from aneurysm rupture. A follow up study at Vanderbilt University (Foster et al 1969) of patients not offered surgery found that 55% of deaths were due to rupture. Even at an institution where surgery was denied only if the patient was very old or had severe coexistent disease,

43% of deaths in patients with unoperated large aneurysms were from rupture (Szilagyi et al 1972).

Small aneurysms 4.0–5.9 cm diameter

Autopsy studies in patients with an abdominal aortic aneurysm showed that more than a third of those less than 6.0 cm in diameter had ruptured and caused death (Szilagyi et al 1966). Follow up studies of patients with aneurysms less than 6.0 cm diameter rejected for surgery have demonstrated a rupture rate of 6% per annum over three years. Rupture rates will tend to increase progressively with the length of follow up as the aneurysms continue to expand. It is known that for aneurysms of 4.0–4.9 cm diameter the mean expansion rate is 0.5 cm per annum increasing to 0.7 cm per annum for aneurysms of 5.0–5.9 cm diameter (Sterpetti et al 1985).

Very small aneurysms < 4.0 cm diameter

The introduction of screening programmes for abdominal aortic aneurysms has presented surgeons with the problem of what to advise the patient with a very small (< 4.0 cm diameter) aneurysm since two-thirds of all aneurysms detected by screening are of this size. The reasons for this are interesting and may be summarized as follows:

1. The longest part of the life cycle of any aneurysm will be when it is small since incremental growth rates increase as the aneurysm enlarges.
2. Large aneurysms are more likely to be detected and present in routine clinical practice.
3. The larger an aneurysm becomes the more likely it is to rupture and remove the patient beyond the benefits of screening.

Very small aortic aneurysms generally enlarge much more slowly than the larger aneurysms which present in routine clinical practice and median growth rates of 0.2 cm per annum are usual (Collin et al 1989b, Nevitt et al 1989). Clinical and autopsy evidence indicates that even these very small aneurysms do sometimes rupture but there is insufficient data for the risk to be accurately quantified. Several follow up studies have shown no case of rupture occurring in such patients while the aneurysms remained very small (Cronenwett et al 1985, Scott et al 1988, Nevitt et al 1989) but ruptures did occur as the aneurysms grew (Cronenwett et al 1985).

WHAT CAUSES IT?

The common abdominal aortic aneurysm of elderly men has been labelled as 'atherosclerotic'. This classification has little justification, has paralysed thinking and needs to be re-examined. In the elderly the aorta, in common with every other artery, will have obvious features of atherosclerosis but this is not enough evidence to make credible a pathological diagnosis which does not fit with many known facts about the disease.

Tilson & Stansel (1980) made a detailed comparison between patients with abdominal aortic aneurysm and those with occlusive aorto-iliac disease. He found that the aneurysm patients were nine times more likely to be male, were on average 11 years older and much less likely to have had previous arterial surgery. Patients with occlusive disease were 16 times more likely to require re-operation after aortic surgery. In addition, aneurysm patients were on average more than 5 cm taller than patients with occlusive arterial disease and had a significantly greater body surface area (Tilson & Dang 1981). In our own experience, aneurysms in patients who have associated occlusive arterial disease are generally smaller and may be less likely to rupture than in patients without severe atherosclerosis. Support for this view is provided by Sterpetti et al (1985) who has shown that mean growth rates for small aneurysms are 50% faster when there is no obvious occlusive arterial disease.

Attention was first drawn to a family of patients with abdominal aortic aneurysm by Clifton in 1977 and the disease has recently been shown to have a prevalence of 29% in male first degree relatives (Collin & Walton 1989). There seems little doubt that abdominal aortic aneurysm has a strong genetic basis and that with the rapid pace of advance in molecular biology a candidate gene may soon be identified.

The ultimate expression of the genetic predisposition is probably determined by environmental influences such as cigarette smoking, diet and hypertension. In experimental animals an atherogenic regimen alone does not usually induce aneurysmal disease but copper deficiency may do so in pigs and poultry (Tilson 1989). Current theories suggest that degradation of collagen (Busuttil et al 1980) or elastin (Brown et al 1985) may be the proximate cause of aneurysm formation and rupture in man and that copper deficiency is not a relevant factor.

WHAT CAN BE DONE ABOUT IT?

The first resection of an abdominal aortic aneurysm was performed by Dubost in Paris in 1951 (Dubost et al 1952). The operation has been modified and simplified since but in essence it remains the only treatment which is known to remove the threat of aneurysm rupture or rescue the patient once rupture has occurred. If the aneurysm has undoubtedly ruptured the only question to resolve is would the patient rather die? If the answer is 'no' then emergency surgery should always be undertaken because even in the least expert hands the operative mortality can never be greater than the 100% mortality of the untreated disease.

An informed decision to undergo elective aneurysm resection can only be made by carefully balancing two risks which ought to be accurately known: the annual risk of rupture for an aneurysm of this size; and the audited operative mortality and morbidity of the surgeon over the last two years and how this average risk will be influenced by any individual health problems of the patient.

The balance of these two variables is such that the following rules can be stated with reasonable certainty for aortic aneurysms which do not extend above the renal arteries.

Aneurysms > 6.0 cm

All patients except for the very old or those with major medical contraindications can be recommended to have surgery in any vascular surgical unit.

Aneurysms 4.0–5.9 cm

The decision requires clinical judgement and depends on individual circumstances. Important considerations are the cardiac and respiratory function and general state of health of the patient together with the quality of surgical, anaesthetic and intensive care facilities available. In an otherwise fit patient, surgery can be confidently recommended provided the operative mortality of the surgeon is less than 5% (Collin 1987).

Aneurysms < 4.0 cm

Elective surgery cannot be recommended while the aneurysm remains this size. The diameter of the aneurysm should be remeasured by ultrasonography every six months to monitor its growth. There are a number of sensible general management decisions to be taken which may influence subsequent aneurysm expansion and its consequences. The patient should stop smoking, take regular exercise and if obese, reduce weight. The physician should control hypertension by appropriate therapy. There is recent evidence that in patients treated with β-adrenergic blockers aneurysm growth rates may be reduced and that this is independent of any effect on blood pressure control (Leach et al 1988)

Thoracoabdominal aortic aneurysms

The surgical treatment of aneurysms involving the whole of the descending thoracic and abdominal aorta has been possible for the last 15 years following the pioneering work of Stanley Crawford (Crawford 1974, Crawford et al 1986) but substantial experience has until recently been limited to very few centres around the world. The reasons for this are firstly that the disease is much less common than infrarenal aortic aneurysm and accounts for only around 5% of all cases seen. Secondly, the operative mortality has been up to 15 times higher than that for abdominal aortic aneurysm surgery in some hands while between 5 and 12% of survivors will have some degree of paraparesis (Hollier et al 1988, Crawford et al 1988).

The number of vascular units undertaking surgery for thoracoabdominal aneurysms has recently begun to increase in the United Kingdom as intraoperative monitoring and surgical results have improved. For every surgical team there is a learning curve which is accompanied by a reduction in operative mortality but even in the best hands this remains around 9% (Cambria et al 1989). For many patients the prospect of developing paraplegia may well seem like a fate worse than death. Indeed there are anecdotal reports that the threat of litigation following paraplegia and the near certainty of the surgeon losing in almost any United States civil court is discouraging a number of American vascular units from undertaking this surgery. In the rather more hospitable medicolegal environment in Britain the patient must at least be informed of the risk and allowed to decide for himself. The incidence of paraplegia is less for aneurysms which do not extend much above the diaphragm (types III and IV) and may be further reduced by routine cerebrospinal fluid pressure monitoring with drainage to maintain the arterial perfusion of the spinal cord during surgery (Hollier et al 1988). It is likely that over the next few years the indications for thoracoabdominal aortic surgery will become better defined and that operative mortality and morbidity will be reduced but this will remain an operation for major specialist units.

IS THIS THE BEST PLACE TO HAVE IT DONE?

How many of us on being confronted by a patient who insists on being operated on by the best surgeon in England would give the reply which I once overheard: 'I am the best surgeon in England'. Those who are tempted should remember that, as in the case I recall, the chances are it will be a lie.

Reported operative mortality for ruptured aneurysm covers a wide range from the extraordinarily low 21% of the Texas Heart Institute (Cooley & Carmichael 1984) to 70% at the University of Rochester (Pasch et al 1984). Considerable caution is required in assessing this sensitive issue of surgical outcome, however, since the type of patients referred and the criteria for selection for emergency surgery vary enormously from one institution to another. Vascular units which depend on secondary referrals for the bulk of their practice generally receive relatively few patients with ruptured aneurysm but operate on a high proportion of those who survive the journey with a low operative mortality. The superior results of such units may be partly explained by the fact that patients fit for transfer and surviving the journey will have contained ruptures and therefore be more likely to survive the operation. This suggestion is supported by comparison of our own predominantly local primary referral practice with that of two

major secondary referral centres in the United States drawing patients from
a large state and international catchment area (Cooley & Carmichael 1984,
Lawrie et al 1979). We operate on 38 patients with ruptured abdominal
aortic aneurysm per annum (Collin et al 1989a) compared with the
combined Houston experience of only 12 patients per annum. On the other
hand, in Houston, 235 patients per annum undergo elective abdominal
aortic aneurysm surgery compared with only 35 per annum in Oxford. The
36% operative mortality for ruptured aneurysm in Oxford is double the
18.4% reported from Houston but elective mortality rates of 1.4% and
3.2%, respectively, suggest that overall standards of care are comparable.
Operative mortality can also be reduced by deciding not to operate on
patients who are very hypotensive on arrival or who have respiratory,
cardiac, hepatic or renal impairment. We operate on all patients under 85
years old unless they have severe degenerative neurological disease or
disseminated neoplasia.

For elective aortic aneurysm surgery the effects of referral and selection
bias will be less marked but reporting bias ensures that the worst results are
never published. Recently reported audits from major vascular referral
centres show elective mortality rates ranging from under 2% to as high as
10%. In a group of district general hospitals without specialist vascular
units a mean operative mortality of 15.8% is known to occur (Guy et al
1990). In districts served by such hospitals the number of patients per
million catchment population being operated on for ruptured abdominal
aortic aneurysm is less than one-third of that for districts with vascular
surgical departments.

It is clearly unacceptable to expose patients undergoing elective aortic
aneurysm surgery to a substantial risk of death from the operation when the
sole justification for the procedure is to prevent premature death from
aneurysm rupture at some unpredictable time in the future. Prophylactic
surgery can only be recommended when morbidity and mortality are low.
Any surgeon whose audited operative mortality remains intractably above
5% for elective aortic aneurysm surgery should seriously question whether
he ought to continue doing this operation.

WILL I BE NORMAL AGAIN AFTERWARDS?

There is a natural tendency for surgeons to underestimate the unpleasant
effects of major surgery on an individual's general state of wellbeing. Even
the patient who makes a totally uncomplicated recovery from aortic
aneurysm resection will usually not feel completely well again for at least
three months. In an elderly man who develops a post-operative
complication the total recovery time after surgery may represent a
substantial proportion of his remaining life expectation. In addition to the
operative mortality risk of 5%, around 10% of patients will experience one
or more substantial complications which will delay recovery while at least

1% will subsequently develop a major graft complication such as graft infection of false aneurysm formation.

It is conventional wisdom supported by follow up studies in Britain (Fielding et al 1981) and the United States (Whittemore et al 1980) that following successful surgery the survival rate of patients treated for an aortic aneurysm approaches that of the general population. Such an outcome seems inherently improbable for a group of patients suffering from a disease linked to other conditions like hypertension and coronary artery disease known to be associated with impaired survival. Follow up studies such as the above are examples of the type III statistical error (Condon 1986) since Ballard (1984) has shown that after elective aneurysm repair survival at 5 years is 77% and at 10 years only 42% of that for an age and sex matched population.

HOW CAN WE PREVENT MY CHILDREN AND OTHERS DYING FROM IT?

The unequivocal answer is by routine ultrasound screening of the abdominal aorta of those at risk. Screening for abdominal aortic aneurysm in all men aged 65–74 was first suggested in 1985 (Collin 1985) and since then screening of this group and others thought to be at special risk has been extensively reported. The gathering of all this epidemiological data has allowed clear conclusions to be drawn about the value of screening and the priority which should be given to different groups at risk (Collin 1990b).

First degree relatives

Abdominal aortic aneurysm is a familial disease and is present in a quarter of the brothers of patients with an aneurysm (Bengtsson et al 1989). Many of the brothers screened in the two studies reported were less than 60 at the time of examination and therefore too young to have developed the disease. It is possible therefore that the total lifetime prevalence in first degree male relatives may be as high as 50%. In practice, screening programmes directed at brothers are unlikely to be productive since many will have moved far from their siblings and all contact with them lost. In addition, since patients treated for aortic aneurysms are usually in their seventies more than half their brothers will be either older or already dead. Nonetheless, it is good practice to ask any patient the number, age, whereabouts and state of health of any brothers and offer to arrange ultrasound examination of the aorta if this seems appropriate.

Most patients will be more concerned for their sons than brothers and will be more likely to have remained in contact with them. The main drawback to screening this group is that on average the sons will not begin to develop the disease for another 20 years although the lifetime prevalence will ultimately be the same as for their fathers' brothers. The best that can be achieved is to advise patients with the disease to impress upon their sons the need to arrange 5-yearly ultrasound examinations of their aorta from the age of 50 onwards.

The general population

Any viable screening programme will necessarily be confined to men since at age 65–69 the disease is 10 times more common in men than women. In designing a screening programme there are three conflicting aims:

1. To achieve a satisfactory detection rate.
2. To avoid detecting aortic aneurysms in those too old or too ill to accept or benefit from treatment.
3. To achieve the lowest operative mortality and maximum benefit for elective aortic aneurysm surgery in patients detected by screening.

In addition, because of inevitable limitations on budgets, equipment and personnel there will always be a fourth aim which need not conflict with the others but will tend to limit the coverage of any screening programme. This objective is to achieve the maximum benefit for the least cost.

All of these considerations point to screening men at the age of 65 and restricting follow up examinations to those discovered to have small subclinical aneurysms when screened. The age of 65 is opportune for screening since it operates various administrative triggers which allow easy identification and recruitment. For example, in the United Kingdom, pensions become payable and capitation payments from the National Health Service to the patients' general practitioners are automatically increased.

In England and Wales, 260 000 men reach the age of 65 each year. With minimal effort, over 50% of these can be recruited for screening and it is likely that with publicity this could be increased to 70%. In comparing costs of screening between countries the main variable is likely to be labour rates for the technicians, secretaries and radiologists. Other fixed costs involved are for the ultrasound machine and imager, room rental, stationery, postage, records and computing. All of these have been the subject of detailed costing and in England have been estimated at £24 000 for 5000 examinations per annum (Russell 1990). Assuming a 70% acceptance rate for screening this would cost £873 000 per annum for England and Wales. With a 5% anticipated detection rate for abdominal aortic aneurysms of all sizes, 9100 would be diagnosed at a cost of £96 each. A relatively trivial additional cost would be incurred by repeat screening every 6 months for patients with small aneurysms not requiring early operation.

It is instructive to compare the screening programme proposed above with that for breast cancer. In Britain, to the end of June 1989, 164 000 women had been invited for breast screening and 110 709 had been screened, a response rate of 67.5%. Of those screened, 8238 (7.4%) had been recalled for further assessment and 733 (0.66%) were found to have breast cancer (Richards 1989). Screening for abdominal aortic aneurysm therefore has a detection rate eight times that for breast cancer but the benefits are even greater since almost all patients with an aortic aneurysm can be completely cured by elective surgery right up to the day when the aneurysm ruptures. Most breast cancers detected by screening will alas already be beyond cure and treatment can at best be only palliative.

CONCLUSIONS

The key facts to remember about abdominal aortic aneurysm are as follows:

1. It is predominantly a disease of elderly men with a male to female incidence ratio at age 65–69 of 10 to 1.

2. It is common, with a prevalence of 5.4% in all men aged 65–74. The prevalence in patients with hypertension or symptoms of occlusive arterial disease in coronary, carotid or peripheral arteries is around 50% greater than in the general population.

3. It is a common cause of death accounting for 1.7% of all deaths in men aged 70–74. It is particularly common as a cause of sudden death and accounts for 4.2% of such deaths in men between 18 and 69 years of age.

4. Aneurysm rupture has an 85% mortality rate since most patients will die before reaching hospital and operative mortality overall is around 50% with only a few specialist units achieving better results.

5. Death from rupture is almost entirely preventable by early diagnosis and elective aneurysm resection. Screening of all men aged 65 would be best but in the absence of this routine abdominal palpation and diagnostic abdominal radiography, ultrasonography, computerized tomography or nuclear magnetic imaging will all diagnose many cases.

6. Diagnosis of an aortic aneurysm is more important than diagnosis of cancer since without treatment aortic aneurysm is as fatal as most cancers and with treatment is almost always completely curable.

7. Elective operative mortality greater than 5% is unacceptable and any surgical unit which consistently fails to achieve this figure should not continue to perform this kind of surgery.

8. One in 20 aneurysms of the abdominal aorta will involve the thoracoabdominal aorta. The mortality and morbidity of surgical treatment of these aneurysms is at best still twice that for infrarenal aneurysms. Their treatment should be confined to a few specialized vascular surgical units.

REFERENCES

Allardice J T, Allwright G J, Wafula J M C, Wyatt P 1988 High prevalence of abdominal aortic aneurysm in men with peripheral vascular disease: screening by ultrasonography. Br J Surg 75: 240–242

Allen P I M, Gourevitch D, McKinley J, Tudway D, Goldman M 1987 Population screening for aortic aneurysms. Lancet ii: 736

Ballard D J 1984 Selective screening for abdominal aortic aneurysms with physical examination and ultrasound. Arch Intern Med 149: 1463–1464

Bengtsson H, Norrgard O, Angquist K A, Ekberg O, Oberg L, Bergqvist D 1989 Ultrasonographic screening of patients with abdominal aortic aneurysms. Br J Surg 76: 589–591

Berridge D C, Griffith C D M, Amar S S, Hopkinson B R, Makin G S 1989 Screening for clinically unsuspected aortic aneurysms in patients with peripheral vascular disease. Eur J Vasc Surg 3: 421–422

Brown S L, Backstrom B, Busuttil R W 1985 A new serum proteolytic enzyme in aneurysm pathogenesis. J Vasc Surg 2: 393–399

Budd J S, Finch D R A, Carter P G 1989 A study of the mortality from ruptured abdominal aortic aneurysms in a district community. Eur J Vasc Surg 3: 351–354

Busuttil R W, Abou-Zamzam A M, Machleder H I 1980 Collagenase activity of the human aorta: a comparison of patients with and without abdominal aortic aneurysms. Arch Surg 115: 1373–1378

Cambria R P, Brewster D C, Moncure A C et al 1989 Recent experience with thoracoabdominal aneurysm repair. Arch Surg 124: 620–624

Clifton M A 1977 Familial abdominal aortic aneurysms. Br J Surg 64: 765–766

Collin J 1985 Screening for abdominal aortic aneurysms. Br J Surg 72: 851–852

Collin J 1987 Elective surgery for small abdominal aortic aneurysms. Lancet i: 909

Collin J 1988 The epidemiology of abdominal aortic aneurysm. Br J Hosp Med 40: 64–67

Collin J 1990a A proposal for a precise definition of abdominal aortic aneurysm. A personal view. J. Cardiovasc Surg 31: 168–169

Collin J 1990b The value of screening for abdominal aortic aneurysm by ultrasound. In: Greenhalgh R M, Mannick J A (eds) The Cause and Management of Aneurysms. W B Saunders, London, pp 447–456

Collin J, Walton J 1989 Is abdominal aortic aneurysm familial? Br Med J 299: 493

Collin J, Araujo L, Walton J, Lindsell D 1988 Oxford screening programme for abdominal aortic aneurysm in men aged 65 to 74 years. Lancet ii: 613–615

Collin J, Murie J, Morris P J 1989a Two year prospective analysis of the Oxford experience with surgical treatment of abdominal aortic aneurysm. Surg Gynecol Obstet 169: 527–531

Collin J, Araujo L, Walton J 1989b How fast do very small abdominal aortic aneurysms grow? Eur J Vasc Surg 3: 15–17

Condon R E 1986 Type III error. Arch Surg 121: 877–878

Cooley D A, Carmichael M J 1984 Abdominal aortic aneurysm. Circulation 1 (Suppl 70): 1.1–1.6

Crawford E S 1974 Thoracoabdominal and abdominal aortic aneurysms involving renal, superior mesenteric and celiac arteries. Ann Surg 179: 763–772

Crawford E S, Crawford J L, Safi J H et al 1986 Thoracoabdominal aortic aneurysm: preoperative and intraoperative factors determining immediate and long term results of operations in 605 patients. J Vasc Surg 3: 389–404

Crawford E S, Mizrami E M, Hess K R, Coselli J S, Safi H J, Patel V M 1988 The impact of distal aortic perfusion and somatosensory evoked potential monitoring on prevention of paraplegia after aortic aneurysm operation. J Thorac Cardiovasc Surg 95: 357–367

Cronenwett J L, Murphy T F, Zelenock G B et al 1985 Actuarial analysis of variables associated with rupture of small abdominal aortic aneurysms. Surgery 98: 472–483

Dubost C, Allary M, Oeconomos W 1952 Resection of aneurysm of the abdominal aorta. Arch Surg 64: 405–408

Estes J E 1950 Abdominal aortic aneurysm, a study of one hundred and two cases. Circulation 2: 258–264

Fielding J W L, Black J, Ashton F, Campbell D J 1981 Diagnosis and management of 528 abdominal aortic aneurysms. Br Med J 283: 355–359

Foster J H, Gobbel W G, Scott H W 1969 Comparative study of elective resection and
    expectant treatment of abdominal aortic aneurysm. Surg Gynecol Obstet 129: 1–9
Graham M, Chan A 1988 Ultrasound screening for clinically occult abdominal aortic
    aneurysm. Can Med Assoc J 138: 627–629
Guy A J, Lambert D, Jones N A G, Chamberlain J 1990 After CEPOD—Aortic aneurysm
    surgery in the Northern Region. Br J Surg (in press)
Hollier L H, Symmonds J B, Pairolero P C, Cherry K J, Hallett J W, Gloviczki P 1988
    Thoracoabdominal aortic aneurysm repair. Analysis of postoperative morbidity. Arch Surg
    123: 871–875
Ingoldby C J H, Wujanto R, Mitchell J E 1986 Impact of vascular surgery on community
    mortality from ruptured aortic aneurysms. Br J Surg 73: 551–553
Lawrie G M, Morris G C, Crawford E S et al 1979 Improved results of operation for
    abdominal aortic aneurysms. Surgery 85: 483–488
Leach S D, Toole A L, Stern H, De Natale R W, Tilson M D 1988 Effect of β-adrenergic
    blockade on the growth rate of abdominal aortic aneurysms. Arch Surg 123: 606–609
Lederle F A, Walker J M, Reinke D B 1988 Selective screening for abdominal aortic
    aneurysms with physical examination and ultrasound. Arch Intern Med 148: 1753–1756
Lilienfeld D E, Gunderson P D, Sprafka J M, Vargas C 1987 Epidemiology of aortic
    aneurysms: I. Mortality trends in the United States 1951–1981. Arteriosclerosis 7:
    637–643
Mortality Statistics Cause 1986 Office of Population Censuses and Surveys, England and
    Wales Series DH2 13 HMSO, London
Nevitt M P, Ballard D J, Hallett J W 1989 Prognosis of abdominal aortic aneurysms. A
    population based study. New Engl J Med 321: 1009–1014
Pasch A R, Ricotta J J, May A G, Green R M, De Weese J E 1984 Abdominal aortic
    aneurysm: the case for elective resection. Circulation 70 (suppl 1): 1.1–1.4
Richards T 1989 Breast cancer screening in Britain. Br Med J 299: 877–878
Russell J G B 1990 Is screening for abdominal aortic aneurysm worthwhile? Clin Radiol 1990
    41: 182–184
Scott R A P, Ashton H A, Kay D N 1988 Routine ultrasound screening in management of
    abdominal aortic aneurysm. Br Med J 296: 1709–1710
Sterpetti A V, Schultz R D, Feldhaus R J, Peetz D J, Fasciano A J, McGill J E 1985
    Abdominal aortic aneurysm in elderly patients. Selective management based on clinical
    status and aneurysmal expansion rate. Am J Surg 150: 772–776
Szilagyi D E, Smith R F, De Russo F J, Elliott J P, Sherrin F W 1966 Contribution of
    abdominal aortic aneurysmectomy to prolongation of life. Ann Surg 164: 678–699
Szilagyi D E, Elliott J P, Smith R F 1972 Clinical fate of the patient with asymptomatic
    abdominal aortic aneurysm and unfit for surgical treatment. Arch Surg 104: 600–606
Thomas A C, Knapman P A, Krikler D M, Davies M J 1988 Community study of the causes
    of natural sudden death. Br Med J 297: 1453–1456
Thurmond A S, Semler H J 1986 Abdominal aortic aneurysm: incidence in a population at
    risk. J Cardiovasc Surg 27: 457–460
Tilson M D 1989 A perspective of research in abdominal aortic aneurysm disease with a
    unifying hypothesis. In: Bergan J J, Yao J S T (eds) Aortic Surgery. W B Saunders,
    Philadelphia, pp 27–35
Tilson M D, Dang C 1981 Generalised arteriomegaly. A possible predisposition to the
    formation of abdominal aortic aneurysms. Arch Surg 116: 1030–1032
Tilson M D, Stansel H C 1980 Differences in results for aneurysms vs occlusive disease after
    aortic bifurcation grafts. Results of 100 elective grafts. Arch Surg 115: 1173–1175
Twomey A, Twomey E, Wilkins R A, Lewis J D 1986 Unrecognised aneurysmal disease in
    male hypertensive patients. Int Angiography 5: 269–273
Whittemore A D, Clowes A W, Hechtman H B et al 1980 Aortic aneurysm repair: reduced
    operative mortality associated with maintenance of optimal cardiac performance. Ann Surg
    192: 414–420

4

Blast injury

S. G. Mellor

INTRODUCTION

There has been a tenfold increase in terrorist incidents around the world over the past 20 years. At least 10 000 people have been killed or injured during this period, many of them by bombs. No part of the world seems to be immune from this problem. All hospital services must therefore prepare themselves in two ways, firstly by being ready to receive mass casualties from such incidents, and secondly by understanding the special problems associated with explosions. The aim of this review is to discuss the pathological effects of blast and their relevance to the clinician.

An explosive device when detonated causes injury in five ways.

1. *Primary injury* is that caused by the blast wave itself, and is all that is implied by the phrase 'blast injury'.

2. *Secondary injury* is caused by the bomb casing and other debris energized and propelled by the explosion: the missiles so produced may cause blunt and penetrating injuries.

3. *Tertiary injury* refers to traumatic amputation caused by the blast wind and those injuries resulting from propulsion of the body by the blast wind.

4. *Flash burns* result from the intense but short-lived heat of the explosion.

5. *Crush injury* may occur if the explosion is sufficient to cause collapse of a building.

Before describing the mechanism and effects of blast, the importance of 'blast injury' to the clinician should be put in perspective. Firstly, survivable injuries from explosions are nearly always a result of secondary missiles accelerated by the explosion. There is a lethal zone around every explosion and within this zone survival from the blast wave itself is not possible. Beyond this there is a zone where victims will die of penetrating injuries from secondary missiles, but may be relatively unharmed by the blast.

Zuckermann (1940) demonstrated experimentally the effect of the blast wave. Various animals were exposed to a 32 kg (70 lb) charge of high explosive such that no secondary missiles were generated. All animals 4 m or less from the explosion were killed. At the lethal limit of the explosion, between 4 m and 5.5 m from the charge, most were killed. Animals between 6 m and 16 m from the explosion were for the most part unharmed, although some showed a reluctance to feed initially. Between 5.5 m and 6 m from the explosion some of the animals displayed signs of respiratory embarrassment but recovered spontaneously over 24–48 hours. None had any sign of external injury. Post mortem examination of the lungs revealed 'bilateral traumatic haemorrhage...varying in degree according to the distance of the animal from the charge'.

It is essential to appreciate that such findings apply only to a pure blast in air where no secondary missiles are produced and no intervening or surrounding structures alter the blast wave.

The significance of the position of victims in relation to the blast wave will be discussed in the next section.

In order to explain the effects of blast injury it is essential to understand the mechanism of blast and its effects. Much new work has recently been published on the pathophysiology of blast. A clearer picture is beginning to form and with that in mind more successful methods of protection from blast can be devised.

MECHANISM OF EXPLOSION

Conventional high explosive, such a trinitrotoluene (TNT), explodes by detonation. This is a more rapid process than combustion and is a shock wave which passes through the explosive substance at about $5000 \, \mathrm{m \, s^{-1}}$, causing rapid chemical decomposition. The force of the explosion for a given weight of explosive depends on its detonation velocity. This is about $4000 \, \mathrm{m \, s^{-1}}$ in the case of commercial gelignite and about $8000 \, \mathrm{m \, s^{-1}}$ in the case of Semtex (Czechoslovakian manufactured plastic explosive). A rapidly expanding sphere of high pressure, high temperature gaseous products is produced, constituting the blast wave. Ground shock, fire and high velocity fragments are produced directly from the explosion. Following the blast wave is the blast wind.

THE BLAST WAVE

The pressure exerted by the blast wave increases to its maximum almost instantaneously. For a 20 kg charge of TNT there might be an effective pressure of 700 kPa over atmospheric, lasting for about 2 ms. Extreme rises of overpressure of shorter duration than this are unlikely to damage human tissue. In the case of a 1500 kg charge of TNT the rise in overpressure might last for up to 10 ms. Figure 4.1 shows an air blast. Although the peak pressure of 550 kPa may be potentially damaging, it lasts for only 0.25 ms and would therefore be quite harmless to humans. Much higher over-

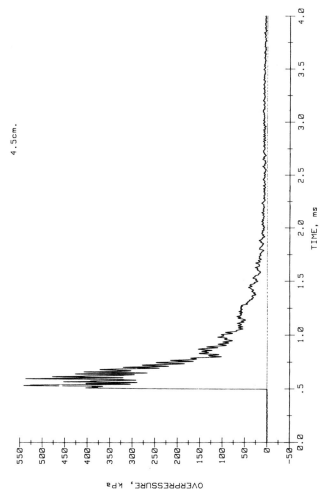

Fig. 4.1   The form of a blast wave. Pressure recordings of an air blast produced in a shock tube.

pressures may be tolerated when the increase is slow (as experienced by deep sea divers). The shock wave produced by the extracorporeal shockwave lithotripter causes no damage to tissue because it is so short. Each pulse lasts for around 0.002 ms and when suitably focused will shatter a renal stone leaving the far more resilient surrounding tissue unharmed. It is interesting to note that even at these short durations repeated shock waves focused on the lung may be damaging (Pode et al 1989).

In air, the blast wave can be considered as an expanding sphere and, like a sound wave, is propagated through and around objects in its path. When the explosion takes place on the ground, some of the shock wave is absorbed by the ground and an earth tremor may be felt (so called 'ground shock'). Much of the shock wave will be reflected off the ground and will reinforce the parent shock wave. Part of the wave will be reflected off objects in its path, reinforcing the wave front many times in these areas. Hence under certain conditions localized areas of overpressure much higher than anticipated from the size of the charge will be encountered. Cooper et al (1983) described in detail the position of victims prior to a number of bombings. Deaths and severe injuries occurred at distances from the explosion where no injury would be expected had the blast been in open air. The dead were against a wall, where local overpressures would be greatest, due to reinforcement of the shock wave. An even more striking example is an incident involving a bomb in a bus, described by Katz et al (1989). The charge involved was 6 kg of TNT. In air, 50% of those within 3 m of the explosion would be at risk of death. In this case, deaths occurred from pure blast 5 m from the explosion where no significant injury in open air would be expected, and again, these were near the sides of the bus where the reinforced blast wave would be at its greatest. Some passengers adjacent to the charge were uninjured, presumably because the seats protected them from the worst of the blast wave and the secondary missiles.

Decay of the blast wave depends on the acoustic impedance of the medium through which it passes. Thus in air, whose acoustic impedance is high, the blast wave front decreases in pressure and velocity in inverse proportion to the cube of the distance from it. When it reaches the speed of sound in air the explosion may be heard. Under water, where the acoustic impedance is very low, the decay of the blast wave is less rapid (linear rather than exponential) and the blast wave is heard and felt much further from its source than it would be in air.

The blast wave is a high energy system. When it encounters a medium of differing acoustic impedance in its path, part of the energy will be reflected at the interface and will reinforce the oncoming blast wave, and part will be transmitted. Three types of wave form have been identified in the body. These are stress waves, shock waves and shear waves. The last of these is a particular characteristic of high speed impact injury (Cooper & Taylor 1989).

Stress waves

These are longitudinal pressure waves, similar to sound waves, which travel through objects at about the same speed as sound but have a much higher amplitude. Very high local forces caused by the passage of the wave produce small but rapid distortions of tissue (stress). In the case of the stress wave, it is not tissue distortion which is important but the peak velocity attained by the small but rapid movements mentioned. Gross laceration of homogenous tissue does not occur. However, at interfaces of media with marked differences in acoustic impedance (e.g. air and water) significant strain occurs resulting in disruption at the interface. Hence the lung is highly susceptible to blast injury. Reflection of the blast wave off solid barriers in its path produces localized areas of very high pressure by reinforcement. In the case of the lung, such areas may be seen around the mediastinum and the larger airways and near the liver and ribcage.

Shock waves

These are a special type of stress wave which cause an almost instantaneous high pressure wave front propagated through the object at a much greater velocity than that at which sound would travel in that medium. They are capable of producing even greater stresses than the stress waves described above.

Shear waves

These are transverse waves of long duration and low velocity which cause gross distortion of the affected object. In the body, they produce asynchronous motion of adjacent connected structures, stretching at sites of attachment and collision of viscera with stiffer structures.

THE BLAST WIND

Following decay of the pressure front there is a period when the pressure falls, sometimes to 100 kPa below atmospheric. The mass movement of air displaced by the expanding sphere of explosive products results in the blast wind or dynamic pressure which follows an explosion. The displacement of bodies by the dynamic pressure may be determined from the equation $(\pi v^2)/2$, where π is the air density and v the air velocity. At its worst, the blast wind can cause total disruption of the human body but is also responsible for traumatic amputation of limbs. The decelerative tumbling and impact with rigid objects experienced by bodies displaced by the blast wind result in varying degrees of injury. Together, these are known as tertiary injury.

The effects of these waves on the body will now be described in more detail.

Table 4.1   Relative effects of overpressures lasting for more than 4 ms

Overpressure (kPa)	Effect
7	Damage to ordinary structures—flying glass and debris
15	Rupture of scarred or inflamed tympanic membrane (Zalewski 1906, Blake et al 1943)
100	50% rupture of tympanic membrane in human cadavers (Blake et al 1943)
175	Threshold lung damage in humans
300	Serious damage to reinforced concrete structures
500	50% chance of severe pulmonary damage and therefore 50% mortality

THE PATHOGENESIS OF INJURY CAUSED BY EXPLOSIONS

The human body is, relatively speaking, remarkably resistant to the primary effects of the blast wave (Table 4.1). Solid or fluid filled organs are rarely damaged by the shock wave. They tend to be damaged by the effects of the shear waves, especially at their mesenteric attachments. Those organs which contain air (ear, lung and bowel) are most readily affected by the blast wave as it stresses the air/fluid or air/tissue interfaces.

The well known clinical effects of the blast wave are death, lung damage and the effect on the ears. The severity of the injury relates directly to the blast loading to which the body was exposed, and its duration. Cause of death from an explosion is usually obvious, but there are special circumstances where the cause of death is obscure and the reasons for this will be discussed in this section.

Specific effects of the blast wave

Ear

Deafness, temporary or permanent, tinnitus, pain and dizziness are well recognized following explosions. Hearing damage is caused by perforation of the tympanic membrane, ossicular fracture or chain disruption and damage to the organ of Corti within the cochlea (Roberto et al 1989). Although vestibular damage may be the cause of dizziness, head injury (from a variety of sources) following explosions is so common that it is more likely to be the prime cause.

Rupture of the tympanic membrane may occur with an incident pressure of less than 15 kPa if the membrane is already scarred or inflamed. About half of exposed individuals will sustain eardrum rupture with an over-pressure of 100 kPa for 10 ms or more. Rupture of the tympanic membrane was noted in 50% of air raid casualties exposed to about 300 kPa for an unspecified duration (Blake et al 1943). Rupture may be caused by the short-lived effect of the shock wave on the air tissue interfaces of the membrane. In addition, the negative pressure following the blast wave is longer lived and is greater than the critical pressure above which soft tissue is forced into the pharyngeal end of the eustachian tube. This renders active opening impossible and presents pressure equalization.

The injury itself varies from a small linear tear to a gross defect in the membrane, and is usually situated in the anteroinferior quadrant. Perforations of the pars flaccida due to blast never occur.

It has been stated that if the tympanic membrane is intact severe blast loading is unlikely to have occurred (Haywood 1988). However, in a recent series, fewer than half of survivors of explosions who were supposedly subjected to a blast loading of more than 500 kPa had ruptured tympanic membranes (Mellor & Cooper 1989). There are two reasons for this observation. Firstly, the orientation of the tympanic membrane towards the incident pressure of the blast wave is critical. With the incident wave normal to the drum, the overpressure measured at the drum will be twice that found if the incident wave is at a right angle to the drum (James et al 1982). Secondly, any survivor from within the theoretical lethal zone of an explosion must have been protected from the full force of the blast wave, if not from the secondary missiles. On the other hand, it is probable that rupture of the tympanic membrane is under reported in survivors with otherwise very severe injuries. Furthermore, the rupture may be entirely symptom free.

Dislocation of the ossicles may occur with or without perforation of the tympanic membrane. Transient deformation of the skull by the advancing blast wave or, indeed, direct trauma may be the explanation in the latter case. Fracture of the handle of the malleus and dislocation of the stapes are the commonest ossicular injuries seen, and imply severe blast loading.

Cochlear injury results in temporary or permanent deafness depending on the incident pressure of the shock wave. The organ of Corti is most at risk. Sensory cell losses continue over several weeks following severe barotrauma, particularly if the underlying reticular lamina is damaged. These injuries may never recover (Roberto et al 1989).

Labyrinthine rupture is also known to occur, affecting the round window, and may be a cause of the dizziness and vertigo experienced by victims of blast. It would be difficult to distinguish this as a cause without very sophisticated investigation as cerebral concussion is so common in victims of explosions.

Lungs

Lung damage in the form of small areas of haemorrhage may occur with blast loading as low as 175 kPa for 4 ms. As the blast loading increases, the lung damage becomes more extensive, until with an overpressure of 500 kPa for 4 ms, 50% of those exposed will die (Bowen et al 1968).

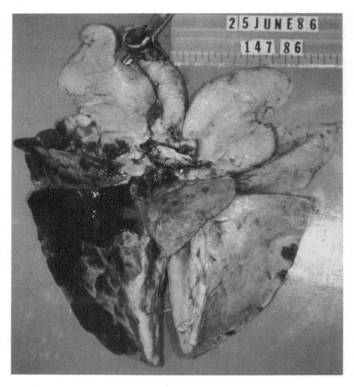

Fig. 4.2   The macroscopic appearance of blast lung. The main area of contusion lies over the liver. In the other lung small areas of contusion corresponding to ribs may be seen.

Although deformation of the ribcage may be seen on high speed cinephotography of the effects of an explosion, this probably does not contribute greatly to blast injury of the lung. The special stress waves described above are the most important cause of lung injury. The stresses are most pronounced at the alveolar/capillary membrane, and result in its disruption if the strain is great enough. This is particularly marked near the mediastinum, liver, ribcage and larger, stiffer airways where reflection and reinforcement set up complex high pressure areas within the lung parenchyma. Disruption of the alveolar/capillary membrane results in haemorrhage and leakage of interstitial fluid into the alveoli. The low velocity waves may cause shearing of lung tissue off the larger more rigid bronchioles resulting in further haemorrhage into the lung. Primary lung injury will therefore range from a few pinpoint haemorrhages in places where the stresses are highest—near the mediastinum and peripherally near the ribs and liver—to complete shock lung. An experimental example of blast lung is shown in Figure 4.2, and its microscopic appearance in Figure

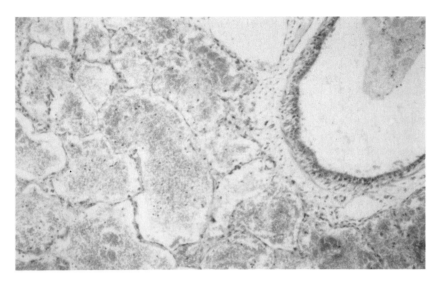

Fig. 4.3   The microscopic appearance of blast lung. Note the haemorrhage into the alveoli.

4.3. Although severe blast injury to the lung is fatal, less severe trauma may have little clinical significance. For example, in a recent study of 828 servicemen killed or injured by explosions in Northern Ireland, only two survivors of explosions required ventilation for blast lung (Mellor & Cooper 1989). In addition, pulmonary insufficiency did not seem to be a problem in those treated for secondary missile injuries who might have been exposed to moderate degrees of blast loading. However, Zuckermann's work quoted earlier suggests that many blast victims will have subclinical bruising of the lung. Varying degrees of bronchopleural fistulae also occur. Many of these will heal, but patients who require assisted ventilation are at a high risk of developing a pneumothorax.

Heart

There is a small percentage of victims of explosions who die with little in the way of either external injury or significant internal injury. Although difficult to prove, it is suspected that passage of the blast wave occasionally causes cardiac dysrhythmia and thereby sudden death. Bradycardia and a variety of ECG changes following the passage of a blast wave have been demonstrated, but often do not become established for some minutes after the explosion. Evidence of right heart strain will be seen where there is lung damage and increased vascular resistance. Bradycardia is abolished in vagotomized animals, and by local anaesthesia of the carotid sinus. In severe blast injury, myocardial haemorrhage and ruptured muscle bundles may be seen. Where there is significant lung injury, alveolar air may enter the circulation and cause coronary artery air embolism.

Solid viscera

Apart from direct trauma from secondary missiles and acceleration of the victim by the blast wind, shear waves cause laceration of solid viscera by gross distortion and tear mesenteric attachments. Solid viscera, especially the liver, are set in motion relative to the body wall by the shear waves. Because its inertia differs from that of the body wall, the liver will collide with the ribcage and may be severely lacerated.

Gastrointestinal tract

Damage to the gastrointestinal tract is probably more common than is clinically appreciated, but in air does not occur without severe concurrent lung injury.

The shear waves can cause submucosal haemorrhage and mesenteric tears. Pockets of air trapped against the bowel wall result in local bruising as the stress wave passes and in more severe cases perforation may occur. The ileocaecal junction is particularly susceptible to perforation and bruising.

Blast injury to the gut with survivable lung injury occurs in victims of underwater explosions. A possible explanation is that the abdomen is submerged but the chest is only partially so. Since the blast wave in water is sustained for so much longer, the submerged abdomen would be more affected by the shock wave, while the partially submerged chest would be less affected.

Nervous system

Apart from head injuries of varying severity due to secondary and tertiary injury, emotional shock, dizziness and disorientation are common findings in relatively uninjured victims of explosions. The symptoms resemble concussion, but in many cases no direct blow to the head will have occurred. The work of Suneson (1989) goes some of the way to explaining this phenomenon. In pigs subjected to peripheral high energy transfer injuries, definite changes to the CNS were revealed by light and electron microscopy studies, although there was no macroscopic evidence of injury. Signs of axon degeneration were seen both peripherally and centrally with damage to the cytoskeleton and microtubules of nerve cells. Functional disturbance of the blood–brain barrier as measured by a reduction in oxygen consumption was also noted.

Fractures may occur around the air sinuses following passage of the blast wave. Cerebral artery air embolism following significant lung injury is also possible. In these cases air emboli may be seen in the retinal vessels (Benzinger 1950, Cooper et al 1983).

Secondary injury

Secondary missiles generated by the explosion may travel at very high velocities causing both blunt and penetrating injuries. These are often very contaminated with much tissue destruction. Tattooing of exposed skin by tiny pieces of dirt is a common problem, and the tattooes are often very deep.

Tertiary injury

Although the pressure exerted by the blast wind is many times less than that exerted by the blast wave, it is longer lived and may be very destructive. It is the dynamic pressure exerted by the blast wind which is responsible for total disruption of a body close to an explosion. In less severe cases, and where the body is partially protected from the blast wind, traumatic amputation of a limb, or even fingers and toes may occur. It must be emphasized that the forces to which the body is subjected to cause any degree of traumatic amputation are very great and those sustaining proximal limb amputation rarely survive (Rignault & Deligny 1989, Mellor & Cooper 1989).

Flash burns

Very high temperatures are generated for relatively short periods during the explosion, resulting in local fires and flash burns to victims close to the explosion.

Cause of death from explosions

Victims close to the explosion will be disrupted by the forces generated by the dynamic pressure and secondary missiles. Further away, in areas where the overpressure is sufficiently high, blast lung will occur without disruption of the body. Its onset is very rapid once an overpressure of 700 kPa for 2 ms or more is reached. These cases will nearly always have concurrent fatal secondary injuries. Under certain circumstances, for example where the victim is in an area of high overpressure but protected from secondary missiles, blast lung may be the only cause of death. The wearing of protective body armour may avoid fatal penetrating injury, but, at present, not the blast wave. In areas where the blast wave has decayed and the secondary missiles are less likely to cause penetration, head injury is the commonest cause of death. Those victims with blast lung who survive long enough to be ventilated may die suddenly from coronary artery or cerebral air emboli. If death occurs in the multiple injured some days after the explosion, the appearance of the lung at necropsy is usually solid, with haemorrhage and oedema. This may be directly due to the blast wave, but by that time other factors such as sepsis, protracted hypovolaemia, fat embolism and smoke inhalation must be considered.

MANAGEMENT OF BLAST INJURY

Triage

Terrorist bombings are intended to produce large numbers of casualties. Of these, some will be killed instantly, some will have very severe injuries and some may die on the way to hospital or during treatment. Many will be deafened, disoriented and emotionally shocked with relatively minor injuries. Clearly, the management of such patients is a considerable drain on resources. Frykberg & Tepas (1988) observed a 59% overtriage rate when all casualties were hospitalized. Whether this refers to admission or simply treatment in the casualty department is not made clear. However, by adopting this policy no serious injuries were missed.

Rignault & Deligny (1989) point to the French experience advocating 'on the spot' triage and resuscitation. They claim this has two advantages. Firstly, the critically injured may be stabilized prior to transfer, with the further advantage of being directed to the most appropriate specialist resource for their injuries. Secondly, hospitals will not be overburdened with hysterical patients with minor injuries. Although superficially appealing, this method is expensive and labour intensive, and may divert much needed medical, nursing and ancillary staff from overstretched hospitals. Furthermore, there is no evidence that survival rates are improved. No victim with a major traumatic amputation (the group in which blood loss is most rapid) survived despite rapid and intensive resuscitation. Of particular relevance in the management of blast injury is the fact that respiratory distress as a result of non-fatal blast lung may not become apparent for some hours after the explosion and may be associated with little in the way of external injury in some cases. Careful assessment in hospital will be necessary in order not to miss this small group of potentially treatable patients.

As a compromise, Frykberg & Tepas (1988) suggest a second echelon where casualty holding and triage can take place away from both the scene of the incident and the receiving hospital. This is the military approach, and is entirely appropriate for the battlefield where there is a long chain of evacuation. However, in urban mass casualty situations, such as isolated bombing incidents, this is not the case. Furthermore, the likely workload is known quite rapidly after the incident and a tailored response can be made. In such an incident setting up second echelon support is more likely to hinder treatment than to enhance it.

My own view is that the most effective triage and resuscitation occurs in hospital, and that valuable resources should not be diverted from a hospital to the site of the incident except in special circumstances, for example, where victims are trapped and in need of urgent treatment while they are freed. Recent experience in major disasters in the UK over the past few years bears out this view. As far as the receiving hospital is concerned, arrangements must be made for all incoming casualties to go through a designated triage point manned by an experienced general surgeon. His only task is to separate those who can wait for treatment from those who cannot. Adequate equipped and manned resuscitation areas must be designated to receive the seriously injured. These areas should be physically separated from the waiting area for the less seriously injured and should not interfere with passage to wards and operating theatres. Accurate documentation of all injuries sustained is essential, and is most likely to be achieved in the hospital environment.

History and examination

Where possible the distance of the victim from the explosion and his position relative to walls, furniture etc. should be recorded. This may alert the examiner to special circumstances where a higher than expected blast loading has occurred, and is vital from the forensic point of view. Many victims will recall their position prior to the blast, but often not their final position in the ensuing noise, smoke and confusion.

Most blast victims will complain of deafness, tinnitus and pain in the ears. The tympanic membrane should always be examined. If it is ruptured, this implies a significant exposure to blast loading and the fact should be recorded to assist in initial management and in future claims for compensation. If the tympanic membrane is uninjured, significant blast loading is not excluded, for the reasons stated above.

A blast loading of greater than 350 kPa for 2 ms can cause significant intra-alveolar haemorrhage and oedema, as described earlier. Signs of lung contusion and pneumothorax should be sought, and an erect chest radiograph should be obtained. Serial chest radiographs are helpful to monitor the development of 'blast lung'. This will happen very rapidly over a few hours in severe cases which are not immediately fatal. Such patients are also at risk of developing a pneumothorax. Depending on the degree of pulmonary contusion, there will be a corresponding fall in arterial oxygen tension. This must be monitored with serial blood gas estimations or the pulse oximeter.

Signs of smoke inhalation should be sought, as this may be an additional cause of developing pulmonary insufficiency.

Colicky abdominal pain, haemetemesis or melaena may occur with blast injury to the abdomen. Increasing constant pain, peritonism and abdominal rigidity indicate that perforation of a viscus has occurred. Persisting hypotension despite adequate resuscitation may indicate intraperitoneal haemorrhage.

All other injuries must be accurately recorded, as compensation is bound to be sought at some stage. In this respect photographs are invaluable and should be obtained if at all possible.

Management

Accurate assessment and effective resuscitation are the cornerstones of management of any seriously injured patient. The following remarks are relevant to the management of patients injured in explosions.

Deafness, tinnitus and dizziness generally pass off in the first few hours after an explosion. Perforations of the tympanic membrane which occupy less than 30% of its area generally heal spontaneously. A detailed review of treatment of blast injury to the ear is provided by Casler et al (1989).

Early administration of oxygen by mask is desirable in the early management of the seriously injured. However, it has been suggested that in the blast injured lung an excessive increase in alveolar oxygen tension may exacerbate bleeding into the lung by dilatation of the vascular bed (von Euler 1946). The use of the pulse oximeter is extremely useful in this respect as it gives an accurate guide to percentage oxygen saturation of the blood allowing oxygen administration to be titrated. Mechanical ventilation should be instituted if oxygen administration by mask is insufficient. However, because of the frequent presence of traumatic bronchopleural fistulae, there is a high risk of pneumothorax in ventilated patients, and therefore prophylactic chest drainage is recommended. Rupture of the alveolar/capillary membrane by the blast wave can result in cerebral, retinal and coronary air emboli which may cause neurological deterioration, transient blindness or sudden death, especially if positive expiratory end pressure becomes necessary. Severe blast injury to the lung is nearly always associated with severe secondary injuries and usually develops very rapidly. Isolated blast injury to the lung may occur where there are few secondary missiles generated and where local conditions reinforce the blast wave (Katz et al 1989). Body armour, as worn by security forces in Northern Ireland, protects against potentially fatal secondary injury, but not against blast injury. Isolated blast lung may also occur in these cases (Mellor & Cooper 1989). Less severe cases of blast lung not requiring ventilation should resolve, providing there is no secondary infection. Active physiotherapy and antibiotic prophylaxis are therefore recommended.

There is no evidence that high dose corticosteroids are of any benefit in these cases.

The abdomen should be carefully examined for signs of intraperitoneal bleeding or perforation of hollow viscera, but it should be remembered that severe injuries to the gastrointestinal tract from blast are rare in the absence of concurrent 'blast lung'. If they do occur in isolation then blunt or penetrating trauma from secondary missiles is more likely to be the cause.

Submucosal and subserosal haemorrhages may cause haemetemesis, melaena and colicky abdominal pain. In the absence of perforation, decompression of the gut via a nasogastric tube and adequate blood and fluid replacement may be all that is required. Laparotomy is indicated if there is severe intraperitoneal haemorrhage or perforation. Perforations of the stomach or small bowel may be oversewn although resection and primary anastomosis may be necessary with more extensive damage. Management of large bowel perforations will depend on the experience of the surgeon, but if in doubt excision and exteriorization is the safest policy. Most large bowel perforations occur at the ileocaecal junction, so resection and anastomosis is feasible in many cases.

Secondary missile injuries are likely to be contaminated and should therefore be treated with adequate debridement and toilet followed by delayed primary suture or skin grafting. External skeletal fixation is a useful way of stabilizing compound fractures of long bones in the first instance.

Although the burns sustained in explosions are often superficial, adequate allowance must be made for them in initial crystalloid and colloid fluid replacement.

Facial tattooing from tiny pieces of grit is a challenging problem to treat due to the depth to which the particles penetrate. The use of the scratch pad made for cleaning diathermy tips has been advocated for immediate treatment of this potentially disfiguring type of injury (Horowitz et al 1988).

Finally, it is becoming clear that psychological counselling of victims of mass casualty situations is vital to their rehabilitation, and should be instituted as soon as possible. It may be of most value to those least injured, particularly if friends or relatives have been more severely injured or killed.

KEY POINTS FOR CLINICAL PRACTICE

Where an explosion takes place mostly in the open, victims with blast injury are likely to have sustained fatal secondary missile injuries.

Body armour can protect the victim from potentially fatal secondary missile injuries, but not from the force of the blast wave. Such casualties should be carefully assessed for blast lung.

Where a relatively small explosion takes place in a confined space there may be a disproportionate number of victims of the blast wave who have few or no other injuries. In these cases, rupture of the tympanic membrane may be a useful guide as to whether significant blast loading has occurred.

The development of blast lung may be monitored with serial blood–gas estimations and chest radiographs. Sudden neurological deterioration and sudden death may occur from air emboli from alveolar/capillary fistulae, and this may be enhanced when assisted respiration becomes necessary. Mechanical ventilation should not be withheld, but chest drains are mandatory due to the likelihood of pneumothorax occurring.

Intra-abdominal visceral perforation and laceration does occur as a result of blast injury but not without severe, probably fatal, blast injury to the lung.

Victims of explosions who suffer major traumatic amputations rarely, if ever, survive. This should be borne in mind if expectant management of severe casualties becomes necessary due to overwhelming numbers.

REFERENCES

Benzinger T 1950 German aviation medicine in World War II. United States Department of the Air Force
Blake P M, Douglas J B W, Krohn P L, Zuckerman S 1943 Rupture of the eardrums by blast. Ministry of Home Security Report BPC 43/169/WS21, Military Personnel Research Committee (Medical Research Council), Department of Human Anatomy, Oxford University, Oxford, England
Bowen I G, Fletcher E R, Richmond D R 1968 Estimate of man's tolerance to the direct effects of air blast. Technical Progress Report, DASA -2113, Washington DC. Defense Atomic Support Agency, Dept of Defense, October
Casler J D, Chait R H, Zajtchuk J T 1989 Treatment of blast injury to the ear. Ann Otol Rhinol Laryngol 98: 13–16
Cooper G J, Taylor D E M 1989 Biophysics of impact injury to the chest and abdomen. J R Army Med Corps 135: 58–67
Cooper G J, Maynard R L, Cross N L, Hill J F 1983 Casualties from terrorist bombings. J Trauma 23: 955–967
Frykberg E R, Tepas J J 1988 Terrorist bombings. Lessons learned from Belfast to Beirut. Ann Surg 208(5): 569–576
Haywood I 1988 The patho-physiology of terrorist violence. Trauma (in press)
Horowitz J, Nichter L S, Stark D 1988 Dermabrasion of traumatic tattoos: simple, inexpensive, effective. Ann Plast Surg 21: 257–259
James D J, Pickette V C, Burdette K J, Cheesman A 1982 The response of the human ear to blast. Part 1: The effect on the ear drum of a "short" duration, "fast" rising pressure wave. Joint AWRE/CDE Report No. 04/82, AWRE, Aldermaston, England
Katz E, Ofek B, Adler J, Abramowitz H B, Krausz M M 1989 Primary blast injury after a bomb explosion in a civilian bus. Ann Surg 209(4): 484–488
Mellor S G, Cooper G J 1989 Analysis of 828 servicemen killed or injured by explosion in Northern Ireland 1970–1984. Br J Surg 76: 1006–1010
Pode D, Lijovetsky G, Landau E L, Shapiro A 1989 Isolated pulmonary blast injury in rats— a new model using the extracorporeal shock wave lithotriptor. Milit Med 154: 288–293
Rignault D P, Deligny M C 1989 The 1986 terrorist bombing experience in Paris. Ann Surg 209(3): 368–373
Roberto M, Hamernik R P, Turrentine G A 1989 Damage of the auditory system associated with acute blast trauma. Ann Otol Rhinol Laryngol 98: 23–34
Suneson A 1989 Distant pressure wave effects on nervous tissue by high energy missile impact. Department of Histology, Neurosurgery and Surgery, University of Goteborg, Goteborg, Sweden (Thesis)
von Euler U S, Liljestrand G 1946 Observations on the pulmonary arterial blood pressure in the cat. Acta Physiol Scand 12: 301–320
Zalewski T 1906 Experimentelle Untersuchungen uber die Resistenz fahigkeit des Trommelfells. Z Ohrenheilkd 52: 109–128
Zuckermann S 1940 Experimental Study of Blast Injuries to the Lungs. Lancet ii: 219–224

5

Recent advances in the treatment of burn injuries

L. F. A. Rossi   P. G. Shakespeare

Burn injuries continue to pose a significant problem in their occurrence and treatment. The scale of the problem is illustrated by the fact that the Wessex Regional Burn Centre (WRBC), serving a population of 3.5 million, expects to treat about 200 cases per year. This probably represents one half of the total number of injuries requiring inpatient treatment in the Wessex Region. Figures for the numbers of burns treated as outpatients are not available to us but will represent a considerable excess over the inpatient admissions. Of the cases admitted to the Wessex Regional Burn Centre some 40% are children under the age of 5 years, the vast majority of whom are scalded in accidents involving kettle spills, hot drink spills and bath accidents. About one-half of these children will require some surgical repair of their wounds and 60% will require therapy after leaving the Burn Centre to help alleviate the effects of scar tissue development.

There is still the potential for the development of improved methods of treating wounds and managing patients. Many of the approaches to the treatment of the different clinical problems faced by the burned patient are empirical and have not been subjected to rational evaluation. Although it is likely that the general principles of successful treatment of the injuries have been formulated there are still major differences in the specific approach to the treatment of clinical problems presenting during the burned patient's recovery. Major historical landmarks in the treatment of burns have been those which have improved the practice of surgery in general, with emphasis particularly on management of circulatory disturbances and infection control.

Above all there remains the goal of reduction in the incidence of burn injuries. The yearly admission rate to this Centre has not changed significantly in the past 15 years. Within the scope of this short review it is the intention of the authors to provide a personal view of the advances which appear to us to be most noteworthy over the last 10 years. It is difficult to approach the subject of burn treatment without making a catalogue list of the perceived problems. We can find no answer to this but will try to keep the listing to general headings rather than specific topics and hope that this will not provide too much discouragement to the reader.

PREVENTION AND FIRST AID TREATMENT

Burn injuries occur predominantly in the home. Perhaps the most notable advance in the prevention of these injuries has been an increased awareness of specific hazards, for example trailing kettle leads, which has led to some manufacturers supplying 'safety' coiled leads as standard equipment on new appliances. The dangers of freshly-made hot beverages and the hazards inherent in the domestic hot-water supply have been more widely recognized. In the work environment, improved safety practices and education of the workforce to burn hazards, for example power cables, inflammable liquids and corrosive chemicals can still be improved. It is now recognized that the application of cold water to a fresh burn for a minimum of 10 minutes is an effective analgesic and reversor of thermal damage to the skin (Davies 1982).

ASSESSMENT OF AREA OF BURN AND DEPTH OF INJURY

The initial assessment of area and depth are critical to the management of the burn injury. This assessment is still open to observer error being largely subjective. The method of the 'Rules of Nine', although not strictly accurate, is still widely used to estimate area of body surface burned. Some modifications to these rules have been introduced for the assessment of burned children. Many thermal injuries are compounded by inhalation injury and recent studies have shown (Clark et al 1986) that mortality probability is significantly increased if the burn is associated with inhalation injury. The authors suggest alterations to the prediction of mortality, (Bull 1971), which consider age and percentage of body surface burned, to take account of this factor. The increase in the probability of mortality can be simply calculated by the combination of a scoring of clinical parameters and laboratory carboxyhaemoglobin estimations. Unfortunately, the assessment of burn depth is still subjective, being made by a combination of history, clinical observation and sensation testing by pinprick. As the detailed requirements of the resuscitation, for example blood administration and subsequent surgical management of the wounds, depend on this there is still a need for an accurate non-invasive objective means of depth assessment (see later).

RESUSCITATION FORMULAE

There has been little change in the past 10 years. The fluids available for resuscitation are: electrolyte solutions (widely used in the USA but not in this country), dextran 110 and Human Plasma Protein Fraction (albumin). These latter two are widely used in this country with Human Plasma Protein Fraction as the fluid of choice. Unfortunately, Fresh Frozen Human Plasma is now not available routinely. All the formulae for

Table 5.1 Proforma for the calculation of fluid requirements in burned adults

Circle requirement

Body weight (kg)	Burn area															Blood vol.
	10	15	20	25	30	35	40	45	50	55	60	65	70	75	80	
40	400	560	760	960	1160	1360	1520	1720	1920	2120	2320	2480	2680	2880	3080	3000
45	440	640	880	1080	1280	1520	1720	1960	2160	2360	2600	2800	3040	3240	3480	3375
50	480	720	960	1200	1440	1680	1920	2160	2400	2640	2880	3120	3360	3600	3840	3750
55	520	800	1040	1320	1600	1840	2120	2360	2640	2920	3160	3440	3680	3960	4240	4125
60	560	840	1160	1440	1720	2000	2320	2600	2880	3160	3480	3760	4040	4320	4600	4500
65	640	920	1240	1560	1880	2200	2520	2800	3120	3440	3760	4080	4360	4680	5000	4875
70	680	1000	1360	1680	2000	2360	2680	3040	3360	3680	4040	4360	4720	5040	5400	5250
75	720	1080	1440	1800	2160	2520	2880	3240	3600	3960	4320	4680	5040	5400	5760	5625
80	760	1160	1520	1920	2320	2680	3080	3440	3840	4240	4600	5000	5360	5760	6160	6000
85	800	1200	1640	2040	2440	2840	3280	3680	4080	4480	4920	5320	5720	6120	6520	6375
90	840	1280	1720	2160	2600	3000	3480	3880	4320	4760	5200	5640	6040	6480	6920	6750
95	920	1360	1840	2280	2720	3200	3640	4120	4560	5000	5480	5920	6400	6840	7320	7125
100	960	1440	1920	2400	2880	3360	3840	4320	4800	5280	5760	6240	6720	7200	7680	7500

1. First period to 8 hours after injury, not after admission.
2. Second period runs from 8–24 hours after injury.
3. Third period runs from 24–48 hours after injury.
4. A fourth period may be given if necessary on clinical grounds 48–72 hours after injury.

$$0-8\,h = \quad cc = \quad cc/h$$
$$8-24\,h = \quad cc = \quad cc/h$$
$$24-48\,h = \quad cc = \quad cc/h$$

Metabolic requirements: No more than 120 cc/h orally if tolerated

Severe burns:

Blood:

Burns less than 25% transfuse blood – average 1% blood volume/1% full thickness burn at end of shock phase.

$$\therefore \frac{BV(\quad)}{100} \times \frac{\%FT}{} = \quad cc$$

Burns greater than 25% give $\frac{1}{2}$ this amount 12 h from burning and other $\frac{1}{2}$ at end of shock phase.

Table 5.2 Proforma for the calculation of fluid requirements in burned children

Circle requirement

Body weight (kg)	Burn area													Blood vol.
	7.5	10	12.5	15	20	25	30	35	40	45	50	60	70	
4	40	60	70	90	100	120	150	180	210	240	270	300	330	300
5	50	70	90	110	130	150	180	220	260	300	330	370	410	375
6	60	90	110	130	150	180	220	270	310	360	400	450	490	450
7	70	100	130	150	180	210	260	310	360	420	470	520	570	525
8	90	120	150	180	210	240	300	360	420	480	540	600	660	600
9	100	130	160	200	230	270	330	400	470	540	600	670	740	675
10	110	150	180	220	260	300	370	450	520	600	670	750	820	750
11	120	160	200	240	280	330	410	490	570	660	740	820	900	825
12	130	180	220	270	310	360	450	540	630	720	810	900	990	900
14	150	210	260	310	360	420	520	630	730	840	940	1050	1150	1050
16	180	240	300	360	420	480	600	720	840	960	1080	1200	1320	1200
18	200	270	330	400	470	540	670	810	940	1080	1210	1350	1480	1350
20	220	300	370	450	520	600	750	900	1050	1200	1350	1500	1650	1500
22	240	330	410	490	570	660	820	990	1150	1320	1480	1650	1810	1650
24	270	360	450	540	630	720	900	1080	1260	1440	1620	1800	1980	1800
26	290	390	480	580	680	780	970	1170	1360	1560	1750	1950	2140	1950
28	310	420	520	630	730	840	1050	1260	1470	1680	1890	2100	2310	2100
30	330	450	560	670	780	900	1120	1350	1570	1800	2020	2250	2470	2250
32	360	480	600	720	840	960	1200	1440	1680	1920	2160	2400	2640	2400
34	380	510	630	760	890	1020	1270	1530	1780	2040	2290	2550	2800	2550
36	400	540	670	810	940	1080	1350	1620	1880	2160	2430	2700	2970	2700
38	420	570	710	850	990	1140	1420	1710	1990	2280	2560	2850	3130	2850

1. First period to 8 hours after injury—not after admission.
2. Second period from 8–24 hours after injury.
3. Third period from 24–48 hours after injury.

∴ 1. 0–8h =   cc =   cc/h
   2. 8–24h =   cc =   cc/h
   3. 24–48h =   cc =   cc/h

Daily metabolic requirements:
   A weight between   4–12 kg = 120 cc/kg   ∴ ÷24 =   cc/h
   A weight between 12–18 kg = 100 cc/kg   ∴ ÷24 =   cc/h
   A weight above 18 kg   = 80 cc/kg   ∴ ÷24 =   cc/h

Severe burns:

Blood:

Burns less than 25% transfuse blood—average 1% blood volume/1% full thickness burn at end of shock phase.

$$\therefore \ \frac{BV(\quad) \times (\quad)\% \, FT}{100} = \quad cc$$

Burns greater than 25% give $\frac{1}{2}$ this amount 12 h from burning and other $\frac{1}{2}$ at end of shock phase.

calculation of volume requirement in common use are still based on the variables of percentage of body surface burned and body weight. All are effective as guides but must be modified by frequent clinical and physiological investigation. At this Centre the formula of Cason (1981) normalized to a body weight of 70 kg is used. The formula suggests that a 70 kg adult patient will require 1.25 l of Human Plasma Protein Fraction per 10% body surface burned over the first 24 hours; half to be given by 8 hours after burn, half in the next 16 hours. An additional period may be added from 24–48 hours, depending upon the condition of the patient. Requirements for patients of higher or lower weights are adjusted on a simple ratio. Suggested requirements for children are somewhat different. The patient is estimated to require one plasma volume (45 ml per kg body weight) for each 15% of body surface burned, with the administration schedule being the same as for adults. To simplify the management procedure a look-up chart for the calculation of fluid requirements has been devised for men, women and children and is incorporated into the Burns Unit admission forms (Tables 5.1 and 5.2). Additional fluid for the normal metabolic requirements is given, orally if possible, but it may be added to the intravenous infusion regimen, especially in children. The minimum area of burn for which resuscitation is recommended is 15% or more of body surface area in adults and 10% or more in children. Physiological monitoring centres mainly on the measurement of urine output and osmolality. Central venous pressure lines are rarely indicated except in cases of incipient renal failure owing to the potential risks of septicaemia.

PAIN CONTROL

One of the most significant advances in the past 10 years has been the increased awareness of the necessity to consider active pain control at all stages of the patient's recovery. In the immediate post-injury stages pain may not be a problem, but where pain control is necessary or appropriate, intravenous opiate analgesia is widely used. Once the patient has been admitted to the treatment centre analgesia can be customized by a dedicated pain nurse according to the patient's needs. This will vary from opiates to paracetamol and the method of administration from patient controlled infusion pump to simple oral or suppository prescriptions (Wilson & Tomlinson 1988). Particular problems arise with pain control for dressings procedures. Many units now have regular theatre sessions for dressings with an anaesthetist in attendance. Where an anaesthetist is not required Entonox may be administered and supervised by a trained nurse. A promising method for control of donor site pain is reported in the technique of transcutaneous nerve stimulation, although this has yet to be substantiated by extensive studies. Another advance has been the recruitment of clinical psychologists to the Burns Team, as it is now widely recognized that burn injury carries significant psychological sequelae both for the patient, and, particularly in children, other members of the family (Mendelsohn 1984).

NUTRITIONAL CARE

The metabolic problems faced by burned patients are still poorly understood. There is, as yet, little agreement on the defined requirements for energy and nitrogen intake after burn injury. Nitrogen excretion, which has been used as the basis for previous calculations of requirements, may not be an appropriate parameter. Dietary supplementation is essential if excessive weight loss is to be avoided. Oral supplementation is still the method of choice, predominantly with proprietary preparations of high energy supplements. A considerable help to the use of oral supplements has been the introduction of the fine-bore silastic nasogastric tube. The place of intravenous feeding has recently been called into question (Herndon et al 1989), but this method has not been in widespread use in this country.

INFECTION

Infection continues to be the major cause of mortality and morbidity after burn injury. The problem is well-summarized by Muir et al (1987). Prevention and treatment of infection are still based on systemic administration of antibiotics and careful wound care using topical antibacterial agents. There have been few significant advances in techniques or substances available. Penicillin still remains the treatment of choice for Lancefield Group A streptococcal infections whilst gram-negative septicaemia is still treated with an aminoglycoside, for example gentamicin. Mixed or gram-positive infections can be treated with semi-synthetic penicillins such as flucloxacillin and latterly the new quinolone antibiotics such as ciprofloxacin.

A significant advance in the recognition of specific problems posed by infections has been the description and investigation of the so-called 'toxic shock syndrome' (TSS) which affects children. In the past this syndrome has been rarely recognized. Only 99 cases were reported in the British literature up to 1984 of which 7 were in burn victims. Since then 15 further cases have been reported in burned children, all under the age of 6 years (Frame et al 1985, Cole & Shakespeare 1990). Toxic shock syndrome is thought to be caused by burn wound colonization with a toxin-producing strain of Staphylococcus. The toxin, one of eight enterotoxins or a related product, enters the systemic circulation. This may have a direct effect on the host or act via toxin-induced mediators such as interleukin-1 and

Table 5.3   Simplified criteria for diagnosis
of toxic shock syndrome in burned
children

Pyrexia, temperature > = 39.0°C
Rash
Shock
Diarrhoea and/or vomiting
Irritability
Lymphopenia

tumour necrosis factor. Toxic shock syndrome carries a 10–20% mortality.

Toxic shock syndrome is diagnosed retrospectively, mainly on clinical grounds. The six criteria can be difficult to apply to small children at an early stage after injury. A simplified set of criteria (Table 5.3) has been proposed in order to establish a provisional working diagnosis (Cole & Shakespeare 1990) and begin immediate therapy. Systemic flucloxacillin (Frame et al 1985) and topical mupirocin have been proposed as prophylaxis against toxic shock syndrome, but may encourage the emergence of resistant strains. Treatment of established toxic shock syndrome involves aggressive monitoring, the use of parenteral anti-staphylococcal beta-lactamase resistant antibiotics, intravenous fluids and rectal paracetamol. Fresh blood or immunoglobulin transfusion may confer passive immunity but no antitoxins are as yet available. A broad clinical spectrum of the condition may exist and staphylococcal toxicoses may be found to be one of the causes of the so-called 'burn-toxaemia'. Staphylococcal colonization of children's burns may be identified in future as a significant cause of morbidity.

WOUND MANAGEMENT

Wounds are still managed by a combination of exposure and closed dressing techniques. The former method is usefully employed for facial and perineal burns. Closed dressings are still primarily based on the materials originally described by Gamgee in the nineteenth century. The burn wound has posed an ongoing challenge to dressing technology development. The 'perfect dressing' still remains to be developed. In addition to the problems of treating the burn wounds themselves, which are complicated by the very variable nature of the injury in both its presentation and area, there exists the problem of dressings for skin–graft donor sites. In this last field there have been significant developments. The donor site is a 'standard' injury and the requirements for performance of the dressings are therefore more restricted. Several promising new materials for this purpose are becoming available. These are either hydrocolloid based (e.g. Granuflex) or calcium alginate based (e.g.

Kaltostat, Sorbsan). There have been encouraging results in particular with alginates which have been reported to decrease donor-site pain and possibly to accelerate healing (Attwood 1989).

SURGICAL REPAIR OF WOUNDS

The present day trend in the surgical repair of wounds is towards early excision and wound cover. This is achieved either by split-thickness skin autograft or full-thickness skin transfer as flaps. The aim is to shorten hospital stay, improve quality of wound repair, both in terms of function and cosmesis, and to rehabilitate the patient to normal life more quickly. With full thickness burns of up to 10% of body surface this is usually possible. Larger areas of burn and mixed thickness areas of burn are still treated more conservatively and may not be grafted until later. Problems may arise from determining the depth of the wound and the availability of donor sites.

A new concept in the early excision and immediate grafting of burns was proposed by Janzekovic (1970) and is widely used especially in deep dermal burns to the dorsum of the hands. The aim of this technique is to obtain sheet split skin graft over those elements of dermis which would otherwise progressively necrose if the burn were left longer than five days. This implies that the wound is in a dynamic state of progression in depth from the time of injury due to thrombosis in the microcirculation at the interface between viable and non-viable tissues. The method requires an accurate identification of the deep dermal burn, is time consuming and requires the use of sheet or unexpanded mesh graft which may not be available in the extensively burned patient. It is a difficult technique which requires a trained burn surgeon.

This difficulty of case selection is highlighted by a recent report on the use of thermography to assess the depth of burns of the hands. This clearly shows that a significant proportion of hands assessed clinically as deep dermal burn will heal spontaneously with good functional result (Cole et al 1990). The technique of thermography has been used in the past to evaluate burn depth but had practical limitations owing to the size and complexity of the equipment. More recent thermographic cameras are portable and contain flexible data acquisition and processing facilities. The use of an infrared transparent but non-water permeable membrane to cover the burn before examination prevents surface cooling due to evaporative water loss in the early stages after burn injury. This technique has the potential to enable selection of cases suitable for early excision and wound repair. More extensive evaluation is needed however, to demonstrate that the results of this justify the expense of purchasing the equipment. Another technique which has the potential to provide an accurate assessment of burn depth is the laser Doppler blood flowmeter (O'Reilly et al 1989). This equipment has not been widely tested for diagnosis of burn depth, and is difficult to use to examine large areas of burn. The basis of preparation of wounds before

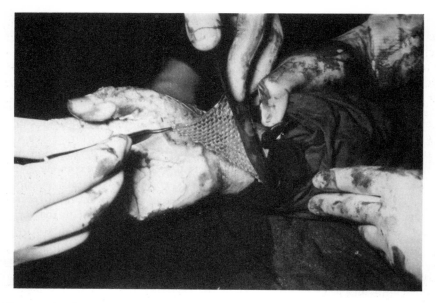

Fig. 5.1   Application of unexpanded meshed skin allows better conformity to the wound and better 'take'.

examination and the timing of the examination, by any physiological measurement technique, need further investigation before the methods can be acceptable as reliable diagnostic tools.

METHODS OF WOUND COVER

The most commonly employed material for closure of wounds continues to be the split thickness skin autograft. In extensive burns all available donor sites are considered, but where selection of donor site is possible the strongest consideration is given to minimizing donor-site deformity by cropping grafts from the buttock areas in females. Attempts are also made to match donor site skin colour to that of the recipient site and encouraging work has shown the usefulness of scalp grafts for resurfacing burns about the face (Finucan et al 1984). The use of meshed skin has become even more widely used in the practice of this Unit (Fig. 5.1). Unexpanded meshed skin shows better conformity to the wound and free drainage of haematoma and exudate is achieved. Machines are now available each of which will offer a range of expansion from 1.5:1 to 6:1. Newer power dermatomes (for example the Zimmer Dermatome) have the capacity to accept blades of different widths, which enable more economical harvesting of skin of consistent thickness from a given donor site.

The problem of obtaining sufficient autograft to cover extensive burns still remains. Tissue culture methods for the production of sheets of epithelial cells have been used to provide material for the repair of burn wounds. This method can be used to provide a several thousand-fold expansion of a small sample of skin. Thus from a 1 cm-square piece of split skin graft approximately 2000–3000 cm² of confluent sheets of epithelia can be produced within 3 weeks. This material can be produced as small sheets and applied to the surface of wounds. The method is technically demanding and produces very thin sheets of epithelial cells only with no dermal element. The method has been used in the United States with some successful results reported (Gallico et al 1984). In the United Kingdom, results have been less encouraging, the experience of most units being that applied cells fail to establish on the surface of the wounds.

Most successful results with cultured epithelial cells have been on patients who had an excision at an early stage after injury and received the cultured cell grafts onto muscle fascia. Application of cells to granulating wounds has not yet proven to be of clinical benefit. The initial studies have not been encouraging but as the culture method has the ability to provide almost unlimited quantities of cells it is certain to find an appropriate role in the treatment of burns and other wounds at some stage in the future. One particularly promising area is the treatment of partial thickness wounds which are difficult to repair with split thickness grafts owing to the presence of viable epidermal elements in the deeper parts. Homograft cells may be usable as temporary, or possibly permanent wound cover, if the potential problems of HIV transmission can be satisfactorily resolved.

In the United Kingdom the use of split or full thickness skin homografts has fallen into abeyance following a reported case of HIV transfer (Clark 1987). Although homograft skin had been in use for many years to provide temporary wound cover the potential for wound repair using this material had been amplified following reports in the Chinese literature of the use of mixed homo/autograft to repair very extensive burns (Yang et al 1982). A promising compromise in this approach has been used in the management of extensively burned children. Widely meshed autograft (6:1) has been applied to the excised burn and covered with parental skin (Clark J personal communication) as a variant of the so-called 'sandwich grafting technique' (Alexander & McMillan 1980). In these circumstances there appears to be considerable 'take' of the parental skin to provide a composite, and apparently permanent, cover to the wound.

Developments in wound adhesives have helped considerably to speed up the fixation of skin grafts in place on the wound. The most widely used adhesive is 'Histoacryl'® (iso-butyl cyano-acrylate). Unlike the formerly used fibrin-based adhesives which were applied at the interface between the wound bed and the graft base, the tissue glue is applied at the edge of the graft in spots overlapping the graft edge and the surrounding area. Use of this material ensures that the graft is fixed immovably in place thus greatly

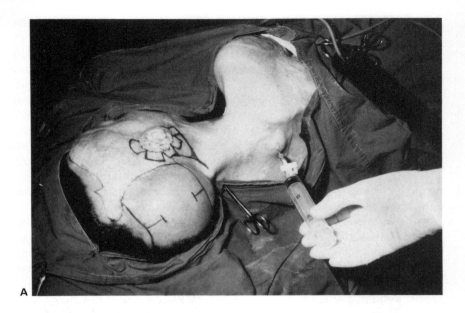

facilitating the application of dressing to the repaired area as well as minimizing the damage caused by shearing in the early stages after application.

A recently introduced topical local anaesthetic cream (EMLA) has

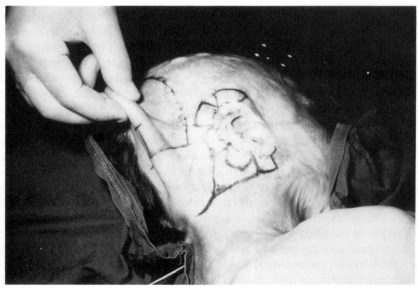

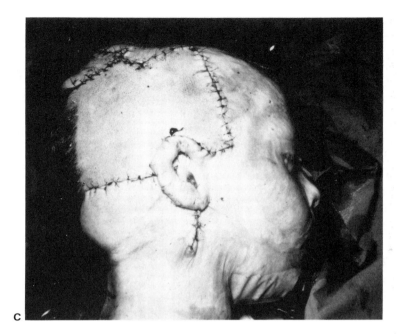

Fig. 5.2   Tissue expanders **A** Inflating the expander through the remote valve;
B Available skin produced by expansion; **C** Expanded flap is moved forward into area
of scar to improve hairline and reconstruct concha.

proved helpful in the harvesting of small area skin grafts. The cream is
applied to the surface of the skin approximately 2–4 hours before the graft
is cut. This procedure has greatly extended the range of small wounds
which can be repaired in the Ward Treatment Room. The cream should not
be applied to raw areas as it may be absorbed into the bloodstream.

Flap repair is still required for the cover of vital structures and situations
where a skin graft would not take, for example over open joints and where
there is loss of perichondrium, paratenon and periosteum. Our new
awareness of the importance of the deep fascia combined with a better
understanding of vascular territories in the skin has provided a wider range
of reliable skin flaps (Ponten 1981). This improved knowledge is
particularly useful in later reconstructive surgery for the relief of
contractures and improvement of cosmesis. The radial forearm flap has
proven particularly useful as a free flap to resurface the neck after excision
of severe contractures (Song et al 1982). This flap can also be used on a
pedicle based either distally or proximally, to resurface the hand or elbow.
Fasciocutaneous flaps have been described in the correction of axillary
contractures and post-burn breast entrapment.

Perhaps the most radical advance in flap design and provision has been
the introduction of the technique of tissue expansion (Radovan 1984). This

method has proven extremely useful in the correction of post-burn alopecia (Leonard & Small 1986). The technique involves the placement beneath the adjacent normal, hair-bearing skin of an empty silastic bag which has either a remote or incorporated self-sealing valve. This bag is filled with saline at intervals until the predetermined expansion is achieved. This expansion and the choice of volume and shape expander is calculated preoperatively using simple measurements and formulae (van Rappard et al 1988). In general the expansion ratio available is at most 2:1 depending upon the shape of the expander. Another common application of this technique is the resurfacing of hypertrophic scars excised from the neck using expanded adjacent neck skin. The technique has also been used successfully to pre-expand flaps for free microvascular transfer (Hallock 1988). This has the combined benefits of providing a large thin flap which gives better cosmesis, and enabling primary closure of the flap donor site.

LATE MANAGEMENT

Management of hypertrophic scarring still depends primarily on the use of pressure as described by Larson et al (1971). This may be achieved using off-the-shelf elasticated tube bandages (Tubigrip) but more often where irregular surfaces are involved custom-made garments are used. Garments may be required for periods of up to two years after the initial injury. The recommended pressure under the garments is 25 mmHg. In practice this is difficult to achieve, especially in those areas of the body with a large radius of curvature such as the manubrio-sternum. Softer areas such as the abdomen also pose a problem and specific problems with inhibition of jaw development have been reported. An alternative treatment in the form of application of silastic gel to the surface of the scar has been described and is still under evaluation (Perkins et al 1982). If the proposed mechanism for the action of silastic is correct, then it is possible that the pressure garments are exerting their effects through mechanical effects on the skin (for example stabilization against shear stress) that are not directly related to pressure.

THE BURNS UNIT

The ideal Burns Unit should provide the right environment for the total care of any burned patient. It requires facilities for resuscitation and ventilation where appropriate. It should have a controlled physical environment to minimize cross infection. Ideally, all surgical procedures should be carried out in the Burns Unit which should have its own operating theatre. Facilities for physiotherapy and dietary supervision together with laboratory space are highly desirable. There is a need for a multidisciplinary approach to the treatment of burn-injured patients since the evolution of the treatment regimes has recognized the importance of clinical problems such as pain control and psychological and dietary support. In the present economic climate it is only to be expected that the necessity for such an expensive, highly specialized unit will be questioned. The authors believe that the arguments of Wallace (1958) for the establishment of the Burn Centre still prevail. These are: the need to achieve good patient care; reduction in the duration of hospital stay after early and skilled treatment; training of medical and nursing personnel in burn care not only for unit staffing but also to train those working in general surgical departments; and the grouping of burn patients to allow research which will lead to advances in care.

CONCLUSIONS

The reader should not regard this review as exhaustive. In the treatment of burns, as in many areas of clinical practice, the views of practitioners will be substantially influenced by their experiences and observations. The authors do not claim immunity to this bias. The rapidly expanding volume of burns literature testifies to the clinical interest in the difficult problem of adequately treating the burned patient. The treatment of burns has witnessed many significant developments since Wallace focused attention on the problems. There still remain, however, many problems for the burn surgeon and the clinical team to solve in the difficult task of treating the burned patient.

REFERENCES

Alexander J W, McMillan B G 1980 Treatment of severe burns with widely meshed skin autograft and meshed skin allograft overlay. J Trauma 21: 433
Attwood A I 1989 Calcium alginate dressing accelerates split skin graft donor site healing. Br J Plast Surg 42: 373
Bull J P 1971 Revised analysis of mortality due to burns. Lancet ii: 1133
Cason J 1981 The treatment of Burns 24 ff. Chapman and Hall, London, p. 24 ff
Clark C J, Reid W H, Gilmour W H, Campbell D 1986 Mortality probability in victims of fire trauma: Revised equation to include inhalation injury. Br Med J 292: 1303
Clark J A 1987 HIV transmission and skin grafts. Lancet i: 983
Cole R P, Shakespeare P G 1990 The toxic shock syndrome in scalded children. Burns (in press)
Cole R P, Jones S G, Shakespeare P G 1990 Thermographic assessment of hand burns. Burns 16: 60
Davies J W L 1982 Prompt cooling of burned areas: a review of benefits and the effector mechanisms. Burns 9: 1–6
Finucan T, Beudo J, Clark J A 1984 Partial thickness scalp grafts. Br J Plast Surg 37: 468
Frame J D, Eve M D, Hackett M E J et al 1985 The toxic shock syndrome in burned children. Burns 11: 234
Gallico G G, O'Connor N E, Compton C C et al 1984 Permanent coverage of large burn wounds with autologous cultured human epithelium. N Engl J Med 311: 448
Hallock G G 1988 Refinement of the radial forearm flap donor site using skin expansion. Plast Reconstr Surg 81: 21
Herndon D N, Barrow R E, Stein M et al 1989 Increased mortality with intravenous supplemental feeding in severely burned patients. J Burn Care Rehab 10: 309–313

Janzekovic Z 1970 A new concept in the early excision and immediate grafting of burns. J Trauma 10: 1103

Larson D L, Abston A S, Evans D B et al 1971 Development and correction of burns scar contracture. In: Research in Burns. Transactions of Third International Congress on Research in Burns. Prague 1970 Bern, Hans Huber

Leonard A G, Small J O 1986 Tissue expansion in the treatment of alopecia. Br J Plast Surg 39: 42

Mendelsohn I E 1984 In: Di Gregorio V R (ed) Clinics in physical therapy, vol. 4, Rehabilitation of the burned patient. Churchill Livingstone, New York, p. 75ff

Muir I H M, Barclay T L, Settle J A D 1987 Burns and their treatment. Butterworths, London, p. 59ff

O'Reilly T J, Spence R J, Taylor R M, Scheulen J J 1989 Laser Doppler Flowmetry evaluation of burn wound depth. J Burn Care Rehab 10: 1

Perkins K, Davey R B, Wallis K A 1982 Silicone gel: A new treatment for burn scars and contractures. Burns 9: 201

Ponten B 1981 The fasciocutaneous flap; its use in soft tissue defects of the lower leg. J Plast Surg 34: 215

Radovan C 1984 Tissue expansion in soft tissue reconstruction. Plast Reconstr Surg 74: 482

Song R, Gao Y, Song Y et al 1982 The forearm flap. Clin Plast Surg 9: 21

van Rappard J H A, Molenaar J, van Doorn K et al 1988 Surface-area increase in tissue expansion. Plast Reconstr Surg 82: 833

Wallace A B 1958 A present (1957) outlook on burns. Plast Reconstr Surg 21: 43

Wilson G, Tomlinson P 1988 Pain relief in burns: how we do it. Burns 14: 331

Yang C C, Shih T S, Xu W S 1982 A Chinese concept of treatment of extensive third degree burns. Plast Reconstr Surg 70: 238

6

AIDS and the general surgeon

A. J. G. Miles   C. Wastell

Acquired immunodeficiency syndrome (AIDS) is the end stage of a progressive state of immunodeficiency following infection by the human immunodeficiency virus (HIV). It is a state of profound suppression of cellular immunity and is characterized by opportunistic infections by organisms normally of low pathogenicity or by the development of secondary malignancies.

The first case of AIDS was reported in 1981 (Gottlieb et al 1981) in Los Angeles following the development of pneumocystis pneumonia in a male homosexual. The causative agent was not identified until 1983 when Barre-Sinoussi and colleagues in Paris isolated a retrovirus from a patient with lymphadenopathy which they called Lymphadenopathy Associated Virus (LAV) (Barre-Sinoussi et al 1983). Simultaneously, a retrovirus isolated by Gallo and colleagues from several patients with AIDS in the USA was named Human T-cell Lymphadenopathy Virus type III (HTLV III) (Gallo et al 1983). These two viruses have been shown to be identical and are now referred to as the Human Immunodeficiency Virus (HIV). HIV has been isolated from blood, semen, saliva, tears, urine and cervical secretions of patients with AIDS (Levy et al 1985).

In the UK to date, 11 676 persons are known to have been infected with HIV and of these 2830 have progressed to AIDS and 1612 have died (CDR HIV/AIDS Update January 1990). At present, male homosexuals are the largest group of persons known to be infected. However, the social implications of undergoing an HIV-antibody test have prevented the vast majority of the population from being tested. It is therefore not known what is the true prevalence of the infection. The median survival from diagnosis to death depends upon a number of factors. In the USA haemophiliacs appear to have the longest survival whilst drug abusing Hispanics have the shortest (Rothenberg et al 1987). Anti-retroviral drugs such as AZT (Zidovudine) can prolong survival for certain groups of patients (Stambuk et al 1989) but infection with HIV remains a fatal disease.

IMPLICATIONS FOR SURGEONS

There have been a number of reports of transmission of HIV from patient

Table 6.1   High-risk groups for
HIV infection

Homosexual males
Intravenous drug abusers
Haemophiliacs
Residents of Central Africa
Sexual partners of the above
Children of infected mothers

to health care worker, usually following a needlestick injury (Neisson-
Vernant et al 1986, Oksenhendler et al 1986). The risk of seroconversion
following a needlestick injury has been estimated as less than 1 in 200
(Marcus 1988). Using this estimate and assuming a 5% HIV-infected
population, the 30-year seroconversion rate for surgeons has been
predicted as less than 2% (Lowenfels et al 1989). Despite this minimal risk
of transmission of HIV from patient to surgeon (CDC MMWR 1988,
Gerdberding et al 1987) some practitioners in the USA have refused to
perform elective surgery on HIV-positive patients (Thompson 1987). In
the UK HIV infection is not regarded as a contraindication to surgery.
    The protection of health care workers from exposure to HIV has led to
the development of a code of practice for operations on 'high-risk' patients
(Jeffries 1987). Although any patient may be infected with HIV, the
number of HIV-infected persons not belonging to one of the recognized

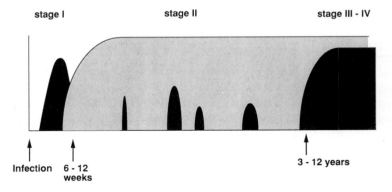

Fig. 6.1   Postulated relationship between HIV antigen and HIV antibody expression in
serum with time.

risk groups is very small (Centres for Disease Registration 1990). Protection of health care workers therefore relies upon identification of these 'high-risk' patient groups (DHSS London 1985) so that clinicians are able to decide when to take extra precautions against transmission of infection from patient to health care worker.

All patients who belong to an at-risk group (Table 6.1) are treated with the same precautions as those taken when treating patients known to be infected with HIV. Precautions should also be considered when dealing with residents of long-stay institutions, prisons and areas of high incidence of HIV in North America. Patients who report a recent negative HIV-antibody test must still be regarded as high-risk for the infection. In a recent study from The Johns Hopkins Hospital, Baltimore, 14.5% of emergency department patients with a history of a recent negative HIV-antibody test were found to be positive on repeat testing (Kelen et al 1989). There are two reasons for this. First, the patient may have been infected with HIV after the test was performed. Second, and of greater clinical importance, the patient may have been infected shortly before the first test and so had not developed antibodies to HIV at the time of testing (Fig. 6.1). This window of HIV seronegativity has been reported to last more than three years in some patients (Imagawa et al 1989) although 95% of cases seroconvert within six months (Horsburgh et al 1989).

Outpatient department

Gloves are not worn when examining HIV-infected patients unless the patient has an open wound. Gloves should be worn for procedures such as proctoscopy and sigmoidoscopy which involve possible exposure to body fluids. Gloves and eye protection are worn for flexible endoscopy. Wherever possible disposable instruments are used. At San Francisco General Hospital the added precaution has been taken of performing almost all flexible endoscopy with video endoscopes. Re-usable instruments such as flexible endoscopes are cleaned in soap and water and then immersed in glutaraldehyde (Working Party of the British Society of Gastroenterology 1988). Specimens and request forms are clearly marked 'risk of infection'. The specimens are then placed in two sealed plastic bags. After double-bagging the specimens are collected with all other specimens in a routine manner. (The pathology porters wear gloves for the collection and handling of all specimens.) No surgical procedure involving sharp instruments is performed outside the operating room.

Operating room

A theatre designated specifically for the use of 'at-risk' cases is not essential but may simplify some of the problems associated with precautions against HIV in a hospital which handles a large number of 'at-risk' cases. The theatre which is to be used for an 'at-risk' patient is first cleared of all unnecessary equipment and the operating table is covered with a single sheet of polythene. The number of theatre personnel is reduced to the minimum required for safe operating. Staff with abrasions or lacerations on their hands are excluded from theatre. The staff who do enter theatre all wear overshoes, gloves and disposable, water-resistant gowns. Staff who need to work in close proximity to the operating table will also wear eye protection, and double gloves are worn by staff directly involved with the operation (surgeon, assistant and scrub-nurse) to reduce the risk of skin exposure to patients' blood (Matta et al 1988).

Surgical technique is modified to minimize risk of sharp injury. A 'no touch' technique is employed whenever possible. Scissors or cutting diathermy are used in preference to scalpel, hand needles are not used and skin clips are used rather than sutures. When sharp instruments do have to be used they are not handed from scrub-nurse to surgeon or *vice versa* but are placed in a receiver. At the conclusion of the operation the patient is not taken to a recovery room but is allowed to recover from anaesthesia in the operating theatre before being taken straight back to the ward. The instruments are cleaned in soap and water and then placed in a clearly marked autoclavable bag. The instruments are then autoclaved in the Central Sterilizing Unit before being unpacked. Subsequently they are re-packed and re-autoclaved.

If parenteral (needlestick or cut) or mucous membrane (mouth or eye) exposure occurs, adherence to CDC guidelines (Centers for Disease Control 1987) for management is advised. This includes serial serologic testing of the source patient and the exposed health care worker. It has been recommended that zidovudine (AZT) should be prescribed for health care workers following sharp injury from patients with AIDS (Clinical Congress, Am Coll Surg; October 1989).

IMPLICATION FOR PATIENTS

The potential risk of exposure to HIV is of importance to all surgical patients. In addition to over 1000 haemophiliacs infected by blood products, at least 39 patients have contracted HIV infection as a result of the administration of contaminated blood. Following the introduction of screening of all blood donations in the UK in 1985, 13 per million donations were found to be positive on antibody testing (Gunsen & Rawlinson 1988). It is hoped that education of the general public and the advice for high-risk groups not to donate will reduce this figure.

The seronegative window which occurs immediately following infection with HIV means that screening of blood donations for HIV-antibodies does not totally exclude the transmission of HIV-antigen (Fig. 6.1). There have been proposals to screen all donations by antigen testing but at present these proposals have not been implemented.

Theoretically, patients can be infected by transmission of HIV from an infected health care worker. To date this has not been reported. Surgeons are not under any obligation to undergo an HIV-antibody test although many of those who work with large numbers of HIV-infected patients have done so. Unfortunately, any person who has had an HIV-antibody test is likely to be penalized by their insurance or mortgage companies. A joint advisory panel of medical and nursing royal colleges and faculties have made proposals regarding the possibility of HIV infection occurring in health care workers* (April 1990). The report states that in the interest of patient safety and public health, an HIV-infected health care worker should not participate in invasive procedures within a patient's open tissues where contact with gloved hands is inevitable and the possibility of puncture and injury cannot be eliminated. The report does not recommend screening of health care workers who routinely participate in these procedures even if they belong to a high-risk group or have been operating in areas of endemic HIV-infection without adequate protection.

RANGE OF SURGERY IN HIV-POSITIVE PATIENTS

Ano-rectal disease

Ano-rectal disease has now become the most frequent reason for surgical intervention in HIV-positive patients. Anal warts, perianal sepsis and anal ulceration are the most frequent conditions encountered. This in part reflects the diseases known to affect male homosexuals irrespective of their HIV status: anal warts and perianal sepsis are known to be more common in male homosexuals than in the general population (Baker & Peppercorn 1982, Johnson et al 1979) but it has also been reported that perianal sepsis is more common at all stages of HIV-infection than it is in healthy male homosexuals (Carr et al 1989). In the UK, 48.5% of persons known to be infected with HIV are male homosexuals (CDR HIV/AIDS Update January 1990), 13–15% of whom will be referred for surgical management of ano-rectal disease whilst they have ARC or AIDS (Miles et al 1990a, Wexner et al 1986) whilst only 4% of other patients with HIV-infection are likely to be affected (Barone et al 1986). There are three important groups to consider in the management of ano-rectal disease in HIV-infected patients: anal warts, perianal sepsis and anal ulceration.

Anal warts

Criteria for surgical referral of HIV-infected patients with anal warts

---

* Report entitled: Guidance for HIV-infected clinical health care workers. Further details available from: The HIV Joint Advisory Panel of Medical and Nursing Royal Colleges and Faculties of the United Kingdom, c/o The Royal College of Surgeons of England, 35–43 Lincoln's Inn Fields, London WC2A 3PN, UK.

include extensive disease, large solitary warts and resistance to medical treatment. Patients with internal anal warts may request surgical management in preference to the repeated proctoscopic examinations required for application of podophyllin. Although the human papilloma virus (HPV) subtypes identified in warts from HIV-infected patients are the same as those found in HIV-negative patients (Ruedlinger et al 1988), the warts tend to be more dysplastic and aggressive than in the HIV-negative patient (Scholefield et al 1989, Frazer et al 1986). The association between anal condylomata and neoplasia ('in situ' as well as invasive squamous carcinoma) is well recognized (Daling et al 1987, Palmer et al 1987). Females should be urged to undergo cervical colposcopic evaluation because of the associated risk of both cervical warts and neoplasia (Reid et al 1982). As in HIV-negative patients, dysplasia is often associated with HPV subtype 16 but the risk of malignant transformation of anal warts in HIV-infected males may be increased in comparison with HIV-negative males (Frazer et al 1986, Scholefield et al 1989). There is also some evidence that there is a greater risk of frank malignancy in this group (Wexner et al 1987).

Anal warts may be more difficult to eradicate in HIV-infected patients (McMillan & Bishop 1989), and healing may be delayed (Hyder & MacKeigan 1988, Wexner et al 1986). We have found that surgical treatment by either electrocautery or laser will effectively eradicate warts. Alternative medical therapy includes podophyllin although it may affect histological changes characteristic of carcinoma in the wart tissue (Goldberg et al 1980). Topical (5%) 5-fluorouracil cream has been proposed as a treatment for warts resistant to electrocautery (Strong & Milsom 1990). Interferon therapy is ineffective in controlling warts in this population (Douglass et al 1986).

There is some discussion of the merits of aggressive control of warts in the relatively healthy HIV-positive patient with biopsy and HPV subtyping to try to predict and prevent the development of invasive squamous or cloacagenic cancers (Northover 1990). However, the mortality from HIV-infection is such that, at present, patients known to have dysplasia are managed conservatively. We are currently following a number of HIV-infected patients with dysplasia including eight with carcinoma-in situ. To date none has progressed from anal dysplasia to invasive carcinoma and the one case of squamous carcinoma in an HIV-infected man which we have treated, occurred with no history of anal warts.

Perianal sepsis

The onset of perianal sepsis in these patients is often slow as many are on long-term antibiotics and the multitude and complexity of other problems means that perianal symptoms are often ignored until they are in extremis.

The sepsis which is encountered is usually straightforward and may be treated in the normal manner (Miles et al 1990a). However, HIV-infected patients may present with a variety of perianal conditions which mimic perianal sepsis, making the differential diagnosis wider for HIV-infected patients than it is for the general population. *Herpes simplex* infection may cause massive ulceration in the anal canal (Siegal et al 1981), non-Hodgkin's lymphoma may be mistaken for perianal abscess (Lee et al 1986, Miles et al 1989) and Kaposi sarcoma in the anal canal can resemble haemorrhoids and may ulcerate and bleed. *Mycobacterium avium intracellulare* infection may cause an indolent, chronic abscess often associated with an intersphincteric fistula.

Reduced sphincter tone and a tendency to incontinence in male homosexuals has been reported (Miles et al 1990b) and therefore these patients should be closely questioned about their ability to control faeces or flatus and warned of the possible disturbances of continence after operation. When operating on perianal conditions it is wise to aspirate perianal lumps with a large bore needle and syringe before attempted incision and drainage. If a solid mass in encountered then Tru-cut needle biopsies may be obtained and no further surgical treatment is required. Perianal or transrectal incisions in this instance have led to fistula formation. Division of the internal anal sphincter should be avoided and a seton should be employed for the treatment of any but the simplest of fistulae.

Anal ulceration

The majority of HIV-infected homosexual patients have a history of previous *Herpes simplex virus* (HSV) infection, therefore patients should have dry microbiology swabs taken from the ulcer for ELISA determination of HSV, and virology swabs for culture, to detect acyclovir-resistant strains of HSV. The infection can then be treated with either oral acyclovir or intravenous foscarnet (Youle et al 1989).

The anal ulceration may be associated with diarrhoea as a result of opportunistic infection. In this situation stool samples are taken both for microscopy (for ova cysts and parasites) and for culture for salmonella and shigella species. Rectal biopsies are also taken from these patients for histological examination (for CMV and cryptosporidium). These infections, if present, can then be treated appropriately.

We have been referred a small number of patients for excision biopsy of persistent anal ulceration following failed medical treatment. The median duration of symptoms prior to surgical referral in these patients was ten weeks (range 4–22). A rapid response to surgical excision of the ulcers in these patients was unexpected. The procedure was carried out primarily to allow histological examination of the ulcer but was followed by complete healing of the wound within ten weeks (median six weeks) in all but one patient (who died two weeks post-operatively from *Pneumocystis carinii* pneumonia). No patient has suffered a recurrence of ulceration after complete healing. Unresponsive lesions such as these have been attributed to either *Herpes simplex* or cytomegalovirus, but these viruses are ubiquitous in the anal canal of AIDS patients and histological examination of the ulcer has rarely shown evidence of infection by these agents.

Abdominal pain

Patients with AIDS often develop abdominal pain as a result of gastrointestinal opportunistic infection (Barone et al 1986). Initially, this frequently resulted in surgical referral or admission with some negative laparotomies being performed. Cytomegalovirus infection of the bowel, biliary tract or spleen is thought to be the commonest cause of abdominal pain in AIDS patients (Potter et al 1984). The biliary tract may also be colonized by cryptosporidium, and either this or cytomegalovirus can cause acute cholecystitis (Pitlik et al 1983, Kavin et al 1986) or sclerosing cholangitis (Kahn et al 1987). The liver and spleen may be infiltrated by lymphoma (Zeigler et al 1984) or *Mycobacterium avium intracellulare*. These rarely cause abdominal pain but can cause obstructive jaundice by involvement of lymph nodes at the porta hepatis. Lymphoma or *Mycobacterium avium intracellulare* infection can also result in small bowel obstruction by infiltration of the mesentery (Steinberg et al 1985). More severe abdominal pain of sudden onset may be caused by perforation of either the large or small bowel as a result of cytomegalovirus infection or infiltration by lymphoma (Foucar et al 1981, Steinberg et al 1985). Kaposi sarcoma has been reported as presenting as acute appendicitis (Baker et al 1986).

The initial investigation of HIV-infected patients presenting with abdominal pain does not differ from that for other patients. In addition to routine investigations, CT scan of the abdomen should be considered at an early stage as it can be useful in detecting focal hepatic lesions, biliary duct dilatation, gallbladder wall thickening or mesenteric adenopathy which may not have been suspected clinically (Jeffrey et al 1986). Rectal biopsy (for CMV) and stool culture (for cryptosporidium) may reveal the presence of an opportunistic infection in the gastrointestinal tract. However these infections are so common in patients with AIDS, that their discovery does not confirm them to be the cause of the abdominal pain.

The indications for emergency surgery in HIV-infected patients are the same as for other patients. At Westminster Hospital appendicectomy has been the most frequent reason for laparotomy in HIV-infected patients. The second commonest reason has been laparotomy for total colectomy in patients with AIDS who had either unremitting haemorrhage or toxic megacolon resulting from CMV colitis, Crohn's disease or infective colitis due to *Shigella* species. As yet we cannot assess the possible therapeutic benefit of these operations but our initial results are more encouraging than others have reported (Wexner et al 1988, Robinson et al 1987). It is of interest that two emergency laparotomies for spontaneous rupture of the spleen have also been performed.

In summary, abdominal pain is a frequent symptom in patients with AIDS. The symptom is now well recognized and rarely results in surgical referral. Severe abdominal pain of sudden onset in a patient with AIDS is a surgical emergency which should be treated in the same way as for any other patient.

Other procedures

In the early stages of the HIV epidemic, open lymph node biopsy was frequently performed for diagnostic purposes. Histological examination of the lymph nodes nearly always revealed benign reactive follicular hyperplasia. Kaposi sarcoma metastasizes to the lymph nodes but the diagnosis is made in the majority of cases from skin or mucous membrane involvement. Lymphomas will cause a disproportionate enlargement of a group or a single lymph node as may mycobacterial infection. In both these situations the diagnosis can usually be made without resorting to surgical lymph node biopsy. Overall increasing familiarity with HIV disease has greatly reduced the need for diagnostic lymph node biopsy (Farthing et al 1986).

'Idiopathic' thrombocytopenic purpura occurs in a number of HIV-infected patients before their progression to AIDS. Splenectomy may be requested for these patients. As previously reported (Ferguson 1988), splenectomy improves the platelet count but it does not appear to delay the progression to AIDS or to prolong survival.

Insertion of Hickman lines is frequently requested for administration of intravenous foscarnet or ganciclovir in the treatment of CMV retinitis. We are currently evaluating the possible benefits of using a totally implantable injection port in an attempt to minimize the infection rates of the catheters.

Insertion of gastrostomy feeding tubes has also been requested for patients with severe opportunistic infection of the oesophagus.

OUTCOME OF SURGERY

There are no prospective studies of morbidity or mortality after surgery in HIV-positive or AIDS patients, but in other situations immunological disorders have been associated with increased post-operative mortality (Johnson et al 1979) and there has been some preliminary work showing that alterations in T cell subsets may adversely affect wound healing (Barbul et al 1989). Major surgery in HIV-negative patients is associated with a depression of cell-mediated immunity for 3–6 days (Ryhanen et al 1984, Ryhanen et al 1985) whereas minor surgical procedures do not appear to affect cell-mediated immunity (Tonnesen et al 1987). Post-operative cell-mediated immunity may also be influenced by the mode of anaesthesia, with spinal or extradural anaesthesia appearing to have less immuno-suppression than general anaesthesia (Tonnesen et al 1987, Tonnesen & Wahlgreen 1988, Ryhanen et al 1985). This post-operative suppression in cell-mediated immunity appears to be transient in the normal population and does not affect clinical outcome (Tonnesen et al 1987, Tonnesen & Wahlgreen 1988) but we cannot say whether these observations will hold true for patients with AIDS. Similarly it is not known whether surgery with regional or general anaesthesia might result in a further impairment of cell-mediated immunity in patients with AIDS or whether the progression of one stage of HIV to the next might be accelerated by surgery in HIV-positive patients (Konotey-Ahulu 1987) or that spinal or extradural anaesthesia may be contraindicated for fear of exacerbating neurological conditions in AIDS patients (Greene 1986). As yet there is no scientific evidence to support or refute these theories.

There are a number of retrospective reviews of the outcome of surgery (Robinson et al 1987, Ferguson 1988, Wakeman et al 1990, Miles et al 1990a) in HIV-infected or AIDS patients. These reports suggest that there is an increased risk of post-operative complications in patients with AIDS, but it is not possible to assess whether survival is adversely affected or not. One study of 51 HIV-positive patients undergoing 73 surgical procedures for ano-rectal disease (Wexner et al 1986) found that 22 (43%) had died within six months and 45 (88%) had poor wound healing at 30 days. More recently a comparable study of 56 HIV-positive patients undergoing ano-rectal surgery (Miles et al 1990a) showed 68% to be symptom-free within one month with a median survival following surgery of 13.5 months. There was no increased morbidity in general surgical procedures in HIV-infected patients in our unit (Wakeman et al 1990). Similar encouraging results have been reported recently from other centres in this country (Carr et al 1989) and suggest either that the outlook has improved since 1986 or that the HIV-infected populations in New York and the UK have different prognoses. Our overall impression is that there is no increased risk for patients infected with HIV at CDC stages I or II and that the risks for patients at CDC stages III and IV are only slightly increased.

The pre-operative nutritional status of HIV-infected patients may be an important factor in wound healing. The progression of HIV-infection to ARC and AIDS is associated with anorexia, weight loss and diarrhoea. These factors may result in protein/calorie malnutrition (Modigliani et al 1985) with effects on healing, post-operative mortality and sepsis (Barbul et al 1989), unrelated to HIV-infection itself. We regard the presence of associated malignancies, hypoalbuminaemia, jaundice or excessive weight loss as more important than suppression of immunological parameters alone.

CONCLUSION

Never before has the causative agent of a newly evolving disease been identified so rapidly. We have discovered more about HIV in the nine years since the first description of AIDS than any other virus in an equivalent period of time. At first in the UK, patients with AIDS tended to be seen only in those centres which were responsible for the health care of either a homosexual population or large numbers of drug abusers. The youth and mobility of these patients has now spread the virus to all parts of the UK. It is therefore curious that surgeons within their ordinary clinical practice appear to ignore the possibility of HIV-infection in their patients. They are perfectly aware of the HIV pandemic but often fail to realize that the patient sitting in front of them may harbour the disease. It is important for surgeons to realize that most of them are treating patients who are HIV-positive. Surgeons must identify patients who belong to high-risk groups for HIV-infection so that they can protect themselves from the infection and prevent its spread to other patients under their care.

REFERENCES

A Working Party of the British Society of Gastroenterology 1988 Cleaning and disinfection of equipment for gastrointestinal flexible endoscopy: interim recommendations. Gut 29: 1134–1151

Baker R W, Peppercorn M A 1982 Gastrointestinal ailments in homosexual men. Medicine 61: 390–405

Baker M S, Willie M, Goldman H, Kim H K 1986 Metastatic Kaposi's sarcoma presenting as acute appendicitis. Milit Med 1: 45–47

Barbul A, Breslin R J, Woodyard J P et al 1989 The effect of in vivo T helper and T suppressor lymphocyte depletion on wound healing. Ann Surg 209: 479–483

Barone J E, Gingold B S, Arvanitis M L, Nealon T F Jr 1986 Abdominal pain in patients with acquired immune deficiency syndrome. Ann Surg 204: 619–623

Barre-Sinoussi F, Chermann J C, Rey F et al 1983 Isolation of a T-lymphotropic retrovirus from a patient at risk for acquired immune deficiency syndrome (AIDS). Science 220: 868–871

Carr N D, Mercey D, Slack W W 1989 Non-condylomatous, perianal disease in homosexual men. Br J Surg 76: 1064–1065

Centers for Disease Control 1986 Classification system for human T-lymphotrophic virus type III/lymphadenopathy-associated virus infections. Ann Intern Med 105: 234–237

Centers for Disease Control 1987 Recommendations for prevention of HIV transmission in health-care settings. MMWR 36: 18–35

Centre for Disease Registration (CDR) 1990 AIDS Weekly Surveillance Report, CDR 90/01

Centres for Disease Control 1988 Update: acquired immunodeficiency syndrome and human immunodeficiency virus infection among health care workers. MMWR 37 (suppl 4): 229–234, 239

Clinical Congress at the American College of Surgeons. October 1989

Daling J R, Weiss N S, Hislop P H T G et al 1987 Sexual practices, sexually transmitted diseases, and the incidence of anal cancer. N Engl J Med 317: 973–977

DHSS 1985 Acquired immune deficiency syndrome (AIDS): general information for doctors. London CMO(85) 7: 3–4

Douglass J M, Rogers M, Judson F N 1986 The effect of asymptomatic infection with HTLV III on the response of anogenital warts to intralesional treatment with recombinant alpha-2 interferon. J Infect Dis 154: 331–334

Farthing C F, Henry K, Shanson D C et al 1986 Clinical investigations of lymphadenopathy, including lymph node biopsies, in 24 homosexual men with antibodies to the human T-cell lymphotropic virus type III (HTLV-III). Br J Surg 73: 180–182

Ferguson C M 1988 Splenectomy for immune thrombocytopenia related to human immunodeficiency virus. Surg Gynecol Obstet 167: 300–302

Foucar E, Mukai K, Foucar K et al 1981 Colon ulceration in lethal cytomegalovirus infection. Am J Clin Pathol 76: 788–801

Frazer I H, Medley G, Crapper R M et al 1986 Association between anorectal dysplasia, human papillomavirus, and human immunodeficiency virus infection in homosexual men. Lancet ii: 657–660

Gallo R C, Sarin P S, Gelmann E P et al 1983 Isolation of human T-cell leukemia virus in acquired immune deficiency syndrome (AIDS). Science 220: 865–867

Gerdberding J L, Bryant-LeBlanc C E, Nelson K et al 1987 Risk of transmitting the human immunodeficiency virus, cytomegalovirus and hepatitis B to health care workers exposed to patients with AIDS and AIDS-related conditions. J Infect Dis 156: 1–8

Goldberg S M, Gordon P H, Nivatvongs S 1980 In: Essentials of Anorectal Surgery. J B Lippincott, Philadelphia: p 156

Gottlieb M S, Schanker H M, Fan P F et al 1981 Pneumocystis pneumonia – Los Angeles. Morbid Mortal Weekly Report 30: 250–252

Greene E R Jr 1986 Spinal and epidural anesthesia in patients with the acquired immunodeficiency syndrome. Anesth Analg 65: 1090–1091

Gunsen H H, Rawlinson V I 1988 AIDS Update. Br Med J 297: 244

Horsburgh C R, Jason J, Holmberg S D et al 1989 Duration of human immunodeficiency virus infection before detection of the antibody. Lancet ii: 637–640

Hyder J W, MacKeigan J M 1988 Anorectal and colonic disease in the immunocompromised host. Dis Colon Rectum 31: 971–976

Imagawa D T, Lee M H, Wolinsky S M et al 1989 Human Immunodeficiency Virus Type I infection in homosexual men who remain seronegative for prolonged periods. N Engl J Med 320: 1458–1462

Jeffrey R B, Nyberg D A, Bottles K et al 1986 Abdominal CT in the acquired immunodeficiency syndrome. AJR 146: 7–13

Jeffries D 1987 ABC of AIDS: control of infection policies. Br Med J 295: 33–35

Johnson W C, Ulrich F, Megvid M M et al 1979 Role of delayed hypersensitivity in predicting postoperative mortality and morbidity. Am J Surg 137: 536–542

Kahn D G, Garfinkle J M, Klonoff D C et al 1987 Cryptosporidial and cytomegaloviral hepatitis and cholecystitis. Arch Pathol Lab Med 11: 879–881

Kavin H, Jonas R B, Chowdury L, Kabins S 1986 Acalculus cholecystitis and cytomegalovirus infection in the acquired immunodeficiency syndrome. Ann Intern Med 104: 53–54

Kelen G D, DiGiovanna T, Bisson L et al 1989 Human immunodeficiency virus infection in emergency department patients. JAMA 262: 516–522

Konotey-Ahulu F I D 1987 Surgery and the risk of AIDS in HIV-positive patients. Lancet ii: 1146

Lee M H, Waxman H, Gillooley J F 1986 Primary malignant lymphoma of the anorectum in homosexual men. Dis Colon Rectum 29: 413–416

Levy J A, Kaminsky L S, Morrow W J et al 1985 Infection by the retrovirus associated with the acquired immunodeficiency syndrome. Clinical, biological, and molecular features. Ann Intern Med 103: 694–699

Lowenfels A B, Wormser G P, Jain R 1989 Frequency of puncture injuries in surgeons and estimated risk of HIV infection. Arch Surg 124: 1284–1286

Marcus R 1988 CDC Co-operative Needlestick Surveillance Group, surveillance of health care workers exposed to blood from patients infected with the human immunodeficiency virus. N Engl J Med 319: 1118–1123

Matta H, Thompson A M, Rainey J B 1988 Does wearing two pairs of gloves protect operating staff from skin contamination? Br Med J 297: 597–598

McMillan A, Bishop P E 1989 Clinical course of anogenital warts in men infected with human immunodeficiency virus. Genitourin Med 65: 225–228

Miles A J G, Mellor C H, Allen-Mersh T G, Wastell C 1989 Anorectal malignancy in HIV-positive homosexual men. J Surg Oncol 15: 1211 (abstract)

Miles A J G, Mellor C H, Gazzard B G et al 1990a The surgical treatment of ano-rectal disease in HIV-positive homosexual males. Br J Surg (in press)

Miles A J G, Allen-Mersh T G, Wastell C 1990b The damaging and cumulative effect of anoreceptive intercourse on ano-rectal function in male homosexuals. Br J Surg (in press)

Modigliani R, Bories C, L'sharpentier Y et al 1985 Diarrhoea and malabsorption in the acquired immunodeficiency syndrome. Gut 26: 179–187

Neisson-Vernant C, Arfi S, Mathez D et al 1986 Needlestick HIV seroconversion in a nurse. Lancet ii: 814

Northover J M A 1990 Allen-Mersh T G (ed) The management of ano-rectal disease in HIV-positive patients (Symposium): Int J Colorect Dis (in press)

Oksenhendler E, Harzin M, Le Roux J M, Rabian C, Clauvel J P 1986 HIV infection with seroconversion after a superficial needlestick injury to the finger. N Engl J Med 315: 582

Palmer J G, Shephard N A, Jass J R et al 1987 Human papilloma virus type 16 DNA in anal squamous cell carcinoma. Lancet ii: 42

Pitlik S D, Fainstein V, Garza D et al 1983 Human cryptosporidiosis: Spectrum of disease. Arch Intern Med 143: 2269–2275

Potter D A, Danforth D N, Macker A M et al 1984 Evaluation of abdominal pain in the AIDS patient. Ann Surg 199: 332–339

Reid R, Stanhope C R, Herschmann B A et al 1982 Genital warts and cervical cancer I. Cancer 50: 377–387

Robinson G, Wilson S E, Williams R A 1987 Surgery patients with the acquired immunodeficiency syndrome. Arch Surg 122: 170–175

Rothenberg R, Woelfel M, Stoneburner R et al 1987 Survival with acquired immuno-deficiency syndrome – experience with 5833 cases in New York City. NEJM 317: 1297–1302

Ruedlinger R, Grob R, Buchmann P et al 1988 Anogenital warts of the condyloma aluminatum type in HIV-positive patients. Dermatologica 176: 277–281

Ryhanen P, Huttunen K, Ilonen J 1984 Natural killer cell activity after open heart surgery. Acta Anaesthesiol Scand 28: 490–492

Rhyanen P, Jouppila R, Lanning M et al 1985 Natural killer cell activity after elective caesarian section under general and epidural anaesthesia in healthy parturients and their newborns. Gynecol Obstet Invest 19: 139–142

Scholefield J H, Sonnex C, Talbot I C et al 1989 Anal and cervical intraepithelial neoplasia: possible parallels. Lancet ii: 765–769

Siegal F P, Lopez C, Hammer G S et al 1981 Severe acquired immunodeficiency in male homosexuals manifested by chronic perianal ulcerative herpes simplex. N Engl J Med 305: 1439–1444

Stambuk D, Youle M, Hawkins D et al 1989 The efficacy and toxicity of azidothymidine (AZT) in the treatment of patients with AIDS and pre-AIDS complex (ARC) – an open and uncontrolled treatment study. Q J Med 70: 161–174

Steinberg J J, Bridges N, Feiner H D, Valensi Q 1985 Small intestinal lymphoma in three patients with acquired immunodeficiency syndrome. Am J Gastroenterol 80: 21–26

Strong S, Milsom J W 1990 Topical 5-fluorouracil cream in the treatment of recurrent anal condyloma acuminata. The American Society of Colon and Rectal Surgeons, 89th Convention, St. Louis, April 29–May 4

Thompson L 1987 Rising tension among health care workers: refusal to treat AIDS patients underscores fears. Washington Post Health June 2: p 6

Tonnesen E, Huttel M S, Christensen N J 1987 Natural killer cell activity in patients undergoing minor gynaecological surgery. Eur J Anaesthesiol 4: 119–125

Tonnesen E, Wahlgreen C 1988 Influence of extradural and general anaesthesia on natural killer cell activity and lymphocyte subpopulations in patients undergoing hysterectomy. Br J Anaesth 60: 500–507

Wakeman R, Johnson C D, Wastell C 1990 Surgical procedures in patients at risk of human immunodeficiency virus infection. J R Soc Med 83: 315–318

Wexner S D, Smithy W B, Milsom J W, Daily T H 1986 The surgical management of anorectal diseases in AIDS and preAIDS patients. Dis Colon Rectum 29: 719–723

Wexner S D, Milsom J W, Dailey T H 1987 The demographics of anal cancer are changing. Dis Colon Rectum 30: 942–946

Wexner S D, Smithy W B, Trillo C et al 1988 Emergency colectomy for cytomegalovirus ileocolitis in patients with the acquired immune deficiency syndrome. Dis Colon Rectum 31: 755–761

Youle M S, Hawkins D A, Collins P et al 1988 Acyclovir-resistant herpes in AIDS treated with Foscarnet. Lancet ii: 341–342

Zeigler J L, Beckstead J A, Volberding P A et al 1984 Non-Hodgkin's lymphoma in 90 homosexual men: Relation to generalised lymphadenopathy and the acquired immunodeficiency syndrome. N Engl J Med 311: 565–570

7

Resection for carcinoma of the pancreas

C. D. Johnson

This chapter looks at the surgical management of patients with localized pancreatic cancer. These tumours are nearly always adenocarcinomas, and usually arise in the head of the gland. For this reason obstructive jaundice is a common clinical feature, and the majority of patients with resectable tumours undergo some form of pancreaticoduodenal resection.

Periampullary tumours and cholangiocarcinomas at the lower end of the common duct may cause diagnostic confusion. These tumours are often resectable, because they cause a recognizable symptom (jaundice) at an early stage. Surgical resection is the generally accepted management for non-pancreatic periampullary tumours, with survival at five years in the range of 30 to 50% (Wise et al 1976, Cuschieri 1986, Robertson et al 1987b, Neoptolemos et al 1987). Careful pathological staging of these tumours demonstrates that many are confined to the ampulla or lower bile duct, and that these tumours have a much better prognosis than those in which invasion into the pancreas is demonstrated (Neoptolemos et al 1987).

Cystic tumours of the pancreas should be distinguished from adenocarcinoma and also from non-mucinous microcystic adenomas. Apparently benign mucinous cystadenomas often contain malignant foci and are said to be always premalignant (Compagno & Oertel 1978). Mucinous cystadenomas are usually found in females in the fifth decade of life. They may be large but are usually well circumscribed and long survival is recorded after resection. For this reason, if the patient is fit, the tumour should be removed (Compagno & Oertel 1978). Nevertheless, in high-risk patients, surgery may be avoided, as these tumours progress very slowly (Smith et al 1990).

DIAGNOSIS AND STAGING OF PANCREATIC CANCER

Currently there are no clinically useful serum markers for pancreatic cancer. Diagnosis depends on clinical suspicion and carefully performed imaging investigations. Cytological examination of pancreatic juice, duodenal aspirates or fine needle aspirates may be helpful if these are positive, but negative results do not exclude carcinoma.

The initial investigation of patients suspected of having pancreatic

99

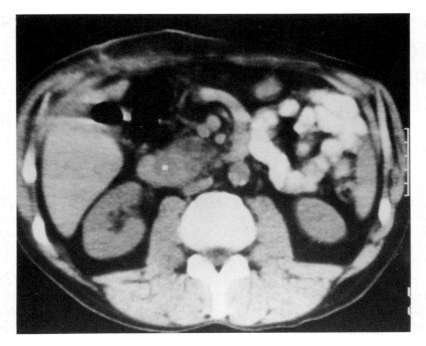

Fig. 7.1   Operable tumour seen on CT scan. There is an area of low density in the pancreatic head, confined within the capsule (marked with white square).

cancer should be an ultrasound examination by a radiologist with expertise in this field. The sensitivity of ultrasound for the detection of pancreatic cancer should now be greater than 90% (Iishi et al 1986, Campbell & Wilson 1988, Lindsell 1990). A full examination of the pancreas using ultrasound should be achieved in three-quarters of patients (Lindsell 1990).

If ultrasound suggests a pancreatic mass or shows distal dilatation of the pancreatic duct, and demonstrates the absence of hepatic metastases, the next investigation should be a CT scan (Fig. 7.1). This should precede endoscopic retrograde cholangiopancreatography (ERCP) for two reasons. First, the CT is necessary to help determine resectability. This information is valuable in helping to plan the endoscopic procedure. In a patient with a resectable lesion, a pre-operative stent is desirable but the endoscopist will not persist if this proves difficult. In the inoperable patient, a more determined effort will be made to stent the bile duct, although the availability of the combined percutaneous/endoscopic technique (Robertson et al 1987a) makes a single endoscopic procedure desirable rather than essential. Second, it is my practice to place an endoscopic stent, if possible, prior to resection in patients with suitable tumours. After stent placement there may be considerable artefact which obscures the detail of

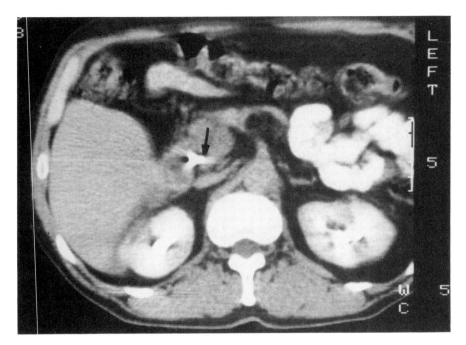

Fig. 7.2   Stent artefact. The radio-opaque stent in the head of the pancreas produces radial streaking which obscures the surrounding pancreas (arrow).

local invasion (Fig. 7.2). ERCP generally follows CT scan, not for diagnosis (Fig. 7.3) but for placement of an endoscopic stent (Fig. 7.4). The justification for stenting is discussed further below.

Two further imaging investigations with potential for the future are endoscopic ultrasound, which may enable earlier diagnosis and easier examination of those patients with gaseous distension of the bowel, and magnetic resonance imaging (MRI) which may allow better distinction between inflammatory and malignant masses.

However, none of these imaging investigations can be applied until the referring physician has considered the diagnosis of carcinoma of the pancreas. Warren et al (1983) found a diagnostic delay in many patients referred to their specialist centre. The delay before referral was much greater in patients found to be inoperable when compared with those who had a resection (8.8 months v 3.4 months). The delay was partly attributed to the patients, who failed to seek medical advice for 3.4 months and 1.9 months, respectively, but patients with inoperable tumour had suffered a delay by their referring doctor of 5.4 months, compared with 1.5 for those who were operable. It is possible that an earlier consideration of the diagnosis might have improved the outlook for some of these patients.

When a patient develops obstructive jaundice the need for investigation

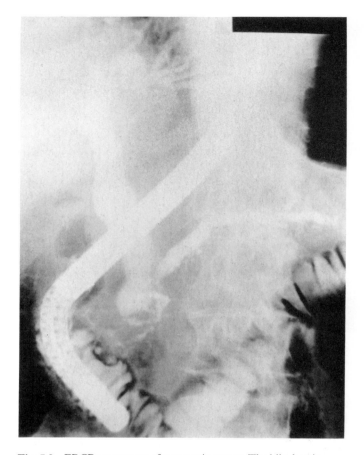

Fig. 7.3 ERCP appearance of pancreatic cancer. The bile duct is
dilated and is abruptly occluded in the pancreas. The pancreatic duct is
also obstructed and dilated.

becomes clear. In fact, weight loss was the commonest symptom in
Warren's patients (90%; 82% had abdominal pain and 76% obstructive
jaundice, painless in 10%). Pain radiating to the back, classically associated
with pancreatic disease, was present in only 30% of cases. Other less
common presentations included diabetes mellitus in ten cases and acute
pancreatitis in six, out of a total of 191 patients. Biochemical investigations
which may help to raise suspicion include a raised alkaline phosphatase
(95%) raised blood sugar (80%) and a low haemoglobin (60%). Serum
amylase *below* the normal range was found in 5% of patients.

Similarly, Moossa (1982) has pointed out that the diagnosis of cancer of
the pancreas must be considered in any middle-aged or elderly patient who
has any of the following features:

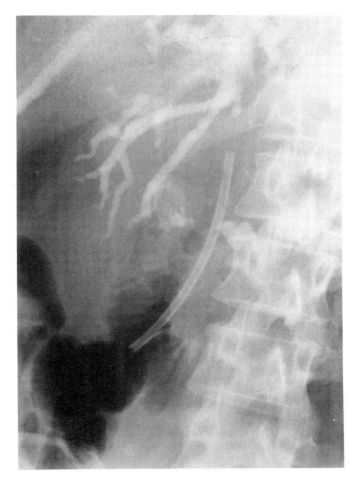

Fig. 7.4   Endoscopic placement of a stent in the bile duct allows drainage of the biliary tree and relief of obstructive jaundice prior to surgery.

1. Recent upper abdominal or back pain
2. Recent vague pain with negative gastrointestinal endoscopies
3. Obstructive jaundice
4. Weight loss greater than 5% of body weight
5. Unexplained acute pancreatitis
6. Recent unexplained diabetes mellitus (i.e. no family history and a non-obese patient).

Staging investigations for carcinoma of the pancreas prior to operation should also include angiography (Mackie et al 1982, Moossa 1982). Selective visceral angiography is useful to predict invasion of the portal

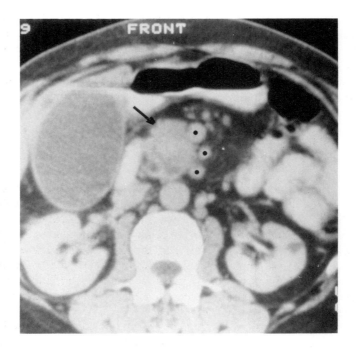

Fig. 7.5   Contrast enhanced CT scan demonstrating the vessels in the mesocolon adjacent to the tumour (vessels, black dots; tumour, arrow).

venous system and arterial encasement, although with contrast-enhanced CT, vascular involvement can often be predicted (Fig. 7.5). Angiography should only be used in patients who are candidates for surgery, after other staging investigations have suggested resectability. Its main purpose is to provide anatomical information on the upper abdominal arterial system (Appleton et al 1989).

It is my practice to stage patients very simply, according to the presence or absence of local invasion and metastases:

Stage I   Tumour confined to the pancreas
Stage II   Local invasion outside the pancreas or lymph node metastases
Stage III   Hepatic, peritoneal, or distant metastases

Stage I tumours are always resectable, and Stage III tumours should not be resected. Stage II tumours may be resectable if local invasion is to the duodenum or soft tissue of the mesocolon for example. Lymph node metastases may also be resectable if these are small and adjacent to the pancreas. Large nodal metastases, particularly around the hepatic artery, bile duct and in the porta hepatis make resection extremely difficult. Local invasion of major vessels (inferior vena cava, portal or superior mesenteric vein) generally indicates a non-resectable tumour, but this vascular invasion may only be demonstrated late in the course of a procedure, with an otherwise favourable tumour. In these cases resection should continue, either leaving a small amount of tumour attached to the vessel, or with a segmental vascular resection and reconstruction, as appropriate.

CARCINOMA OF THE HEAD OF THE PANCREAS

Justification for resection

There are three main reasons for advocating resection of pancreatic cancer if this is possible. First, patients who undergo resection live longer than those who do not. This is a commonplace observation in every unit which regularly practises resection, and is clearly in part due to selection of patients with less advanced tumours for surgical resection. Nevertheless, Russell's group has recently shown (Chandiramini et al 1990) that there was a significant survival advantage for resection even after age and tumour size had been standardized in 31 patients treated by resection compared with 117 patients treated by surgical bypass.

Second, I believe that palliation is better with a successful resection than with other forms of treatment. Resection usually relieves the pain of pancreatic cancer (which I believe is largely due to obstruction of the pancreatic duct). Recurrent tumour after resection is usually pain free. The jaundiced patient who undergoes resection will not experience recurrence of jaundice unless multiple liver metastases develop. In both these areas resection offers better palliation than either surgical or endoscopic drainage of the biliary tree. Quality of life is difficult to measure, nevertheless Trede (1987) has written that 'the quality of survival in our experience weights the scales in favour of resection'.

Finally, there is the question of a possible cure of pancreatic cancer. Some surgeons (Chandiramini et al 1990) report that all their patients with pancreatic cancer die within three years of resection. Nevertheless, others have had more encouraging results. Trede (1987) found nine survivors in 37 patients operated on more than five years previously, although even then he hesitates to talk of cure, as three of these subsequently died from recurrent tumour. Others have found a five-year survival rate in the order of 10 to 20% (Dunn 1987, Kairaluoma et al 1987, Edis et al 1980, Andren-Sandberg & Ihse 1983). I have seen only one report of a patient (Dunn 1987) who survived longer than five years (73 months) following palliative treatment.

It is my belief, and that of others (Cuschieri 1986, Moossa 1982, Trede 1987) that these arguments offer sufficient reason to attempt resection of any pancreatic tumour which is technically resectable, provided that the patient is fit to withstand the operation.

Operative mortality

Resection can only be offered if there is a reasonable expectation that the patient will survive the procedure. Whipple's pancreatectomy has traditionally been regarded as one of the most lethal procedures in surgery. This view was summarized by Gudjonsson et al (1978) who reviewed all the available reports at that time and found an operative mortality of 22%.

Since that time there have been many advances in surgical technique, anaesthesia, intensive care, and the state of health of patients selected for surgery. Operative mortality has been reported consistently below 10% for the last 15 years (Sato et al 1977, Kairaluoma et al 1987, Trede 1987, Edis et al 1980, Dunn 1987, van Heerden 1984, Ishikawa et al 1988, Tashiro et al 1987, Cooper & Williamson 1985, Grace et al 1986, Braasch et al 1986, Bradbeer & Johnson 1990).

Although it is generally accepted that elderly patients represent a poor risk group for extensive pancreatic resection, the surgeon must take account of the patient's general condition and fitness for surgery rather than absolute age. Kairaluoma et al (1987) compared operative mortality in 21 patients aged 70 years and more with that seen in 40 patients younger than 70 years. Two (10%) of the older patients and four (9%) of the younger patients died as a result of surgery. My own experience with smaller numbers confirms that with careful selection of patients, even those in their late 70s can undergo resection with good results.

Radical pancreatic resection for carcinoma of the pancreas can now be considered the most appropriate treatment for resectable tumours, with a similar operative mortality to radical gastrectomy for carcinoma of the stomach, and a lower mortality than many reports of oesophageal resection.

Table 7.1   Long-term survival after resection for pancreatic cancer

First author	Number of patients	Mean or median survival (months)	% survival		
			1 year	2 years	3 years
Andren-Sandberg & Ihse 1983	61	14		13	
Braasch et al 1986	14	18	85	18	
Bradbeer & Johnson 1990	19	13		22	
Chandiramini et al 1990	31	16			0
Dunn 1987	22	18.5	42	21	11
Edis et al 1980	133		54	29	12
Ishikawa et al 1988	37 (R1)		45	18	13
	22 (R2)		66	38	38
Kairaluoma et al 1987	21 (> 70 yr)	11	87	50	34
	47 (< 70 yr)	11	56	49	33
Sato et al 1977	19		37		21
Trede 1987	91	15.5			27
van Heerden 1984	21	13			9
Warren et al 1983	27	20.4	56		15

Long-term results

The possibility of five-year survival has been discussed above. The occurrence of late tumour recurrence after this time suggests that we should not talk about cure in terms of five-year survival. Unfortunately this survival will be denied to many patients with apparently favourable tumours. Table 7.1 shows the median survival and percentages surviving at one, two and three years in several recent series using the type of pancreatectomy generally practised in the UK. It can be seen that about half the patients can expect to survive 12 to 15 months, but that only about one in five are currently surviving to two years or more. There are one or two exceptions to this which will be discussed below.

Choice of operation

There are three reasonable, and one unreasonable, procedures to choose from. Cephalic pancreaticoduodenectomy with distal partial gastrectomy, commonly called the Whipple procedure, is probably the most widely practised. Some authors favour total pancreatectomy, in an attempt to remove invasive tumour within the pancreas, and to reduce the morbidity from the pancreatic anastomosis. Pylorus preserving pancreaticoduo-denectomy (PPPD) enables removal of the tumour in some patients, with better long-term nutritional results (Braasch et al 1986). Fortner proposed regional pancreatectomy, with multiple vascular resections in continuity. These operations often take ten hours or more, have a high mortality, and are no longer practised.

Whipple or total?

Whipple's operation is likely to be ineffective in the removal of tumour in 15–20% of patients who have intrapancreatic spread up to and beyond the resection line (Ihse et al 1977, Tryka & Brooks 1979). Much of the morbidity associated with pancreatectomy is related to leakage from the pancreatic anastomosis. This complication occurs in 14% of cases and has a mortality of about 24% (Grace et al 1986, Herter et al 1982, Jones et al 1985, Levet et al 1984, Lygidakis et al 1989, Neoptolemos et al 1987, Obertop et al 1982, Papachristou & Fortner 1981, Piorkowski et al 1982, Prevost et al 1987, Tarazi et al 1986, Tashiro et al 1987, Trede & Schwal 1988). Pancreatic leakage accounts for 40% of deaths after Whipple resection (Moossa et al 1984). For these reasons, some authors recommend routine total pancreatectomy (Moossa et al 1984). In practice however, the more extensive total pancreatectomy not only fails to lower operative mortality, but in fact increases it (Edis et al 1980, van Heerden 1984, Trede 1987). In addition, the five-year survival curves of patients who undergo these two procedures are identical (Edis et al 1980). All patients become diabetic after total pancreatectomy, and will require pancreatic enzyme supplements.

A reasonable policy therefore, is to plan to carry out a Whipple resection. The resection margin at the pancreatic neck should be examined by frozen section histology, and if tumour is present, a total pancreatectomy should be performed.

Whipple or PPPD?

The pancreas drains to lymph nodes in the pyloric region and around the right and left gastric arteries. While it may be feasible to perform a PPPD in patients with small tumours, especially those on the lower part of the pancreatic head, is this justified? There is a school of thought which suggests that as more extensive operations have failed to improve prognosis, then a less extensive operation may not impair it. Early experience appears to support this view. Grace et al (1986) report similar 'long-term survival' in two groups of 13 patients undergoing Whipple's resection or PPPD. Braasch et al (1986) reported 14 patients who underwent PPPD for pancreatic carcinoma. Median survival time was 18 months with two patients alive at three and five years.

Care must be taken, however, to exclude microscopic tumour invasion of the duodenum, even in macroscopically localized cases. Frozen section examination of the duodenal margin is recommended (Boerma & Coosemans 1990).

It is possible that in selected patients with no obvious lymph node enlargement, PPPD with lymph node clearance might be as effective as the Whipple procedure currently practised by many surgeons. Is this because the PPPD is adequate or is the standard Whipple procedure inadequate?

Is there a place for lymphadenectomy?

There is no doubt that pancreatic cancer spreads to local lymph nodes. It is debatable whether a systematic attempt at resection of all potentially involved lymph nodes may influence the outcome of the disease. It is likely that the standard Whipple resection as practised by most surgeons is inadequate for this purpose (Fortner et al 1977). Is it feasible to remove potentially involved lymph nodes without going to the lengths of Fortner's regional pancreatectomy? Nagai et al (1986) reported an autopsy study of eight patients with localized cancer of the pancreas. Four of these tumours showed no direct extension of the primary tumour beyond the pancreas, and four showed limited direct extension to the duodenum, bile ducts or stomach. The non-invading tumours were all less than 1.5 cm in diameter. The locally invasive tumours measured from 3 to 5.5 cm in diameter. One of the patients also had hepatic metastases.

In the small localized tumours the authors examined over 600 lymph nodes. One patient had one involved lymph node in relation to the superior body (outside the range of Whipple resection), and one patient had one involved node in the superior body and two in the para-aortic nodes. In four patients with locally invasive tumours, there were always involved lymph nodes in relation to the head of the pancreas and in the pancreaticoduodenal area. Perigastric nodes were involved in one patient. All four patients had involved lymph nodes in the juxta-aortic region, that is adjacent to the aorta and the celiac and superior mesenteric arteries. Three patients also had involved nodes in the wider para-aortic region which included all nodes related to the aorta and vena cava.

Several interesting conclusions can be drawn from this work. If the pattern of lymph node spread in these patients is typical of all patients with localized pancreatic tumours, then involvement of perigastric nodes appears to be uncommon and PPPD would therefore appear to be a reasonable alternative to the Whipple resection in appropriate patients. The frequent involvement of lymph nodes well outside of the usual field of resection probably explains the failure of pancreatectomy to control the disease. Although half of these patients had lymph nodes related to the body of the pancreas, the juxta-aortic lymph nodes were involved in two further patients. This would suggest that total pancreatectomy might still not remove these nodes. Para-aortic nodes were involved in four patients, at or below the level of the renal arteries and in one patient adjacent to the interior mesenteric artery.

Can this knowledge be used to improve survival? Ishikawa et al (1988) have reported the effect on survival of a change of surgical technique from the standard procedure to a more extensive lymphadenectomy. From 1971–1981, 37 patients underwent curative pancreatectomy with localized lymph node resection (R1). A further 22 patients were operated on in the period from 1981–1983. These patients had a more extensive pancreatic resection, to the left of the aorta, and lymphatic connective tissue clearance to include juxta aortic nodes and retroperitoneal tissue (R2). All patients had frozen section examination of the cut end of the pancreas, and total pancreatectomy was performed if tumour was present at this margin. Operative mortality fell from 14% to 5% in the second period. Three-year survival was significantly greater at 38% in the R2 group compared with 13% in the R1. There may therefore be some advantage in a more radical lymph node dissection, but it is impossible to determine from this report the contribution made by increasing surgical experience, changes in patient selection, and other undefined variables.

Pancreatic anastomosis

Most surgeons reconstruct the pancreas by pancreaticojejunostomy. This may be either end to end, or end to side, with various modifications described to reduce the risk of leakage ('dunking' the pancreas into the bowel, or mucosal suture with serosal overlay of the pancreas, for example). Pancreatic proenzymes are activated by enterokinase which occurs in the small bowel mucosa. They remain inactive at low pH. Activation of pancreatic enzymes may account for the high leak rate and high mortality from leakage reported by some surgeons.

Pancreaticogastrostomy overcomes these problems (Bradbeer & Johnson 1990). The low pH and absence of enterokinase in the stomach prevent activation of pancreatic enzymes. In 41 patients we had one pancreatic fistula, which closed spontaneously after five days. Our operative mortality was 5%. The technique is straightforward: the pancreatic capsule is sutured to the gastric serosa, then a small incision is made in the stomach to match the pancreatic duct. A few fine sutures approximate gastric and pancreatic duct mucosa, then the serosal suture is completed to enclose the anastomosis.

Adjuvant therapy

It is beyond the scope of this chapter to consider adjuvant radiotherapy and chemotherapy in detail. Nevertheless an alternative response to the evidence of lymph node micrometastases outside of the field of excision is to offer all patients adjuvant treatment following surgery. This approach avoids the need for extensive dissection in the retroperitoneum, but there is as yet little evidence in favour of either radiotherapy or chemotherapy used in this way. There may be some benefit in post-operative combination adjuvant therapy, consisting of radiotherapy to the pancreatic bed and systemic 5-fluorouracil (Gastrointestinal Study Group 1987). A study of this treatment is currently under way in the UK.

Management of jaundice

Major surgery in jaundiced patients is well recognized as carrying a greater risk of complications than similar surgery in non-jaundiced patients. The risk is greater in patients with pre-operative anaemia, low serum albumin, very high elevation of bilirubin, and malignancy (Blamey et al 1983, Dixon et al 1983). The major complications are renal failure, coagulation disorders, gastrointestinal haemorrhage and delayed wound healing. This last at least may be due to poor nutrition (Armstrong et al 1984) but Pain et al (1985) have suggested that the underlying pathological process is endotoxaemia.

Little can be done to change the patient's nutritional status prior to surgery, although the prudent surgeon will take care that this does not deteriorate during investigation. All jaundiced patients should receive a daily injection of 10 mg vitamin K prior to any intervention. If any abnormality of coagulation is demonstrated this must be corrected, with fresh frozen plasma if necessary, prior to surgery.

Renal failure associated with the management of jaundiced patients is one area where careful attention to detail has greatly improved results. It appears that close supervision of the peri-operative fluid balance may be more important than the use of a diuretic such as mannitol (Gubern et al 1988). All authors are agreed that it is essential to maintain good hydration before, during and after surgery, and many routinely use the osmotic diuretic, mannitol, or diuretic doses of dopamine. Pain et al (1985) proposed the use of bile salts or lactulose to alter the intestinal flora and diminish endotoxaemia. A randomized trial of these agents in over 100 patients with obstructive jaundice has shown an extremely low incidence (1%) of clinical renal failure (Pain et al 1990). The control group received pre-operative hydration and per-operative mannitol. There were six patients in this group who developed post-operative biochemical evidence of renal impairment. This occurred in only one or two patients each in the groups given either bile salts or lactulose pre-operatively, in addition to hydration and mannitol. It is therefore clear that careful fluid management is the most important factor in the prevention of clinical renal failure, but there may be some additional benefit from pre-operative administration of lactulose or bile salts.

Percutaneous biliary drainage

Theory based on the observation that an elevated bilirubin increased the risk of complications led to the suggestion that pre-operative biliary drainage might improve the results of surgery. Unfortunately this was not borne out by controlled studies designed to test this. The initial report of percutaneous drainage by Nakayama et al (1978) described 104 patients in whom successful percutaneous drainage was established. The authors claimed a significant reduction in complications after surgery when compared with historical controls. Others have found only a slight benefit, or none at all, with pre-operative percutaneous drainage (Table 7.2). Three randomized studies demonstrate that pre-operative percutaneous drainage has no effect on mortality.

Several explanations for this failure of a theoretical concept have been put forward. The drainage is percutaneous and bile is lost to the outside,

Table 7.2   Operative mortality in six studies of pre-operative percutaneous transhepatic biliary drainage in patients with obstructive jaundice

Reference	Pre-op drain	Controls	Type of comparison
Nakayama et al (1978)	4/69(6%)	36/148(28%)	Historical
Denning et al (1981)	4/25(16%)	8/32(25%)	Non-randomized
Hatfield et al (1982)	4/28(14%)	4/27(15%)	Randomized
Gundry et al (1984)	1/25(4%)	5/25(20%)	Non-randomized
McPherson et al (1984)	11/34(32%)	6/31(19%)	Randomized
Pitt et al (1985)	3/37(8%)	2/38(5%)	Randomized

rather than entering the gut, so protein and bile salts are lost and the enterohepatic circulation of bile salts remains interrupted. Infection may be introduced, converting an obstructed but sterile system into a partially-obstructed infected system. Bile leakage may occur around the catheter into the peritoneal cavity. Percutaneous drainage cannot be recommended as a routine practice prior to resection of pancreatic cancer.

Endoscopic placement of an internal biliary stent

Endoscopic placement of an internal biliary stent overcomes many of these supposed disadvantages of external drainage. Bile returns to the lumen of the bowel, there is good drainage of the biliary tree and infection is unusual in the short term. Lygidakis et al (1987) demonstrated that preliminary endoscopic biliary drainage could lower the biliary pressure and the incidence of bacteraemia in patients with distal bile duct obstruction. Published results of the effectiveness of pre-operative endoscopic drainage are not available, but it is my practice to use this technique whenever possible. Following placement of a stent and a delay of three weeks, the patient usually becomes non-jaundiced. His appetite returns and he feels very much better. It is not yet possible to say whether this approach offers a material benefit in terms of reduced complications from resection.

CARCINOMA OF THE BODY OF THE PANCREAS

Tumours away from the head of the pancreas are usually diagnosed at a very late stage. The symptoms may have been vague, the patient may have had no abdominal pain until invasion of an adjacent structure or the development of ascites calls attention to the tumour, or else the first sign of the disease may be a palpable abdominal mass. For these reasons the tumour is usually well advanced at the time of diagnosis. I have found no exception to the rule that a palpable carcinoma of the body of the pancreas is always unresectable.

Moossa (1982) commented on the dismal prognosis of carcinoma of the body of the pancreas. Apart from the original report in 1935, he could find no reference to a patient surviving more than one year after resection of carcinoma of the body of the pancreas. I have seen only two patients in whom it was possible to remove a carcinoma of the distal pancreas. One man of 72 years presented with gastrointestinal bleeding. He required emergency operation which revealed a 6 cm tumour of the pancreas, adherent to the stomach, with bleeding from the gastric fundus. The tumour was removed with en bloc resection of the distal pancreas, spleen, and upper half of the stomach. The other patient was a woman in her fifties, undergoing surgery for a gynaecological condition. At operation an unsuspected 3 cm mass was found in the tail of the pancreas. This was removed by distal pancreatectomy and splenectomy. It is too early to say whether these patients will fare any better than others with symptomatic tumours.

CAN WE IMPROVE THE RESULTS?

A significant contribution to long-term survival has already been made by improvement in operative mortality. If fewer patients die at the time of surgery, then more have the opportunity to benefit from a successful resection. Nevertheless this contribution is a relatively minor one. It must not be forgotten that up to 90% of patients are not operable at the time of presentation. If by earlier diagnosis one in ten of these patients could be moved into the operable group, the operability rate would double.

There is so far no evidence that improved diagnostic techniques have contributed to better diagnostic accuracy, or earlier diagnosis (Warren et al 1983, Gillen & Peel 1986, Dunn 1987). Warren et al (1983) demonstrated that delay between the onset of symptoms and correct diagnosis was much greater in patients with inoperable tumours. Furthermore, the doctor who was initially consulted contributed two-thirds of the delay in the inoperable group compared to less than half in the operable group. There is therefore clearly a responsibility on all surgeons dealing with abdominal complaints to take careful note of any suggestive symptoms, even in the absence of jaundice. The symptoms and the patients who merit careful investigation have been outlined above. At present, the only hope for earlier diagnosis and therefore for improved outcome from surgery lies with greater clinical awareness of the diagnosis, and a readiness effectively to investigate all patients who could possibly have an early cancer of the pancreas.

Key points for clinical practice

Earlier diagnosis is probably the most effective way to improve outcome in pancreatic cancer. Consider the diagnosis and investigate the pancreas carefully in all patients with suggestive symptoms: unexplained abdominal pain, weight loss, diabetes or acute pancreatitis.

Pancreatic resection offers the best treatment for pancreatic cancer if this can be achieved. Resection gives the best palliation, increases length of survival, and is the only hope of cure. For tumours in the head of the pancreas a pancreaticoduodenectomy is recommended. Pylorus preserving operation may be done if the tumour is small and in the lower part of head.

Always get a frozen section of the neck of the pancreas. If there is tumour here, perform a total pancreatectomy.

Reconstruction of the pancreas is easy and safe using a pancreatico-gastrostomy.

An attempt should be made to drain the jaundice with an internal stent pre-operatively. If there is difficulty with this, the patient should proceed directly to surgery without delay.

REFERENCES

Andren-Sandberg A, Ihse I 1983 Factors influencing survival after total pancreatectomy in patients with pancreatic cancer. Ann Surg 198: 605–610
Appleton G V, Bathurst N C G, Virjee J et al 1989 The value of angiography in the surgical management of pancreatic disease. Ann R Coll Surg Engl 71: 92–96
Armstrong C P, Dixon J M, Duffy S W et al 1984 Wound healing in obstructive jaundice. Br J Surg 71: 267–270
Blamey S L, Fearon K C H, Gilmour W H et al 1983 Prediction of risk in biliary surgery. Br J Surg 70: 535–538
Boerma E J, Coosemans J A R 1990 Non-preservation of the pylorus in resection of pancreatic cancer. Br J Surg 77: 299–300
Braasch J W, Rossi R L, Watkins E et al 1986 Pyloric and gastric preserving pancreatic resection. Ann Surg 204: 411–418
Bradbeer J, Johnson C D 1990 Pancreaticogastrostomy after pancreaticoduodenectomy. Ann R Coll Surg Engl 72: 266–269
Campbell J P, Wilson S R 1988 Pancreatic neoplasms: how useful is evaluation with US? Radiology 167: 341–344
Chandiramini V A, Theis B A, Russell R C G 1990 Role of resection in the management of pancreatic cancers. Gut 31: A488
Compagno J, Oertel J E 1978 Mucinous cystic neoplasms of the pancreas with overt and latent malignancy (cystadenocarcinoma and cystadenoma). Am J Clin Pathol 69: 573–580
Cooper M J, Williamson R C N 1985 Conservative pancreatectomy. Br J Surg 72: 801–803
Cuschieri A 1986 Carcinoma of the pancreas. Hospital Update 12: 543–558
Denning D A, Ellison E C, Carey L C 1981 Preoperative percutaneous trans-hepatic biliary decompression lowers operative morbidity in patients with obstructive jaundice. Am J Surg 141: 61–65
Dixon J M, Armstrong C P, Duffy S W, Davies C G 1983 Factors affecting morbidity and mortality after surgery for obstructive jaundice: a review of 373 patients. Gut 24: 845–852
Dunn E 1987 The impact of technology and improved perioperative management upon survival from carcinoma of the pancreas. Surg Gynecol Obstet 164: 237–244
Edis A J, Kiernan P D, Taylor W F 1980 Attempted curative resection of ductal carcinoma of the pancreas. Review of Mayo Clinic Experience 1951–1975. Mayo Clin Proc 55: 531–536
Fortner J G, Kim D K, Cubilla et al 1977 Regional pancreatectomy. En bloc pancreatic portal vein and lymph node dissection. Ann Surg 186: 42
Gastrointestinal Study Group 1987 Further evidence of effective adjuvant combined radiation and chemotherapy following curative resection of pancreatic cancer. Cancer 59: 2006–2010
Gillen P, Peel A L G 1986 Failure to improve survival by improved diagnostic techniques in patients with malignant jaundice. Br J Surg 73: 631–633
Grace P A, Pitt H A, Longmire W P 1986 Pancreatoduodenectomy with pylorus preservation for adenocarcinoma of the head of the pancreas. Br J Surg 73: 647–650
Greig J D, Krukowski Z H, Matheson N A 1988 Surgical morbidity and mortality in one hundred and twenty nine patients with obstructive jaundice. Br J Surg 75: 216–219
Gubern J M, Sancho J J, Simo J, Sitges-Serra A 1988 A randomized trial on the effect of mannitol on postoperative renal function in patients with obstructive jaundice. Surgery 103: 39–45
Gudjonsson B, Livstone E M, Spiro H M 1978 Cancer of the pancreas. Cancer 42: 2494–2506
Gundry S R, Strodel W E, Knol J A et al 1984 Efficacy of preoperative biliary tract decompression in patients with obstructive jaundice. Arch Surg 119: 703–708
Hatfield A R W, Tobias R, Terblanche J et al 1982 Preoperative external biliary drainage in obstructive jaundice. Lancet ii: 896–899
Herter F P, Cooperman A M, Ahlborn T N, Antinori C 1982 Surgical experience with pancreatic and periampullary cancer. Ann Surg 195: 274–281

Ihse I, Lilja P, Arnesjo B, Bengmark S 1977 Total pancreatectomy for cancer. Appraisal of 65 cases. Ann Surg 186: 675–680

Iishi H, Yamamura H, Tatsuta M et al 1986 Value of ultrasonographic examination combined with measurement of serum tumour markers in the diagnosis of pancreatic cancer of less than 3 cm diameter. Cancer 57: 1947–1951

Ishikawa O, Ohigashi H, Sasaki Y et al 1988 Practical usefulness of lymphatic and connective tissue clearance for carcinoma of the pancreas head. Ann Surg 208: 215–219

Jones B A, Langer B, Taylor B R, Girotti M 1985 Periampullary tumours: which ones should be resected? Am J Surg 149: 46–52

Kairaluoma M I, Kiviniemi H, Stahlberg M 1987 Pancreatic resection for carcinoma of the pancreas and the periampullary region in patients over 70 years of age. Br J Surg 74: 116–118

Lerut J P, Gianello P R, Otte J B, Kestens M D 1984 Pancreaticoduodenal resection. Ann Surg 199: 432–437

Lindsell D R M 1990 Ultrasound imaging of pancreas and biliary tract. Lancet i: 390–394

Lygidakis N J, Brummelkamp W H, Huibregtse K, Tytgat G N J 1987 Different response to preliminary biliary drainage in proximal versus distal malignant biliary obstruction. Surg Gynecol Obstet 164: 159–162

Lygidakis N S, van der Hyde M N, HoutHoff H S et al 1989 Resectional procedures for carcinoma of the head of the pancreas. Surg Gynecol Obstet 168: 157–165

Mackie C R, Moossa A R, Frank P H 1982 The place of angiography in the diagnosis and management of pancreatic tumours. In: Moossa A R (ed) Tumours of the pancreas. Williams and Wilkins, Baltimore, pp 355–380

McPherson G A D, Benjamin I S, Hodgson H J F et al 1984 Pre-operative percutaneous transhepatic biliary drainage: the results of a controlled trial. 71: 371–375

Moossa A R 1982 Pancreatic cancer. Approach to diagnosis, selection for surgery and choice of operation. Cancer 50: 2689–2698

Moossa A R, Scott M H, Lavelle-Jones M 1984 The place of total and extended total pancreatectomy in pancreatic cancer. World J Surg 8: 895–899

Nagai H, Kuroda A, Morioka Y 1986 Lymphatic and local spread of T1 and T2 pancreatic cancer. Ann Surg 204: 65–71

Nakayama T, Ikeda A, Okuda K 1978 Percutaneous transhepatic drainage of the biliary tract. Gastroenterology 74: 554–559

Neoptolemos J P, Talbot I C, Carr Locke D L et al 1987 Treatment and outcome in 52 consecutive cases of ampullary carcinoma. Br J Surg 74: 957–961

Obertop H, Bruining H A, Eeftinck Schattenkerk M et al 1982 Operative approach to cancer of the head of the pancreas and the peri-ampullary region. Br J Surg 69: 573–576

Pain J A, Cahill C J, Bailey M E 1985 Perioperative complications in obstructive jaundice: therapeutic considerations. Br J Surg 72: 942–945

Pain J E, Cahill C J, Gilbert J E et al 1990 A multicentre study of the prevention of renal failure in obstructive jaundice. Br J Surg (in press)

Papachristou D N, Fortner J G 1981 Management of the pancreatic remnant in pancreatoduodenectomy. J Surg Oncol 18: 1–7

Piorkowski R J, Blievernicht S W, Lawrence W et al 1982 Pancreatic and periampullary carcinoma. Am J Surg 143: 189–193

Pitt H A, Gomes A S, Lois J F et al 1985 Does preoperative percutaneous biliary drainage reduce operative risk or increase hospital cost? Ann Surg 201: 545–553

Prevost F, Roos J, Rousset J F 1987 Traitement chirurgical des adenocarcinomes de la tete du pancreas et de la region peri-ampullaire. Ann Chir 41: 12–17

Robertson D A F, Ayres R, Hacking C N et al 1987a Experience with a combined percutaneous and endoscopic approach to stent insertion in malignant obstructive jaundice. Lancet ii: 1449–1452

Robertson J F R, Imrie C W, Hole D J et al 1987b Management of periampullary carcinoma. Br J Surg 74: 816–819

Sato T, Saitoh Y, Noto N, Matsuno S 1977 Follow-up studies of radical resection for pancreaticoduodenal cancer. Annals of Surgery 186: 581–588

Smith A C, Chandiramini V A, Ainley C C et al 1990 Characteristics and management of cystic pancreatic tumours. Gut 31: A488

Tarazi R Y, Hermann R E, Vogt D P et al 1986 Results of surgical treatment of periampullary tumours: A 35-year experience. Surgery 100: 716–722

Tashiro S, Murata E, Hiraoka T et al 1987 New techniques for pancreaticojejunostomy using a biological adhesive. Br J Surg 74: 392–394

Trede M 1987 Treatment of pancreatic carcinoma: the surgeon's dilemma. Br J Surg 74: 79–80

Trede M, Schwal G 1988 The complications of pancreatectomy. Ann Surg 207: 39–47

Tryka A F, Brooks J R 1979 Histopathology in the evaluation of total pancreatectomy for ductal carcinoma. Ann Surg 190: 373–381

van Heerden J A 1984 Pancreatic resection for carcinoma of the pancreas: Whipple versus total pancreatectomy—an institutional perspective. World J Surg 8: 880–888

Warren K W, Christophi C, Armendariz R, Basu S 1983 Current trends in the diagnosis and treatment of carcinoma of the pancreas. Am J Surg 145: 813–819

Wise L, Pizzimbono C, Dehner L P 1976 Periampullary cancer. A clinicopathologic study of sixty-two patients. Am J Surg 131: 141–149

8

Treatment of cutaneous malignant melanoma

R. D. Rosin

There have been many changes in the management of patients with malignant melanoma since surgical excision was described by Pemberton in 1855.

The interest in this malignancy far outweighs its importance as it is not common, accounting for only 2% of all malignancies. However, in Caucasians, it has the steepest increase in incidence of all malignant tumours. This alone warrants scrutiny. There has been a revolution in recent years towards a more conservative surgical approach. For more than 75 years, the standard surgical management has been wide and deep excision, at least 5 cm around the lesion. The rationale of the 5 cm margin is usually accredited to W. S. Handley, who in 1907 reported a single autopsy of a patient with metastatic melanoma. In that study, he dealt only with the spread of malignant melanoma around the metastasis. Handley acknowledged that he had never studied the skin around any primary cutaneous malignant melanoma, using these words: 'no other opportunity of investigating the spread of permeation around a primary focus of melanotic growth has fallen to me'.

Because there was no evidence of local recurrence near the primary excision scar, Handley stated that 'permeation of the lymphatics is the principal agent in this local centrifugal spread'. He noted that the spread of the disease 'occurs primarily and most extensively in the plane of the deep fascial lymphatic plexus'. He recommended that the margins of excision be 1 inch (2.5 cm) of normal skin and an additional inch of subcutaneous tissue. As a consequence of Handley's publication, surgeons began to recommend 5 cm margins of excision around primary malignant melanomas, and some continue to advocate this extent today.

Improvement in prognosis is coming about in two ways. People in general are now more aware of the disease, so hopefully it will be diagnosed earlier. For neglected lesions, great strides in therapies other than surgery have been made.

The problem

Mortality from malignant melanoma is rising more rapidly than from any other malignancy in Caucasians, doubling every 7–10 years in countries close to the Equator, and every 10–15 years in more temperate zones. In 1980 the incidence was 40:100 000 in Queensland, Australia while only 4:100 000 in Scotland. The incidence has quadrupled in Australasia and doubled in Norway, Britain, America and Canada over the last 30 years. This increase in incidence is not observed amongst other skin cancers. At the present rate of increase, melanoma will be more common than breast cancer by the year 2000 (Shukla & Hughes 1990).

In America, the age adjusted annual incidence is 4.2 per million population. The most commonly affected age group is 40–49 years with females outnumbering males. There are approximately 9000 patients with melanoma per year in the USA. The incidence of other skin cancers is 300 000, compared to 600 000 cases of cancers of all other sites. Malignant melanoma accounts for almost all the deaths from skin cancer.

Aetiology

There is now strong evidence that increased exposure to sunlight is mainly responsible for the rapid increase in this skin cancer. It has to be asked if the increased incidence is true or merely due to an artefact from greater diagnosis. The observed trends suggest that it is a true increase. It is well known that solar irradiation is associated with all skin cancers. Ethnic origin, climate, socioeconomic status and lifestyle are all risk factors, interacting with sun exposure. Furthermore, patients with pathological conditions such as albinism and xeroderma pigmentosa are susceptible to forming melanomas.

Approximately 50% of melanomas arise in a pre-existing mole. The development of malignancy in a mole should be suspected if any of the following changes occur:

1. Change in size
2. Change in outline
3. Change in colour
4. Change in elevation
5. Change in the surface characteristics
6. Change in the surrounding tissues
7. Itching
8. Bleeding.

CLINICO-PATHOLOGICAL TYPES OF MELANOMA

Clinical Stage I cutaneous malignant melanomas are confined to the skin with no evidence of spread. Different clinical types are described:

1. *Lentigo maligna* (Syn. melanoma arising in Hutchinson's melanotic freckle). This is the least common type (7%) and also the least malignant. It

occurs most frequently on the face of the elderly who have been subjected to chronic sun exposure.

2. *Superficial spreading.* The most common type (65%), it occurs on any part of the body, is variegated in colour and has an irregular edge. Its characteristic is that it has a horizontal growth phase first.

3. *Nodular.* Nodular melanoma is the most malignant type, invasive from the outset. It may occur on any part of the body. Its colour is commonly uniform and it is characterized by an immediate vertical growth phase.

4. *Acral lentiginous.* These lesions are found on the palms, soles and digits. Subungual malignant melanomas come under this heading. They usually have a horizontal growth phase to begin with, but as they present late, by the time they are diagnosed they are usually nodular.

5. *Amelanotic.* These rare malignant melanomas are non-pigmented, usually nodular and difficult to diagnose.

CLINICAL FACTORS WHICH INFLUENCE SURVIVAL

Younger patients fare better than the old. Dominant prognostic factors related to the lesion itself include anatomical site, presence or absence of ulceration, clinical stage of the disease and the histological features (depth of invasion and thickness). Upper extremity lesions have a better prognosis than those on the legs. Extremity lesions carry a better prognosis than head and neck or truncal lesions. The presence of ulceration in the primary site is

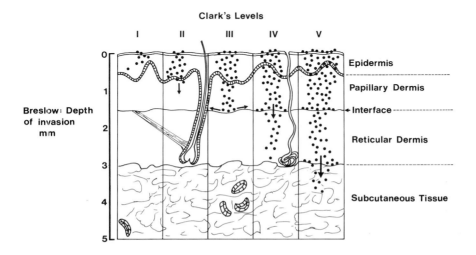

Fig. 8.1   Clark's levels and Breslow thickness. Black dots represent melanoma cells.

a particularly ominous sign, significantly altering survival. Lymph node metastases similarly affect survival adversely. Lentigo maligna has a good prognosis regardless of the site of melanoma or the age of the patient.

Clinical staging

Stage I is where cutaneous malignant melanoma has been defined.

Clinical Stage II disease is subdivided into IIa and IIb. The presence of satellites or in-transit metastases make a lesion IIa, whilst enlarged regional lymph nodes constitute stage IIb. A lesion can of course be IIab with both satellites and enlarged regional lymph nodes.

Clinical Stage III disease is that when the disease has spread further than the regional lymph nodes resulting in widespread metastases.

Pathological staging

Two main parameters (Fig. 8.1) are now used in assessing the invasiveness of melanomas: the anatomical level of invasion, and the thickness of tumour as measured with an optical micrometer.

Mehnert & Heard (1965) have the credit for introducing a system of four levels of micro-invasion: intraepidermal (in situ); invasion into the papillary dermis; invasion into the reticular dermis; and invasion into the subcutaneous tissues. Mortality rates were proportional to depth of invasion. Later, Clark et al (1969) modified the system by introducing a special Level III in which tumour cells accumulate along the interface between papillary and reticular dermis without invading the latter. In 1970,

Table 8.1 Prognostic variables in malignant melanoma

Stage of the disease	Maximum diameter Level of invasion (Clark et al 1969) Tumour thickness (Breslow 1970) Regional metastasis Distant metastasis
Tumour characteristics	Histogenic type Mitotic rate Vaso-invasive properties Amelanosis Ulceration Tumour shape (cross-sectional profile) Evidence of partial regression Satellitosis
Host characteristics	Sex (hormonal status) Age Anatomical site Inflammatory reaction around primary
Iatrogenic factors	Maltreatment (incisional procedures)

Breslow showed that tumour thickness as measured with an optical micrometer provides an objective method of predicting prognosis. Evidence is accumulating that the level of invasion is an indirect measure of tumour thickness. Balch et al (1979) found that maximum tumour thickness is a more powerful parameter than level of invasion. The same conclusion was reached by the WHO and the Melanoma Study Group. Breslow in 1979 reviewed the benefits of the two systems. The major disadvantage of Clark's levels is a subjective description of Level III. The subjectivity of Clark's staging is underlined by the unsatisfactory overall agreement between pathologists in the classification and grading of histological criteria. The only other histological prognostic factor is the number of mitotic figures per high power field.

The prognostic variables for malignant melanoma both clinically and pathologically are summarized in Table 8.1.

Investigations

There is no method of diagnosing malignant melanoma except by histological examination. Studies in the use of computers to interpret photographs of the lesions are at present being assessed.

At present we have no methods of establishing the presence of micrometastases. Evaluations for metastatic melanoma begin with a careful

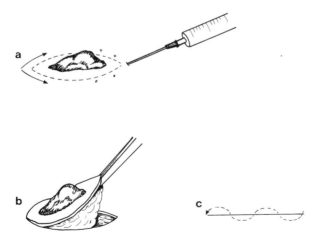

Fig. 8.2 Excisional biopsy performed under local anaesthetic: **a** infiltration around tumour; **b** excision of an ellipse of skin with a wedge of subcutaneous tissue. The forceps grasp normal skin, not the tumour; **c** closure of the wound with a subcuticular stitch.

history and physical examination. The most common sites of distant metastases are the skin, lungs, liver, bone and brain. Scans are often ordered as part of a routine metastatic evaluation, although their yield for occult metastases is very low. Lymphangiography has been tried but there are too many false positives and false negatives. Recently, we have used labelled monoclonal antibodies to demonstrate deposits. However, in our institution, this has not proved useful. CT scanning and ultrasonography also have a low specifity and sensitivity, except for established disease. The diagnosis must be made histologically.

Establishing a diagnosis

It is our practice to perform an excisional biopsy of the lesion and if the lesion is impalpable, this is carried out following Taylor & Hughes' (1985) policy with a 1 cm clearance, which may prove to be curative. Incisional biopsy is deprecated as it does not allow the pathologist to perform a full histological examination—some areas may be thicker than others. For very large lesions such as a Bathing Trunk tumour, an incisional biopsy of the thickest part clinically is indicated. Electrocoagulation, curettage and shave biopsies must be avoided. If the histopathologist is experienced in interpreting frozen sections, then this is acceptable. Clark's level of invasion and Breslow's maximal thickness should be reported in every case.

Excisional biopsy is performed under local anaesthetic, and a policy of minimal handling of the tumour is observed (Fig. 8.2). The deep fascia is not excised. In a study of Landthler et al (1989), it was shown that the five-year disease-free rate and five-year survival rate of 319 melanoma patients with a narrow excisional biopsy performed under local anaesthetic as the first procedure, followed by delayed wide excision, was not different from 635 primarily radically-treated patients. The time interval between the excisional biopsy, whether less than 21 days or greater than 21 days, also had no influence on the outcome of the patient.

TREATMENT OF CLINICAL STAGE I MALIGNANT MELANOMAS

Early recognition and curability

Misconceptions about the curability of melanoma exist because the current high survival rates are not widely known. Dismal older data no longer reflect the spectrum of disease. The surgical treatment has hardly changed during the last few decades and no generally acknowledged effective adjuvant therapy has been developed, so that the present improved survival rates must reflect earlier diagnosis. Day et al (1983) reported that in 1966,

70% of patients were not diagnosed until their melanomas were at least Clark Level III depth of invasion. By contrast, ten years later 50% presented before their melanomas reached this level of invasion.

Thickness, specific location and survival

The thickness of the primary melanoma is the dominant prognostic factor for clinical Stage I disease and in the relation between thickness and survival there is a step function in which the risk of death increases sharply the thicker the lesion. Day et al (1983) have shown the eight-year survival rate to be 99% if the thickness is less than 0.85 mm, 93% where the thickness is between 0.85–1.69 mm, 69% if it is between 1.7–3.64 mm and only 38% if it is greater than 3.65 mm. The survival rates are approximately the same whether histological evidence of regression is present or absent and whether regional lymph nodes are electively removed or left intact.

Day has also stated that these survival rates vary markedly with the location of the primary. The combination of specific location and measurement of thickness predicts recurrence and death better than any other combination of two variables. Nearly all metastases from melanomas 0.85 to 1.69 mm in thickness are associated with lesions located on the upper back, postero-lateral arm, posterior and lateral neck and posterior scalp (the BANS region).

Radiation or surgery?

For a short time radiation was used (1917–1934) as the primary mode of therapy in some countries, but it is now accepted that Clinical Stage I melanoma should be treated surgically.

Resection margins and survival (How wide and deep is wide and deep enough?)

The evidence that most melanomas should be excised with a border of normal skin at least 5 cm from the edge of the melanoma giving a specimen over 10 cm in diameter is unacceptable. This practice is sanctioned by two standard surgical textbooks and has been endorsed in recent state of the art publications, although exceptions were made for Clark Level II lesions.

Following Sampson Handley's Hunterian lectures, Petersen et al (1962) widened the recommended margin to 15 cm for some melanomas after identifying 19 patients with recurrences within 15 cm of the primary tumour. Other evidence supporting a margin of at least 5 cm has come from the studies of Cochran (1969) and Wong (1970). The former found that two-thirds of primary melanomas had an increased number of melanocytes in the area of adjacent grossly normal skin; however, he did not mention the limit of this change or comment on the atypicality of the melanocytes. Wong found an occasional morphologically bizarre melanocyte in grossly normal skin 5 cm from the edge of some primary melanomas. However, in 1983, we reviewed 75 malignant melanomas treated by wide excision and could find no abnormal melanocytes further than 2.6 mm away from the scar (Rosin et al 1984). Modern studies using tumour thickness as the most important prognostic factor have shown that the margin of resection has no effect on the length of survival, which implies that an arbitrary radius of 5 cm is almost certainly unnecessary. Breslow & Macht (1977) determined that of 62 patients with primary melanomas less than 0.75 mm thick excised with a margin of 0.1 to 5.15 cm, all survived for five years without relapse. Balch and his associates (1979) have reported no five-year recurrences for 36 patients with primary melanomas less than 0.75 cm thick. A randomized prospective study to assess the efficacy of narrow excision of primary melanomas no thicker than 2 mm was carried out by the World Health Organization. Narrow excision (1 cm margin) was performed on 305 patients, and wide excision (3 cm + margin) was performed on 307 patients. The major prognostic criteria were well balanced in the two groups. The mean thickness of the melanomas was 0.99 mm in the narrow excision group and 1.02 cm in the wide excision group. The subsequent development of metastatic disease involving regional nodes and distant organs was no different in the two groups. Disease-free survival rates and the overall survival rates were also similar in the two groups. Only three patients had a local recurrence as a first relapse. There was no local recurrence in patients with a primary melanoma thinner than 1 mm. It must be pointed out that in the study there were more than twice as many women than men, although the numbers were equal in each group. Though this study showed no correlation between the magnitude of surgical margins and mortality rates, I would have expected a higher mortality rate with thicker melanomas. Similar data have come from the Lahey Clinic and other centres. Historically, facial and digital melanomas have often been excised with narrower margins for cosmetic reasons, yet there is no evidence that the number of local recurrences has increased for patients with these melanomas.

Depth of excision and survival

The optimum depth of excision of Stage I melanomas has received less attention than the width of margin. Olsen (1966) showed that melanomas without any associated clinical evidence of metastases had more lymph node metastases when the primary excision extended through the underlying fascia than when this was left intact. Of 36 melanomas excised down to the fascia but not through it, lymph node metastases only developed in five cases (14%). In contrast, of 31 excised together with underlying fascia, lymph node metastases subsequently developed in 14 (45%). This finding did not exclude the possibility that fascia was taken more often for the thickest melanomas. It has been our policy to leave the fascia unless, as in the back, it is not evident in places or has to be removed to facilitate primary closure.

Recommendations for excision of Stage I cutaneous malignant melanoma

Taylor & Hughes (1985) have suggested a policy of selective excision for primary melanoma. They recommend that thin melanomas are excised with a 1 cm margin, intermediate ones with 2 cm and the thicker ones greater than 1.5 mm in thickness with a 3 cm margin. They showed no adverse effect on outcome in terms of both local and regional recurrence. The recommendations of Day et al (1983) are for excision of no more than 1.5 cm of clinically normal skin bordering melanomas that rarely metastasize (melanomas less than 0.85 mm thick) located anywhere and those of 'non-BANS' situation measuring 0.85 to 1.69 mm thick. All other melanomas should be excised with a 3 cm radius. No rationale was given for the figures 1.5 cm and 3 cm.

The goal of surgery of primary malignant melanoma is obviously the complete eradication of local disease and thus the elimination of the risk of local recurrence. However, the term 'local recurrence' has never been defined precisely. To some, local recurrence means reappearance of biopsy proven malignant melanoma within or contiguous to the scar of the previous excision. With others, however, the term local recurrence is synonymous with local metastases (satellites or in-transits). A true local recurrence is persistence of the malignant process at the site of excision because the primary had been incompletely removed. This is rare in cases of malignant melanoma of any thickness even when narrow margins have been taken. Wide excision is not associated with improvement in survival. Numerous studies have questioned this hypothesis and have concluded that for all malignant melanomas, survival is independent of the width of margins of surgical resection. Ackerman & Scheiner (1983) have even suggested that surgery for primary cutaneous malignant melanoma should be no different from surgery for any other malignant primary neoplasm in the skin.

It is recommended that a lesion which is a possible malignant melanoma should be excised under local anaesthetic. If it is impalpable, a 1 cm clearance is performed as this may be definitive with a thin malignant melanoma. If it is palpable but not nodular, then a 2 cm clearance is performed and all other melanomas are excised with a 3 cm clearance. There is no benefit in using a split skin graft and therefore all wounds should be closed primarily whenever possible. Should a melanoma turn out to be thicker than expected, one must return to take out a wider area of skin depending on its Breslow thickness.

Lentigo maligna melanomas do not have to be widely excised as they are extremely slow growing with a low potential for change.

Prophylactic isolated limb perfusion

Isolated limb perfusion was first designed by Creech et al (1959) at Tulane University, New Orleans, USA. It is well established as a treatment for recurrent disease in a limb and this will be described later. It is used in poor prognosis extremity malignant melanomas in certain centres, where, compared to historical controls, patients have had a longer disease-free interval and survived longer (Le Jeune et al 1989). According to the European Organization for Research and Training in Cancer (EORTC) conventional surgery allows a disease-free survival of 60% and a survival of 70% in high-risk Stage I melanoma. Our experience involves no randomized control group so it can only be suggested that our figures are very encouraging and show isolated limb perfusion to be superior to conventional surgery. To assess the value of this form of therapy properly as a prophylactic treatment for high-risk primary extremity melanomas, a randomized trial has been initiated by the EORTC Malignant Melanoma Co-operative Group and the World Health Organization Melanoma Programme. Comparison has been made between isolated limb perfusion plus conventional surgery and conventional surgery alone. A similar study (Ghussen et al 1988) included too few patients.

A similar trial was commenced in the UK with the MRC and the Melanoma Study Group, but this has been slow to accrue patients.

Tumours thicker than 1.7 mm with no evidence of nodal disease are selected for isolated limb perfusion as a prophylactic measure. The single drug melphalan is used and the perfusion is carried out usually at a temperature greater than 40°C (see below).

Follow-up examinations

The follow-up examination of patients after completion of the first treatment is of great importance. Studies of follow up procedures for patients with breast cancer and colon cancer have suggested that there is nothing to be gained from regular examination, but this has not been our experience with malignant melanoma. Asymptomatic recurrences, usually in the regional lymph nodes, have been discovered frequently. Patients are seen three-monthly for the first year, four-monthly for the second, six-monthly until five years and then yearly. Local recurrence, in-transit and regional lymph node metastases and distant metastases should be looked for at each visit. Early identification of metastases will often permit successful further treatment. The patient is also educated to look for signs of recurrent disease and a further primary lesion. Approximately 80% of metastases become evident in the first two years and 90% by the end of five years. All patients are advised to avoid sunburn.

Influence of pregnancy

The survival rate for patients with malignant melanomas removed during pregnancy does not differ from the non-pregnant women of the same age (Beral 1987). The treatment policy should not be altered in pregnant women. Women who have had poor prognosis melanomas should be advised against pregnancy for three years, not because of any alteration to the risk of metastases, but to carry them past the time of most recurrences before increasing their parental responsibilities.

TREATMENT OF STAGE IIa DISEASE

Various modalities have been used with varying success. Local treatment either with a scalpel, laser or cryoprobe are all effective if the disease load is not too large. Superficial electron radiotherapy can also be beneficial.

In our hands, isolated limb perfusion has proved the most effective form of treatment for this stage of disease. We have had 45% complete response,

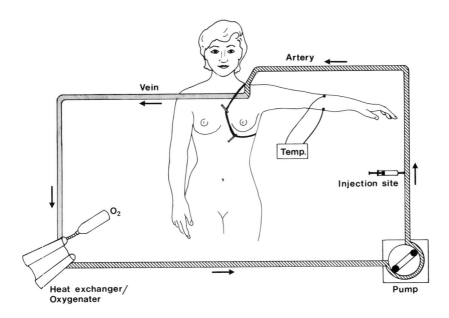

Fig. 8.3 Upper extremity isolated limb perfusion (for explanation see text).

40% partial response, 10% stable disease and only 5% who did not respond and had progressive disease.

Technique of isolated limb perfusion

Upper limb perfusion (Fig. 8.3)

An incision is made in the subclavicular region. The clavicular and sternal portions of the pectoralis major are separated and the pectoralis minor is detached from the coracoid process. This exposes the intermediate and superior levels of the axilla. The latter are radically dissected and all collateral vessels are ligated. The patient is then fully heparinized following which first the axillary vein and then the artery are cannulated. An Esmarch's bandage is then tightened around the shoulder, anchored with Steinman pins inserted into the subcutaneous tissue around the root of the limb. After one hour perfusion, and subsequent washout of the vasculature

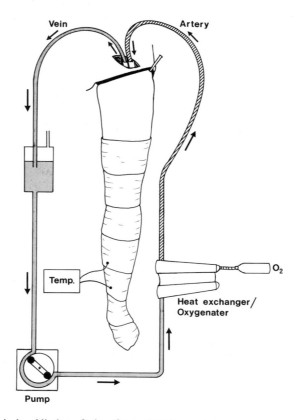

Fig. 8.4   Iliac isolated limb perfusion (for explanation see text).

with approximately 2 l of Hartman's solution, the tourniquet is removed, the cannulas are taken out of first the artery and then the vein and the arteriotomy and then the venotomy are repaired with continuous Prolene sutures.

A full axillary block dissection is performed as it is extremely difficult to assess this region following isolated limb perfusion. Perfusion is carried out for recurrent disease usually with three drugs: melphalan, actinomycin D and nitrogen mustard. If a repeat perfusion is being performed then vindesine or DTIC are used.

Lower limb perfusion (Fig. 8.4)

A skin crease incision is made in the iliac fossa and the external iliac vessels are approached extraperitoneally. An ilio-obturator lymph node clearance is performed up to the bifurcation of the common iliac artery. All collateral vessels situated behind the inguinal ligament are controlled and/or divided following which the patient is heparinized. The internal iliac artery and vein are then cross clamped. The external iliac vein is cannulated followed by cannulation of the external iliac artery as for an upper limb perfusion. A Steinman pin is inserted into the anterior superior iliac spine and a tourniquet made of an Esmarch's bandage strongly tightened around the root of the limb over the Steinman pin.

In older patients who have disease confined to below the knee, a femoral isolated limb perfusion may be performed placing an inflatable tourniquet above the mid-thigh incision. With this type of perfusion, there is rarely any leak at all.

Preparation of the limb to be perfused. In the operating theatre Thermistor probes are inserted into the subcutaneous tissue on the distal part of the limb and into the forearm or calf musculature. The limb is then wrapped in silver foil to insulate it.

Extracorporeal circulation in isolated perfusion. The extracorporeal circuit consists of a roller pump, a membrane oxygenator with 2 cm silicone tubing. The pump is primed with Hartman's solution and on occasion, the leg is drained to prime the pump. Perfusate flow is set as high as possible, that is with blood levels in the reservoir at equilibrium. Leakage is measured with radioactive albumin which is injected into the circuit and assessed centrally. The input temperature is kept at 41°C and the drug(s) is given once the skin temperature has reached 40°C, in divided doses at 0, 15 and 30 min. This method is used in case the leak should be too high when the second and/or third dose can be omitted.

Results

There has only been one in-hospital death following isolated limb perfusion in over 200 patients. This was from cardiac and renal failure. No amputations had to be performed during the peri-operative period.

Pain is transient and tolerable, and related only to the redness and burning of the skin. Ten cases of deep vein thrombosis occurred and required long-term anticoagulants. Two of the patients developed pulmonary emboli and both responded to long-term anticoagulation. There were no problems with retroperitoneal haemorrhage. One intimal flap had to be repaired. Thrombo-granulocytopenia was always secondary to leakage greater than 15%. Severe oedema was only present in one patient but mild oedema was found in 20%.

Recurrences. There were only 12 local recurrences in those patients who did respond. All these reappeared within three years. The disease-free survival was 38% after five years. Survival was over 90% for prophylactic perfusions and approximately 30% five-year survival for Stage II disease.

Discussion

My experience of more than 13 years with over 200 isolated limb perfusions confirms the validity of regional treatment of melanoma for patients with extremity recurrences (Rosin & Westbury 1980). It may well have a place as stated above in Stage I poor prognosis melanomas as well. Vaglini et al (1987) have shown response using hyperthermic antiblastic perfusion with DTIC in Stage IIa and IIab melanoma. We have used this drug if the first perfusion has been ineffective.

In patients with Stage IIab disease, it is our practice to perform an iliac isolated limb perfusion together with an ilio-obturator-inguinal block dissection. The incidence of oedema following this operation is approximately 35%, of which 5% have marked oedema.

Prognosis for recurrent Stage I malignant melanoma

The outcome of patients with Stage I melanoma has been well assessed in terms of prognostic factors and their effect on survival. However, little is known of the recurrence patterns of cutaneous melanoma and survival subsequent to recurrence. A retrospective computer-aided chart review by Reintgen et al (1987) identified 4185 patients with melanoma who had Stage I disease clinically. During a follow-up period of 1–14 years, 35.9% suffered a recurrence. Melanoma of the trunk (37.8%) and head and neck (46.1%) had an increased incidence of recurrent metastases compared with melanoma of the extremities (29.8%). Local/regional metastases accounted for 62.5%, 77.3% and 85.6% of the recurrences in the head and neck, trunk and extremity primary sites, respectively, with 65% of the relapses occurring within the first three years. Actuarial five-year survival rates of patients who had recurrent disease were significantly decreased compared with those of patients who had no evidence of metastases during their clinical course. Multifactorial analysis was performed to estimate the survival of patients after recurrence. This mathematical model to predict the outcome of individual patients after recurrence may provide a more rational prognosis for patients and their families.

Regional lymph nodes

It is universally accepted that when regional lymph nodes are enlarged and firm, such as in clinical Stage IIb melanoma, a therapeutic regional lymph node dissection is indicated. Radical neck dissection with superficial parotidectomy is recommended for a primary tumour of the head and neck. Axillary dissection en bloc with the pectoralis minor muscle is recommended for involved axillary nodes, and for involved groin nodes, inguino-femoral and ilio-obturator node dissection are generally recommended. Pelvic node dissection (ilio-obturator) is performed only in the presence of histologically proven metastases in the groin nodes. In the absence of metastases in the inguino-femoral lymph nodes, the probability of pelvic lymph node involvement is low. If one is unsure of the nature of an enlarged node, perhaps in the early post-operative phase or if there has been some infection, then a fine needle aspirate for cytological examination is recommended.

The treatment approach for the clinically uninvolved regional lymph nodes has been a highly controversial issue since the first reported node dissection was published in the middle of the nineteenth century. The problem has not been satisfactorily resolved despite the large number of published studies. Indications for and timing of prophylactic lymphadenectomy remain the subject of much debate. Those in favour of 'prophylactic' or 'elective' node dissection base their conviction on the following argument. Approximately 5% of clinically negative nodes contain microscopic metastatic foci. Because of the inadequacy of clinical assessment of the regional nodes it is safer to remove them, even if they are negative, than to leave behind occult cancer. The survival rate of patients who undergo elective node dissection is superior to that of patients who receive therapeutic node dissection, probably because the minimal residual nodal disease is the starting point for further metastatic dissemination. Histological staging in the high-risk patient may point to the need for adjuvant therapy. A major argument is that definitive treatment can be carried out during the stage of minimal tumour burden in the regional lymph nodes.

Those who favour delayed or 'therapeutic' dissection of nodes claim that with this approach, unnecessary major surgery with its complications can be avoided in four out of five patients without a significant difference in survival; the survival figures are not influenced by treating the nodal areas expectantly, according to the 'wait and see' policy. There is some evidence that removal of the regional nodes may favour local recurrence and 'in-transit' metastases. Furthermore, some investigators state that the regional nodes are an important immunological defence mechanism, and that their removal may be detrimental.

Most of these arguments are based on retrospective studies. There is now agreement resulting from the introduction of microstaging that elective lymph node dissection is not justified in low-risk melanoma patients (less that 1 mm or Clark Levels I and II) (Balch 1987).

Two prospective studies have been carried out to determine the efficacy of elective lymph node dissection in Stage I melanoma of the extremities—the WHO Melanoma Study Group (1977) and the American Melanoma and Sarcoma Study Group. The WHO study includes 553 patients with Stage I melanoma of the limb; 286 patients had wide local excision and node dissection at the time of the appearance of node metastases; 267 patients had local excision, complemented by immediate node dissection. By careful statistical analysis of these data, it was concluded that in Stage I melanoma of the limbs, delayed dissection of the nodes is as effective in controlling the disease as is immediate dissection. None of the factors of level, thickness, sex, site of tumour or maximum diameter of the tumour influenced the survival for patients who had had excision alone.

The conclusion of the WHO study was criticized for several reasons. The number of patients allocated to the trial from the various European centres was unbalanced, resulting in significant geographic differences, a factor which may have affected the results of treatment. Second, the pre-dominance of women to men (4.5:1) is another factor known to influence treatment results because the survival statistics are better for women. It was also stated that the randomizing procedure was not stratified according to the thickness and level of invasion of the tumour. For nearly half of the patients in the study, there was no information regarding Clark/Bres-low microstaging. Furthermore, various subgroups showed clinically impressive results. For example, among patients with melanomas 1.6–4.5 mm thick, the survival rate was 78.5% in the group that had an immediate dissection and 69.7% in those who did not have lymphadenectomy.

The second prospective randomized study that considered the efficacy of elective node dissection in Stage I malignant melanoma of the extremities is that of Sim et al (1978). A total of 173 patients were included and they too found that elective node dissection was not beneficial. Critics of this report emphasize that 64% of the patients had melanomas less than 1.5 mm thick, that only 7% of the elective lymph nodes contained occult meta-stases and the follow-up period was limited.

Although the mortality following lymphadenectomy is low, the complication rate is considerable. Morbidity is especially pronounced in patients with groin dissection when removal of the inguinal nodes is combined with dissection of the ilio-obturator group of nodes. Complications include skin flap necrosis (40%) and lymphoedema (30%) in some series. We have had no skin flap necrosis in our series which is, I am sure, due to the technique of excision of the skin edges after block dissection. Lymphoedema and lymphocyst formation are encountered.

Pack (1959) introduced the concept of lymph node dissection in continuity with the primary lesion. Their idea was that an en bloc resection prevented in-transit metastases from viable tumour foci in the intermediate lymphatics between the primary lesion and its lymph node basin. This has been called an integumentectomy. We do not accept this operation as we feel one cannot excise lymphatic deposits. If the lesion is on an extremity, we would prefer an isolated limb perfusion.

Surgical technique for bloc dissection

It is not in the remit of this chapter to detail the operative technique. However, certain principles should be mentioned.

Just as one should never perform a shave biopsy or an incisional biopsy on a melanoma, so removal of one lymph node from a region must be denigrated. If there is any uncertainty about whether a node is positive or not, fine needle aspiration cytology should be performed. There is no doubt that once a node has been 'picked' there is greater spread of malignant cells outside the lymphatics within the region.

In all regions, one must be careful to remove all lymphatic tissue and the deep fascia. Adventitial tissues of the vessels are best removed. When vessels are exposed such as the carotid in the neck and the femoral vessels in the femoral triangle, they should be covered by transposition of a nearby muscle. All bloc dissections should be drained using suction drains and a pressure dressing applied. It is sensible to give peri-operative antibiotic cover. There is no doubt that there is a higher incidence of complications in those patients who are overweight.

Present policy

It is our policy to perform prophylactic lymph node dissection only if the melanoma has poor prognostic histological factors and is within 5 cm of a regional lymph node group. Prophylactic dissection is not recommended for any patient where the primary lesion is situated on the trunk and not immediately adjacent to a lymph node field. These patients require careful follow-up and operation based on clinical changes. Balch et al (1985) feel that there is a subgroup of melanoma patients of high risk for regional node micrometastases but at low risk for distant micrometastases which have been identified. There are at present two prospective trials being carried out, one under the auspices of the NCI in Washington DC, and the second which is confined to trunk melanomas being conducted by the WHO Melanoma Group in Europe.

METASTATIC MALIGNANT MELANOMAS – STAGE III DISEASE

The prognosis for patients with metastatic malignant melanoma is poor. In the Queensland series 51.5% of these patients were dead within one year of the first metastasis: 64.5% of metastases occur within 12 months of treatment of the primary lesion, 16% present between one and three years, whilst 19.5% present between three and eight years. The site of the first metastasis is usually regional lymph nodes (65%) with local recurrence, retrograde cutaneous spread and in-transit metastases occurring in another 11.8%. Distant visceral metastases occurred as the first metastasis in 18% of patients in Queensland (O'Rourke & Emmett 1982). Metastases are found also in the liver, brain, bone and lungs.

Surgical excision may be appropriate for some symptomatic metastases. Radiotherapy has a place in the treatment of fixed inoperable lymph nodes, brain metastases, and for cutaneous recurrences not responsive to other forms of treatment using superficial electrons.

For widespread disease, chemotherapy has been used both with single and multiple agents. Vindesine has a 25% response rate which is similar to that of DTIC when used alone. When these drugs are combined there is a response rate of approximately 30%. The addition of interferon has improved the response rate.

As vindesine has so few side effects in comparison to DTIC, this is used as the first line of treatment for systemic disease. If there is no response, interferon is added and failing this combination, DTIC as well.

Rosenberg et al (1989) at the NCI have used high dose interleukin-2 (IL-2) either alone or in conjunction with activated immune cells such as Lymphokine Activated Killer (LAK) cells or tumour infiltrating lymphocytes, or with other lymphokines such as alpha-interferon and tumour necrosis factor (TNF). Monoclonal antibodies and cyclophosphamide have also been used in combination.

The toxic side effects include malaise, nausea, vomiting, hypotension, fluid retention and organ dysfunction. Treatment-related deaths were seen in 1% of all treatment courses and 1.5% of the 652 patients treated. These patients had a number of different types of metastatic malignancy. A response was considered to be complete if all measurable tumour disappeared. Partial response was defined as a 50% decrease in the sum of the product of the longest perpendicular diameters of all lesions after at least one month with no increase in any tumour and no new tumour. A total of 270 patients with disseminated malignant melanoma were treated by a variety of different combinations with IL-2. Approximately 50% of patients with metastatic melanoma showed objective responses. There was one complete response in the patient treated with TNF and IL-2 and three complete responses with a combination of alpha-interferon with IL-2. There would appear to be a response rate of somewhere in the region of 21% in disseminated melanoma. The response appears to be all or none, which is different from chemotherapy in which there are often many partial responses in some metastatic sites.

CONCLUSION

Statistics from around the world reveal an unexplained increase in the incidence of and rate of death from melanoma. As a result of public education and awareness, cutaneous melanomas are being diagnosed earlier.

Classification of the disease has undergone radical changes as a result of better appreciation of the differences in the biological evolution of different types of melanomas and the correlation between these patterns and the prognosis. Recognition of the prognostic value of microstaging of the individual lesions has had a major effect on planning of more rational therapy. The combined determination of the level of invasion and the tumour thickness has resulted in a more logical approach to the surgical management of melanoma. Reliable prognostic indices are now used to define the high-risk groups and to fashion the therapy according to the risk factors and the patient's individual needs. No ideal prognostic profile exists and the clinician is without doubt the best equipped to predict survival with increasing accuracy. Thin melanomas have an excellent prognosis and the chance for regional or distant tumour spread is very low. We must therefore strive to manage this disease successfully by earlier detection.

Surgery is the only curative treatment of malignant melanoma. The patient's best chance for cure is adequate surgery on an early lesion. The rationale of wide local excision of the primary tumour has been contested over the last decade and the classical recommendations challenged. We believe that the dimensions of the excision should be determined by the thickness of the lesion. It is accepted that a node dissection is indicated when the regional nodes are clinically involved (Stage IIb). In the case of the lower limb, the inguino-femoral lymphadenectomy should be complemented with ilio-obturator clearance if the groin dissection contains histologically proven diseased nodes. This procedure is also useful for staging. There appears to be no difference whether the lymph node dissection in Stage IIb disease is performed at the time of removal of the primary or six weeks later.

The question of the surgical management of clinically uninvolved regional lymph nodes is not settled yet. It seems to be agreed that in thin melanomas of less than 1 mm, the probability of regional node involvement is very low and therefore elective node dissection is not recommended.

The sad fact at the present time is that there is no effective adjuvant or even therapeutic systemic therapy. In view of this, it is even more important that the tumour is diagnosed as early as possible.

REFERENCES

Ackerman A B, Scheiner A M 1983 How wide and deep is deep and wide enough? A critique of surgical practice in excisions of primary cutaneous malignant melanoma. Hum Pathol 14: 743–744

Balch C M 1987 Cutaneous melanoma: a review of clinical management. Cancer Update 83: 70–78

Balch C M, Murad T M, Soong S J et al 1979 Tumour thickness as a guide to surgical management of clinical stage I melanoma patients. Cancer 43: 883–888

Balch C M, Cascinelli N, Milton G W et al 1985 Elective lymph node dissection: Pros and cons. In: Balch C M, Milton G W (eds) Cutaneous melanoma: Clinical management and treatment. Results Worldwide. Lippincott, Philadelphia, pp 131–157

Beral V 1987 Hormonal and other metabolic factors. In: Veronesi U, Cascinelli N, Santinami M (eds) Cutaneous melanoma: State of knowledge and future perspective. Academic Press, New York, pp 319–324

Breslow A 1970 Thickness, cross-sectional areas and depths of invasion in the prognosis of cutaneous melanoma. Ann Surg 172: 902–908

Breslow A, Macht S D 1977 Optimal size of resection margin for thin cutaneous melanoma. Surg Gynecol Obstet 145: 691–692

Clark W H Jr, From L, Bernardino E A, Mihm C 1969 The histiogenesis and biologic behavior of primary human malignant melanomas of the skin. Cancer Res 29: 705–726

Cochran A J 1969 Histology and prognosis in malignant melanoma. J Path 97: 459–468

Creech O, Ryan R, Krements E T 1959 Treatment of malignant melanoma by isolation perfusion technique. JAMA 169: 339–345

Day C L, Milton M C, Sober A J et al 1983 Narrower margins for clinical stage I malignant melanoma. N Engl J Med 306: 479–482

Ghussen F, Kruger I, Groth W, Stutzer H 1988 The role of regional hyperthermic cytostatic perfusion in the treatment of extremity melanoma. Cancer 61: 654–659

Landthler M, Braun-Falco O, Leitl A et al 1989 Excisional biopsy and the first therapeutic procedure versus primary wide excision of malignant melanoma. Cancer 64: 1612–1616

Le Jeune F J, Lienard D, El Douaihy M et al 1989 Results of 206 isolated limb perfusions for malignant melanoma. Eur J Surg Oncol 15: 510–519

Mehnert J H, Heard J L 1965 Staging of malignant melanoma by depth of invasion: a proper index to prognosis. Am J Surg 110: 168–176

Olsen G 1966 The malignant melanoma of the skin: junctional activity. Acta Chir Scand 365: 137–142

O'Rourke M G F, Emmett A J J 1982 Malignant Skin Tumours. Churchill Livingstone, Edinburgh

Pack G T 1959 End results in the treatment of malignant melanoma. Surgery 46: 447–460

Petersen N C, Bodenham D C, Lloyd O C 1962 Malignant melanomas of the skin: a study of the origin, development, aetiology, spread, treatment and prognosis. Br J Plast Surg 15: 97–116

Reintgen D S, Vollmer R, Tsocy et al 1987 Prognosis for recurrent stage I malignant melanoma. Arch Surg 122: 1338–1342

Rosenberg S A, Lotz M T, Yang J C et al 1989 Experience with the use of high dose Interleukin-2 in the treatment of 625 cancer patients. Ann Surg 474–485

Rosin R D, Westbury G 1980 Isolated limb perfusion for malignant melanoma. Practitioner 224: 6

Rosin R D, Longhurst H, Boylston A 1984 Saucer plate five centimetre clearance is unnecessary for the majority of stage I malignant melanomas. Clin Oncol 10: 79–89

Shukla V K, Hughes L E 1990 Naevi and melanomas. Surgery 79: 1888–1895

Sim F H, Taylor W F, Iving J C et al 1978 A prospective randomized study of the efficacy of routine elective lymphadenectomy in management of malignant melanoma: preliminary results. Cancer 41: 948–956

Taylor B A, Hughes L E 1985 A policy of selective excision for primary cutaneous malignant melanoma. Eur J Surg Oncol 11: 7–13

Vaglini M, Belli F, Marolda R et al 1987 Hyperthermic antiblastic perfusion with DTIC in Stage IIIA and IIIAB melanoma of the extremities. Eur J Surg Oncol 13: 127–129

WHO Melanoma Study Group 1977 Inefficacy of immediate node dissection in stage I melanoma of the limbs. N Engl J Med 297: 627

Wong C K 1970 A study of melanocytes in the normal skin surrounding malignant melanomata. Dermatologica 141: 215–225

9

Adjuvant chemotherapy in surgery

J. A. Smallwood

The realization that optimum surgery can only cure a limited number of patients with operable cancer has stimulated the adjunctive use of other anticancer therapies. Cytotoxic drugs have been attractive in this situation because their systemic distribution ensures that occult cancer cells, wherever secondarily sited, can be treated.

In general, the selection of adjuvant drugs follows proven worth in advanced disease; whereas cure in this situation is rarely achieved, important cell kinetic differences with small tumour loads make cure a realistic possibility. This review will briefly outline the scientific basis for

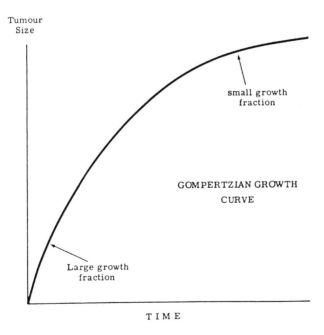

Fig. 9.1 Tumour growth rate. Many tumours grow fast initially, and the growth fraction is large. However, as the size of the tumour increases, the growth rate and growth fraction fall. This is described as Gompertzian growth kinetics.

adjuvant chemotherapy and then summarize results of its application in the four common solid epithelial tumours.

CELL KINETICS AND ADJUVANT THERAPY

Experimental animal–tumour studies by Skipper, Schabel and Bruce in the 1960s (Priestman 1979) showed that tumour growth follows a Gompertzian model with exponential growth only in the earliest phase of individual tumour development (Fig. 9.1). As tumours prosper the proportion of proliferating (chemosensitive) cells or growth fraction decreases and with cell crowding, particularly in solid tumours, there is a relative hypoxia that further reduces sensitivity to cytotoxic agents.

The smallest tumour load or micrometastasis is not only vulnerable in cell kinetic terms it is also more likely to be totally eradicated by chemotherapy since most agents kill by first-order kinetics i.e. for a given drug dose a constant proportion of a total tumour population is killed, regardless of size. A drug kill of 99.9% would totally destroy a tumour load of 100 cells but would fail to kill 10^6 cells in a larger metastasis of 10^{10} cells. In order to cure patients with the larger tumour load, effective drugs would need to be given in repeated courses for a prolonged period of time.

The most effective drug regimes in advanced malignant disease use drug combinations that kill malignant cells by different mechanisms and have different targets of toxicity. Such combinations are chosen for 'synergy' in that their combined activity exceeds the sum of their separate activity. For example, chlorambucil and vincristine separately produce remissions of 25% in Hodgkin's disease; when combined these drugs produce remissions in 65% of patients.

These same principles apply in adjuvant therapy where drug combinations, if effective in advanced disease, are usually the most effective in an adjuvant role.

The overwhelming dilemma in accepting these principles of adjuvant chemotherapy (high dose, combination regimes, prolonged exposure and early treatment) is that of treating 'fit' people, many of whom have already been cured by surgery alone.

ETHICAL ISSUES IN ADJUVANT CHEMOTHERAPY

Few clinicians doubt the scientific basis for adjuvant therapy and the need for large controlled trials with adequate statistical power. The practical problems of running large multicentre trials are many but are often shadowed by moral and ethical dilemmas; these differ according to the country of origin. In the UK, a central ethical issue has been that of informed consent particularly where studies have included a control group given no treatment. Informed consent is an absolute requirement of the Helsinki declaration, which by its nature in cancer patients may cause

Table 9.1 Adjuvant chemotherapy of breast cancer

Study	Drug	Effect
	Peri-operative	
NSABP	Thiotepa	None overall; advantage for premenopausal women with node positive disease
OSLO	Cyclophosphamide	Overall advantage in survival (10%)
	Post-operative	
NSABP	Melphalan	None overall; advantage for premenopausal women with positive nodes
Milan	Cyclophosphamide Methotrexate, 5-fluorouracil	Overall survival advantage only for premenopausal women with 1–3 positive nodes
	Meta-analysis	
61 trials (29 000 women)		Improved survival *only* in premenopausal women with 1–3 positive nodes

distress, which leads to poor accrual and trial failure; some workers have argued strongly that a more beneficent approach (Baum et al 1989) is appropriate in these circumstances and have called for a far stronger ethical leadership to advise. The present, parochial and idiosyncratic ethical committee system is less than adequate to fulfil such a role.

There is unquestionably a need for central guidance and a high profile national ethical committee; it would advise and guide all major patient studies and liaise with the media and government agencies.

ADJUVANT CHEMOTHERAPY AND BREAST CANCER

The problem

Breast cancer is the most common malignant tumour of women with over 21 000 new cases reported each year in the UK and 12 000 deaths; it is the most common cause of death in women between the ages of 35 and 55 years.

About two-thirds of patients with potentially curable local disease will eventually die from systemic disease whatever optimum local measures have originally been undertaken. Not surprisingly, the potential value of additive, systemically delivered anticancer therapy has been extensively examined in Europe and the USA.

A wide range of agents has been tested both singly and in combination but a relatively few major, randomized, controlled trials are worthy of critical review; these few can conveniently be divided into early and late (Table 9.1).

Peri-operative therapy

Two important studies were performed in the 1960–1970 period. Both were initiated on the basis that short courses of peri-operative treatment may eradicate cancer cells released into the circulation at the time of operation, rather than as an attempt to destroy established micrometastases. All 'operable' cases without distant metastases were included.

In the first study, launched by the National Surgical Breast and Bowel Project (NSABP), post-operative thiotepa was given for three days. This was compared to no treatment in the early phase and 5-fluorouracil at a later stage. The late results of these studies showed no overall survival advantage in favour of treatment but a strong survival advantage (20%) in one subgroup of premenopausal women with more than three axillary nodes involved (Fisher et al 1975).

The second study from Oslo (Nissen-Meyer et al 1982) employed a six-day peri-operative regime of intravenous cyclophosphamide and has continued to show a 'significant' survival advantage of 10% in favour of treatment even after 15 years. This difference did not become apparent for the first four years which supports a genuine treatment effect on minimal residual disease.

The concept that peri-operative adjuvant therapy of short duration may influence cancer recurrence has been seriously questioned (Henderson & Canellos 1980) but the results of these two studies produce a compelling case for further examination of peri-operative therapy.

Post-operative therapy

The more recent studies of adjuvant chemotherapy have been based on an attempt to eradicate remote micrometastases rather than systemically released cells at the time of surgery. Accordingly, drugs have been used in combinations for prolonged periods and because of toxicity, the patient groups studied have had to be refined. Those with locally advanced disease have been excluded and generally only those with node positive early disease have been selected (i.e. $T_1T_2(T_3)$, $N_0N_1M_0$).

In 1972, the NSABP undertook a second study (protocol B-05) designed to examine the effect of two years melphalan (L-pam) after radical or modified radical mastectomy had demonstrated node positive early disease. Early reports showed an overall treatment benefit but this was lost at five years; the only subgroup that continued to show a benefit was the patients with minimal nodal involvement (1–3 nodes) and premenopausal status but the numbers were small (Fisher et al 1984).

At about the same time, the Milan group began their major study of 12 cycles of adjuvant combination chemotherapy combining cyclophosphamide, methotrexate and 5-fluorouracil (CMF). Between 1973 and 1975, 391 patients with node-positive early disease were randomized to either treatment or control. After ten years (Bonnadonna & Valagussa 1985) the relapse-free survival rates continue to show a significant benefit in favour of treatment; subgroup analysis shows this to be entirely confined to premenopausal women with minimal node involvement (1–3 nodes). It has been suggested that since this survival benefit was seen from the first analysis, fewer cycles of therapy may be needed to achieve the equivalent effect. This question remains open.

A consistent effect in trials on premenopausal women has generated much debate as to the possible influence of drug-induced ovarian ablation. In the Milan study, those achieving long-term survival after chemotherapy contained equal numbers of those with normal menstrual cycles and those rendered amenorrhoeic. Evidence would suggest, therefore, a primarily non-endocrine cytotoxic effect but complex modes of action may yet exist and further research is required.

Outside of these two trials there have been many studies of drug regimes using various selection criteria; because comparisons and deductions have been difficult to make, the Early Breast Cancer Trialist Collaborative Group in 1988 undertook a statistical review of 61 randomized trials involving 29 000 women in order to establish the value, if any, of adjuvant therapy; this is often referred to as the Peto overview or meta-analysis.

Adjuvant therapy meta-analysis

This overview restricted itself to the end-point of survival, and examined two subsets, those over and those under 50 years. Log rank analyses were used to estimate any effect of treatment on the annual odds of death. For each trial, deaths observed (O) were compared with deaths expected (E) in each treatment group. For the majority of trials, O-E values were negative suggesting that overall about 140 deaths were avoided by treatment i.e. 14% reduction in the odds of death. The annual odds of death in women aged less than 50 was reduced by 22% but there was no similar effect in the over 50s; the benefit in younger women was statistically significant. The review also noted that polychemotherapy had greater benefit than single agents alone and that treatment longer than six months' duration did not appear to offer an advantage.

The value of meta-analysis has itself been a subject of critical review (Lancet 1989) but most workers in the UK currently accept the potential value of adjuvant chemotherapy in the specific subset of premenopausal node-positive women; it is however the experience of many, that relatively few such patients elect to undergo therapy when faced with the side effects.

Adjuvant therapy in node-negative disease

Because patients with node-negative disease were regarded as having a good chance of survival (70%), adjuvant therapy with its often severe side effects was considered unethical. When the early results of adjuvant therapy in node-positive patients were seen to be so good, these reservations became less important and a small number of prospective studies were established; these had not been reported at the time of the meta-analysis.

Many would say that patients with node-negative disease were the most likely to benefit from adjuvant therapy because their micrometastatic load should be least of all; alternatively many more patients who had been cured by surgery would be exposed to unpleasant therapy unnecessarily.

The early results of these major studies have recently been published. The NSABP study (Fisher et al 1989) in node-negative early breast cancer included only those patients with oestrogen receptor negative tumours; these were selected for their worse prognosis. After four years, those who underwent a sequential regimen of methotrexate, 5-fluorouracil and then leucovorin had no overall survival advantage when compared to controls but there was a trend towards improved relapse-free interval.

In The Ludwig Breast Cancer Study Group (1989) of a regime of cyclophosphamide, methotrexate, fluorouracil and leucovorin, there was no overall survival advantage but again an increasing trend with time of improved relapse-free interval. The final study from the West Midlands Oncology Association (UK) showed no benefit whatsoever from a regime of fluorouracil, methotrexate and chlorambucil after a median follow-up of seven years (Morrison et al 1989).

In response to these results a number of editorial reviews have appeared with differing interpretations (N Engl J Med 1989) but few oncologists in the UK would advocate cytotoxic adjuvant therapy for node-negative patients at the moment. There may well be subgroups with node-negative disease who are very much more at risk of recurrence and would benefit from treatment. Such groups have yet to be identified.

ADJUVANT HORMONAL THERAPY IN BREAST CANCER

Hormonal manipulation is a well-established and valuable manoeuvre in the treatment of advanced breast cancer; its use as an adjuvant is a logical choice. Although not strictly a cytotoxic agent, in breast cancer hormonal manipulation is a major form of adjuvant therapy.

Early studies looked exclusively at adjuvant oopherectomy but none of the five major studies performed (NSABP, Oslo, Manchester, Toronto, Boston) showed any long-term survival benefit; one subgroup from the Toronto study of premenopausal women over 45 years did show a survival advantage. A review of these studies (Henderson & Canellos 1980) concluded that adjuvant oopherectomy confers no obvious survival benefit. Unfortunately oestrogen-receptor analysis was not available for these trials and it is unknown whether receptor-positive patients would benefit. With the availability of hormone receptor analysis came a new generation of prophylactic (and therapeutic) hormonal agents. One of these, tamoxifen, had such minimal side effects that it was regarded as an ideal adjuvant, and not surprisingly has replaced oopherectomy in studies of hormone therapy.

Adjuvant tamoxifen

The Nolvadex® Adjuvant Trial Organization (NATO) was the first to report a significant survival advantage for women who took adjuvant tamoxifen 20 mg/day for two years (Baum et al 1985). In 1987 the Scottish Cancer Trials Office reported their study of adjuvant tamoxifen for five years and confirmed the NATO results. This second study also confirmed without doubt that this benefit could not be realized if tamoxifen were given on first relapse in the control group and secondly that this benefit was paradoxically independent of oestrogen receptor status.

Other important studies failed to show such clear results but most have demonstrated some benefit in favour of tamoxifen. In order to rationalize the world experience, adjuvant tamoxifen was submitted to meta-analysis as part of the Peto overview (1988). In 28 trials involving 16 500 women there were 3782 deaths. Comparison of observed with expected deaths revealed that 300 deaths were avoided or delayed by tamoxifen treatment but only in the over-50 age group. This represents a statistically significant reduction of 20% in the odds of death.

The optimum length of time for tamoxifen therapy is unknown but two years is generally accepted as the norm; the long-term side effects appear minimal but there is a small risk of endometrial cancer which is balanced by a reduction in second primary breast cancers (Fornander et al 1989).

In conclusion, adjuvant tamoxifen confers a survival advantage in postmenopausal women following surgical treatment of early breast cancer. The case for its use in premenopausal women is unproven.

ADJUVANT THERAPY IN COLORECTAL CANCER

The problem

After bronchogenic carcinoma, colorectal cancer is the most common malignant disease in the USA and in the majority of European countries. In the UK, 26 000 new cases are seen each year, with about 18 000 deaths.

Although 75% of new cases are amenable to 'curative' resection only 50% of these will survive five years. Individual prognosis or five-year survival correlates well with Dukes' stage: Dukes' A—90%, Dukes' B—60% and Dukes' C—30%. The realization that surgery by whatever technique is unlikely to modify these results has further led to trials of adjuvant therapy aimed at the two major patterns of disease recurrence: pelvic recurrence in rectal cancer patients (radiotherapy) and liver metastases for all colorectal cases (chemotherapy).

Local recurrence and adjuvant radiotherapy

Almost one in three patients after successful resection of a rectal tumour will develop local pelvic recurrence; about half of these will present within

Table 9.2   Reported local recurrence rates in randomized trials of adjuvant radiotherapy for operable rectal cancer. (For references see Buyse et al 1988)

Trial (reference)	Dose	No of patients randomized	Local recurrences Radiotherapy control		P-value	Endpoint
Pre-operative radiotherapy						
MRC 1	5 or 20 Gy	824	235/549	112/275	NS	Local
EORTC 2	34.5 Gy	466	5/152	21/166	**	Local only
			17/152	42/166	**	Local + distant
VASOG 2	31.5 Gy	361	37/180	40/181	NS	Residual or recurrent disease
Stockholm	25 Gy	694	23/271	54/274	***	Pelvic recurrence
MRC 2	40 Gy	261	41/129	50/132	NS	'Local' recurrence
ICRF	25 Gy	478	'Significant difference'		*	'Local recurrence'
North-West	25 Gy	284	26/143	58/141	***	'Local recurrence'
Post-operative radiotherapy						
GITSG	40 Gy	202	15/96	27/106	NS	Local as the first sign of recurrence
Denmark	50 Gy	494	18/244	20/250	NS	Local only
			38/244	44/250	NS	Local + distant
NSAPB	46.5 Gy	368	30/184	45/184	NS	Local + distant
MRC 3	40 Gy	369	14/180	42/189	***	'Local recurrence'

NS = not conventionally significant: * $p < 0.05$, ** $p < 0.01$, *** $p < 0.001$

one year and three-quarters by two years. This is much sooner than presentation with liver secondaries. If it is assumed that the bowel ends are tumour-free at the time of surgery, and steps are taken to eradicate exfoliated cells, then local recurrence relates well to Dukes' stage, local fixation and tumour involvement of lateral resection margins (Umpleby 1989).

Since radiotherapy is of proven worth in locally advanced disease, its use as an adjuvant in the management of earlier disease has been studied in at least 16 randomized trials; rather more studies have used pre-operative irradiation, possibly because it requires shorter courses and is generally regarded as safer. Post-operative treatment allows refined selection of patients based on histology and laparotomy but there is a greater potential morbidity and treatment requires longer overall fractionization (4–5 weeks).

The results of irradiation have been assessed according to local recurrence rates and overall patient survival. There is little doubt that there is a significant beneficial effect of treatment on local recurrence. Of the 11 prospective randomized trials, five have shown a statistically significant benefit in favour of radiotherapy with the remainder showing a trend in favour of treatment (Table 9.2), particularly with pre-operative regimes.

Analysis of those randomized studies which compare overall survival have generally been disappointing with not one showing a statistically significant benefit (Buyse et al 1988). In order to address the possibility that poor numbers may hide a small but genuine benefit, the results of relevant trials

Table 9.3   Mortality in published trials comparing prolonged adjuvant systemic chemotherapy with no chemotherapy (including trials with identical radiotherapy for both treatment and control)

Trial (reference)	Treatment & Duration	Deaths / No. Entered Chemo.	Deaths / No. Entered Control	O–E	Var.	Odds Ratio* Comparing Treatment with Control Mortality Rates (& 95% c.i.)
Prolonged single–agent CTX						
Chicago	N Mustard 1 year	5/31	7/31	−1.0	2.5	
VASOG–19a	5FU 7 weeks	129/193	148/205	−5.3	21.1	
VASOG–19b	5FU indefinitely	40/42	41/42	−0.5	0.7	
VASOG–FUDR	Floxuridine 5 weeks	233/352	239/352	−3.0	38.9	
Richmond	5FU 1 year	31/102	33/101	−1.2	11.0	
VASOG–23	5FU indefinitely	218/334	242/343	−8.9	36.9	
Glasgow	5FU 1 year	3/16	2/19	0.7	1.1	
COG	5FU 1 year	69/151	81/168	−2.0	19.9	
Sweden	5FU 3 months	104/216	98/205	0.4	26.3	
Slough	Razoxane indefinitely	75/139	75/133	−1.7	16.9	
Exeter	5FU 8 weeks	30/68	28/68	1.0	8.4	
Leicester*	5FU 6 months	22/42	20/45	1.7	5.5	
■ Subtotal: single agents		959/1686	1014/1712	−19.8	189.2	10% ± 7
Prolonged multiple–agent CTX						
VASOG–27	5FU+MeCCNU 1 year	148/327	160/318	−8.1	40.3	
GITSG–6175	5FU+MeCCNU 16 months	70/156	71/159	0.2	19.5	
Vienna	5FU+MMC+AraC 3 months	25/59	21/62	2.6	7.2	
GITSG–7175	5FU+MeCCNU 18 months	30/58	37/62	−2.4	7.5	
SWOG–7510	5FU+MeCCNU 1 year	48/95	48/94	−0.3	11.9	
NSABP R–01	5FU+V+MeCCNU 18 months	78/187	95/184	−9.2	23.1	
NSABP C–01	5FU+V+MeCCNU 18 months	141/358	162/383	−5.4	44.8	
■ Subtotal: multiple agents		540/1240	594/1262	−22.6	154.3	14% ± 7
■ TOTAL: All published trials		1499/2926	1608/2974	−42.4	343.4	12% ± 5

```
                          0.0      0.5      1.0      1.5      2.0
                          Treatment better | Treatment worse
```

Treatment effect 2P < .02

Test for heterogeneity: X^2_{18} = 8.5; NS

*   only deaths due to colorectal cancer published

have been subjected to two meta-analyses, one totalling 3000 patients (Buyse et al 1988) and, more recently, 5000 patients (AXIS protocol 1989). Both suggest that there could be a 10% reduction in mortality in favour of the treatment arms, irrespective of radiation dose. The question of radiotherapy as an adjuvant to improve survival in rectal cancer must therefore remain open until a larger study with effective statistical power has been completed. The current national UK study of adjuvant radiotherapy and 5-fluorouracil infusion (AXIS) promises to resolve this issue. Outside of the pelvis, adjuvant radiotherapy for colonic lesions has generally been regarded as dangerous compared to the known low risk of recurrence. The one exception may be tumours of the splenic flexure, where high local recurrence rates of up to 20% have been reported (Phillips et al 1984). The use of adjuvant radiotherapy for this site has not been studied.

Adjuvant chemotherapy and colorectal liver metastases

In one-third of cases undergoing curative resection, distant metastases will eventually occur, invariably in the liver and sometimes elsewhere. Trials of adjuvant cytotoxic chemotherapy have generally been confined to patients with tumours in Dukes' stages B and C, where there is significant risk of dissemination at the time of primary treatment.

Cytotoxic agents have been administered singly or in combinations, for the most part based on 5-fluorouracil which has the greatest single agent activity in advanced disease. Other agents which show activity in advanced disease and which have been studied in adjuvant therapy include nitrogen mustard, thiotepa, razoxane, fluoroxuridine and methyl-CCNU.

The results of the major prospective, comparative controlled studies are summarized in Table 9.3; none has shown a statistically significant survival advantage in favour of therapy. As with radiotherapy, the trials so far have not included large numbers and are therefore likely to miss a small benefit. With meta-analysis, there appears to be a reduction in the odds of death of about 10% for those given 5-fluorouracil and this increases to 15% when 5-fluorouracil is given for prolonged courses (Table 9.3). Analysis of subgroups within this statistical overview is confounded by differences in criteria of selection but one group which merits particular attention in future studies is patients with rectal cancer, who seem to have benefited more than patients with colonic cancer.

There is as yet no proven advantage of adjuvant systemic chemotherapy alone in colorectal cancer but there is a suggestion that a modest benefit may exist. This requires assessment in prospective studies with adequate patient numbers.

Adjuvant chemotherapy and immunotherapy

Following on from several smaller studies which showed a survival benefit when 5-fluorouracil and levamisole were combined as adjuvant therapy for colonic cancer, the National Intergroup (USA) undertook a large prospective randomized study which has recently reported (Moertel et al 1990).

This study included patients with Dukes' B and C lesions who were randomized to either one year of 5-fluorouracil and levamisole or to no treatment. In addition, Dukes' C patients were randomized to a third arm of levamisole only. At a median follow-up of three years there has been a 33% reduction in deaths for Dukes' C patients on the combination regime; this is highly statistically significant. This difference was not realized for patients with Dukes' B lesions but the recurrence rate has been smaller.

The mechanism of the beneficial effect of levamisole is unknown. It has a wide spectrum of activity, from the modulation of many cellular enzyme systems to the potentiation of human interferon and interleukin-2. Whatever its mode of action, it appears to potentiate the action of 5-fluorouracil in a way that demands urgent resolution.

Adjuvant hepatic perfusion with cytotoxic agents

Although established liver metastases take their blood supply mainly from the hepatic artery, it is theoretically unlikely that micrometastases, which gain access to the liver via the portal vein, would have an arterial blood supply. It is logical therefore, to use the portal venous route for cytotoxic delivery, as it targets the organ of interest and limits the potentially toxic effects seen with systemic routes. This is particularly relevant for 5-fluorouracil, which is metabolized in the liver. More effective, larger doses can be delivered to this organ via the portal vein, with minimal effects elsewhere.

Most studies have started treatment the day following surgery. At operation, an indwelling cannula is placed in a venous radicle of the mesenteric circulation or in the umbilical vein. Other studies have preferred to delay treatment for 4–6 weeks to enable recovery from surgery, but there is theoretical logic in beginning therapy early in order to treat tumour cells shed at the time of surgery. Following the original study by Taylor et al (1985), which showed a statistically significant survival benefit at four years with this technique, seven other multicentre studies have been undertaken, but none of these has published more than preliminary data.

The technique of portal delivery of cytotoxics is clearly an exciting approach to the problem but harder data from larger studies are required before this mode of adjuvant therapy can be finally accepted as beneficial. The current AXIS study in the UK should be sufficiently large to enable firm conclusions to be made.

ADJUVANT THERAPY FOR GASTRIC CANCER

In Britain, gastric cancer is falling in incidence but is still the third commonest cause of death from cancer in men and the fourth commonest in women. Only 20% of all new cases have apparently local disease for which radical surgery alone can offer any chance of cure; 80% will present with advanced Stage IV disease and in these, adjuvant therapy cannot be considered.

Of those who undergo resection for presumed local disease, about half will die within the next two years. There is a very good case for adjuvant therapy in these patients. Unfortunately, radiotherapy has not performed well in advanced disease, which suggests that gastric cancer is essentially radio-resistant; responses have been observed in patients with minimal residual disease after resection (Gunderson & O'Conell 1989) but this has never been extrapolated to occult disease.

Adjuvant chemotherapy following surgery has been extensively investigated. Two early and encouraging studies from Japan were followed by numerous others with both single and multiple agents, but the majority have failed to show a survival advantage (Clark & Slevin 1987).

The three most active agents, 5-fluorouracil, adriamycin and mito-mycin C have been combined in a number of studies but the 40% response rates with advanced tumours have not been translated into improved survival after adjuvant therapy following surgery (Fielding 1983).

Cytotoxic agents have been combined with the immune-enhancer levamisole, with early encouraging results (Mira et al 1980). However no obvious survival advantage could be detected in a recently published large randomized trial (Italian GI Tumour Study Group 1988). A similar approach, using the antiulcer drug cimetidine in its 'immune-enhancer' role has however shown promising results. In a prospective randomized study from Denmark (Tonneson & Kaup-Jersen 1986), cimetidine 400 mg twice daily for two years significantly prolonged median survival but there were very few survivors at five years. A similar regime is currently being studied by the British Stomach Cancer Group.

The results of both radiotherapy and chemotherapy have so far been disappointing in gastric cancer but the disease is invariably advanced at presentation; new anti-cancer agents and different approaches are badly needed.

ADJUVANT THERAPY OF PANCREATIC CANCER

Like gastric cancer, pancreatic cancer presents in most patients at an advanced stage; only 15–20% of cases in most series are resectable. The distinction must be made between adjuvant chemotherapy where significant residual disease remains, and occult micrometastatic disease. Most 'adjuvant' studies have been undertaken with advanced disease.

As a single agent, 5-fluorouracil has been of limited benefit if any (Davis et al 1974) but when combined with radiotherapy has shown a modest prolongation of life but no increased long-term survival (GI Tumour Study Group 1979). Further studies confirm this (GITSG 1987). Combinations of agents have shown response rates of up to 40% but no increase in median survival.

The finding that pancreatic cancer contains oestrogen receptor-positive cell lines (Theve et al 1983) has led to the interesting notion that tamoxifen may be tumoricidal. Early reports have been encouraging (Tonneson & Kaup-Jersen 1986) but the results of definitive studies are awaited.

CONCLUSION

Adjuvant chemotherapy has a sound theoretical basis and is effective in animal models, but its application in solid human tumours has been generally disappointing; this in some ways is not surprising as the residual tumour burden cannot be accurately assessed, nor can the individual chemosensitivity of tumours. These two areas stand out for further study. The development of new cytotoxic agents and drugs that exploit immune antitumour effects may offer better prospects in the future.

REFERENCES

Axis Protocol UK Coordinating Committee on Cancer Research 1989 (UKCCR) MRC Cancer Office pp 1–6
Baum M, Brinkley A, Dossel J A et al 1985 Controlled trial of tamoxifen as single adjuvant agent management of early breast cancer. Br J Cancer 87: 608–611
Baum M, Zilkha K, Houghton J 1989 Ethics of clinical research: lessons for the future. Br Med J 299: 251–253
Bonnadonna G, Valagussa P 1985 Adjuvant systemic therapy for resectable breast cancer. J Clin Oncol 3: 259–275
Buyse M, Zeleniuch-Jacquotle A, Chalmers T C 1988 Adjuvant therapy of colorectal cancer. Why we still don't know. JAMA 259: 3571–3578
Clark P, Slevin M L 1987 (leader) Chemotherapy for stomach cancer. Br Med J 295: 870
Davis H L, Ramirez G, Ansfield F J 1974 Adenocarcinomas of the stomach, pancreas, liver and biliary tracts. Survival of 328 patients treated with fluorouracil therapy. Cancer 33: 193–197
Early Breast Cancer Trialists Collaborative Group 1988 Effects of adjuvant tamoxifen and of cytotoxic therapy on mortality in early breast cancer—an overview of 61 randomised trials among 28896 women. N Engl J Med 319: 1681–1692
Fisher B, Slack N, Katrych D 1975 Ten-year follow up = results of patient with carcinoma of the breast in a co-operative clinical trial evaluating surgical adjuvant chemotherapy. Surg Gynecol Obstet 140: 528–534
Fisher B, Redmond G, Fisher E R et al 1984 A summary of findings from NSABP trials of adjuvant therapy. In: Jones S E, Salmon E S (eds) Adjuvant therapy of cancer IV. Grune and Stratton, New York, pp 185–194
Fisher B, Redmond C, Dimitrov N V et al 1989 A randomised clinical trial evaluating sequential methotrexate and fluorouracil in the treatment of patients with node-negative breast cancer who have oestrogen-receptor negative tumours. N Engl J Med 320: 473–478
Fielding J W L 1983 An interim report of a prospective, randomised, controlled study of adjuvant chemotherapy in operable gastric cancer. Bristol Stomach Cancer Group. World J Surg 7: 390–399
Fornander T, Cedermark B, Mattsson A et al 1989 Adjuvant tamoxifen in early breast cancer: occurrence of new primary cancers. Lancet i: 117–119

GI Tumour Study Group 1979 Comparative therapeutic trial of radiation with or without chemotherapy in pancreatic carcinoma. Int J Radiat Oncol Biol Phys 5: 1643–1647

GI Tumour Study Group 1987 Further evidence of effective adjuvant combined radiation and chemotherapy following curative resection of pancreatic cancer. Cancer 59: 2006–2010

Gunderson L L, O'Conell H 1989 Adenocarcinoma of the stomach: Areas of future in adjuvant therapy. Int J Radiat Oncol Biol Phys 8: 1–11

Henderson I C, Canellos G P 1980 Cancer of the breast: the past decade. N Engl J Med 307: 17–30, 78–90

Italian Gastrointestinal Tumour Study Group 1988 Adjuvant treatments following curative resection for gastric cancer. Br J Surg 75: 1100–1104

Lancet 1989 (editorial) Adjuvant systemic treatment for breast cancer meta-analysed. Lancet i: 80–81

Mira H, Ono F, Moriyania M et al 1980 Immunochemotherapy of gastric cancer with levamisole. Acta Med Okayam 34: 257–281

Moertel C G, Fleming T R, Macdonald J R et al 1990 Levamisole and fluorouracil for adjuvant therapy of resected colon carcinoma. New Engl J Med 337: 352–358

Morison J M, Howell A, Kelly K A et al 1989 West Midlands oncology association trials of adjuvant chemotherapy in operable breast cancer. Results after a median follow up of seven years. II Patients without involved axillary lymph nodes. Br J Cancer 60: 919–994

N Engl J Med 1989 Editorials V De Vitta, N L McGuire 320: (8) 525–529

Nissen-Meyer R, Kjellgren K, Massun B 1982 Adjuvant chemotherapy in breast cancer. Cancer Res 80: 142–148

Phillips R K S, Hitlinger R, Blesovsky et al 1984 Local recurrence following 'curative' surgery for large bowel cancer. The overall picture. Br J Surg 71: 12–16

Priestman T J 1979 Cancer chemotherapy—an introduction. Montedison Pharmaceuticals Ltd (England) pp 62–84

Scottish Cancer Trials Office 1987 Adjuvant tamoxifen in the management of operable breast cancer. The Scottish Trial. Lancet ii: 171–175

Taylor I, Machin D, Mullee M et al 1985 A randomized controlled trial of adjuvant portal vein cytotoxic perfusion in colo-rectal cancer. Br J Surg 72: 359–363

The Ludwig Breast Cancer Study Group 1989 Prolonged disease-free survival after one course of perioperative adjuvant chemotherapy for node-negative breast cancer. N Engl J Med 30: 491–496

Theve N O, Poussette A, Carlstrom K 1983 Adenocarcinoma of the pancreas, a hormone sensitive tumour? A preliminary report on treatment. Clin Oncol 9: 193–197

Tonneson K, Kaup-Jersen M 1986 Antioestrogen therapy in pancreatic carcinoma: a preliminary report. Eur Surg Oncol 12: 69–70

Umpleby H 1989 The development and treatment of local recurrence in colorectal surgery. In: Taylor I (ed) Progress in Surgery Volume 3, pp 59–75

10

Management of thoracic trauma

D. Weeden

The effect of thoracic trauma depends on the structures injured and the pre-existing respiratory state and varies in severity from minor to rapidly fatal. In the UK, injury is the commonest cause of death in the 15–35 age group. Road traffic accidents are the commonest cause of major trauma with a quarter of the victims sustaining chest injuries. A total of 20–33% of deaths are theoretically preventable (Anderson et al 1988). The majority of deaths occur within four hours and are related to uncontrolled haemorrhage, uncorrected hypoxia or delay in surgical intervention.

GENERAL MANAGEMENT

Assessment and management should proceed simultaneously. It is essential to assess immediately the adequacy of the airway, ventilation and circulation. Physical characteristics of the accident may lead to suspicion of particular injuries and a fatality in the same accident increases the probability of significant injury. One should avoid excessive volume replacement. A standard postero-anterior erect chest X-ray and a lateral view are obtained. Antero-posterior supine films cause apparent mediastinal widening and obscure haemothoraces. Early estimation of arterial blood gases is mandatory. Clinical parameters are assessed regularly as rapid deterioration can occur. Most major injuries require invasive monitoring with central lines inserted on the side of injury.

Hypoxia

Significant hypoxia is present when the Pao_2 is below 8 kPa with the patient breathing room air or below 40 kPa on 100% oxygen (FIo_2 1.0). With Pao_2 below 8 kPa there is a rapid fall in oxygen saturation and carriage. Signs of hypoxia are tachypnoea above 35, laboured respiration using accessory muscles, tachycardia, agitation and disorientation. Patients with severe head injuries are more hypoxic than their respiratory pattern suggests. Major causes of hypoxia are outlined in Figure 10.1.

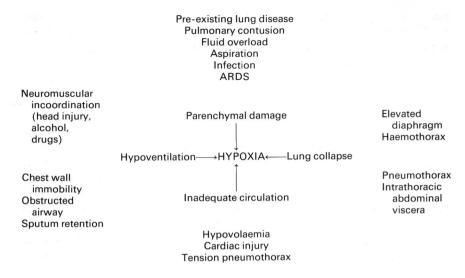

Fig. 10.1   Aetiology of hypoxia.

Airway management

Upper airway obstruction can be caused by massive facial swelling, fractured mandible, tongue displacement, aspiration, inhalation of foreign bodies and laryngo-tracheal injuries. The upper airway should be cleared by suction and by lifting the jaw. However, it should be noted that this does not move the tongue forward when bilateral mandibular fractures are present. Intubation should not be performed until hypoxia is corrected by mask ventilation. Over-insertion of the tube should be avoided as this leads to intubation of the right main bronchus. With suspected cervical fractures, manipulation of the airway is dangerous but fewer than 10% of significant chest injuries have cervical fractures so the danger of hypoxia is greater (Pepe 1989). The cervical spine should be immobilized by a second person stabilizing the head during intubation.

Ventilation can be provided by a jet system via the cricothyroid membrane if there is no proximal obstruction, as expiration is by passive recoil. The cricothyroid membrane lies 1.5–2 cm below the thyroid notch above the cricoid ring. The larynx is stabilized between finger and thumb of the non-dominant hand and the skin and membrane infiltrated with local anaesthetic. The membrane is incised with a shielded blade, the introducer is passed into the trachea and the tube is advanced. A 14-gauge needle with a side hole, mounted on a syringe containing saline, may be inserted through the membrane at 45° to the skin heading caudally whilst aspirating. The presence of bubbles indicates entry into the trachea. Cricothyroid puncture may be life-saving when there is extreme urgency because tracheostomy cannot be performed quickly enough to relieve critical airway obstruction. In other cases tracheostomy gives complete control of the airway if endotracheal intubation cannot be achieved.

Ventilation

Tissue oxygenation requires ventilation, gas transfer and an adequate cardiac output. Indications for mechanical ventilation are tachypnoea above 40, Pao_2 below 8 kPa, $Paco_2$ above 8 kPa, a progressive fall in Pao_2, extensive pulmonary contusion or diffuse infiltrative change on chest X-ray, or a severe flail chest. There are many modes of ventilatory support and these are beyond the scope of this review. The aims of ventilation are to increase Pao_2 above 8 kPa and saturation above 95%, to achieve a FIo_2 below 0.6 to prevent oxygen toxicity and absorption atelectasis, and to maintain physiological $Paco_2$ (3.5–5.5 kPa) and pH (7.35–7.45), and an intrapulmonary shunt below 20%.

Circulation

Immediate circulatory failure following thoracic trauma may be due to exsanguination, tension pneumothorax, cardiac tamponade or myocardial damage. Following major chest trauma, particularly with exsanguination, external cardiac massage is ineffective. If an effective output is not achieved within five minutes by internal massage, there is no chance of survival (Mattox 1989).

Myocardial contractility, heart rate and afterload can all be optimized but significant improvement in output can only occur with adequate venous return which is often impaired. Young fit adults with hypovolaemia cope well until sudden decompensation occurs. One should aim for a haematocrit of 30% which provides adequate oxygen carriage and lowers viscosity. Do not raise systolic blood pressure above 100 mmHg before a chest X-ray has confirmed the absence of major vascular injury.

In cardiogenic shock, myocardial contractility is impaired. It may respond to manipulation of preload (venous pressure), afterload (vasodilators) or contractility (inotropes). Intra-aortic balloon counter-pulsation can be used when pharmacological support fails but is only occasionally beneficial.

Cardiac tamponade decreases diastolic ventricular filling, because intra-pericardial pressure exceeds venous pressure, thus reducing stroke volume. Surgical intervention is always required.

Autotransfusion can be used with massive blood loss but requires special apparatus, takes time to set up, and is most useful when there are major vascular or liver injuries.

Table 10.1   Features of pneumothorax, haemothorax and ruptured diaphragm

	Simple pneumothorax	Tension pneumothorax	Haemothorax	Ruptured diaphragm
Tracheal position	Normal	Displaced	Displaced	Displaced
Percussion note	Normal	Increased	Decreased	Variable
Jugular pressure	Normal	Elevated*	Normal*	Normal*
Breath sounds	Normal (Unless large)	Decreased	Decreased	Decreased basally
Bowel sounds (chest)	Absent	Absent	Absent	Sometimes
Respiratory distress	Variable	Severe	Variable	Severe

* = unless hypovolaemic when decreased

Pneumothorax

A closed pneumothorax occurs in about 30% of significant chest injuries (Carrero & Wayne 1989) and in 80% is associated with some haemothorax. Rib fractures are present in 90% of adults with pneumothoraces (Carrero & Wayne 1989) but less often in children. Clinical features are outlined in Table 10.1. An erect expiratory chest X-ray should be obtained. In 10% of cases the initial chest X-ray appears normal and the pneumothorax becomes apparent over the first eight hours (Fig. 10.2). All traumatic

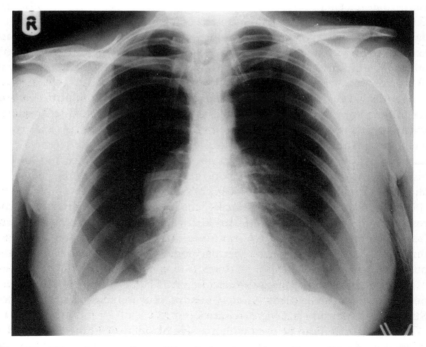

Fig. 10.2   Bilateral pneumothorax. There is almost complete collapse of both lungs but the dense residual lung tissue is seen at both hila.

pneumothoraces should be drained. This prevents a tension pneumo-thorax, encourages early full lung expansion and evacuates any haemo-thorax. Without drainage half of all traumatic pneumothoraces will increase over the first 24 h. Failure to expand the lung may be due to inadequate drain size, to the position of the drain (not reaching the apex), kinking (especially with small anterior drains), inadequate suction, excessive air leak or bronchial obstruction. Failure to expand with effective drainage is an indication for bronchoscopy and often thoracotomy.

Surgical emphysema originates either from the lung with disruption of both pleurae, via the hilum to the mediastinum, from mediastinal air-containing structures or via external wounds and drain sites. It is rarely physiologically significant and usually reabsorbs slowly. Emphysema without a pneumothorax can be observed with repeated chest X-rays unless the patient is ventilated when one or both hemithoraces must be drained. Mediastinal emphysema may indicate tracheo-bronchial or oesophageal injury.

A full thickness defect in the chest wall produces an open pneumothorax with complete lung collapse and paradoxical mediastinal movement. This decreases venous return and ventilation of the contralateral lung. When the cross-sectional area of the defect is greater than that of the trachea, air enters the open hemithorax leading to asphyxia. Management is by occlusive dressing and chest drainage to prevent tension pneumothorax. This is followed by reconstruction.

A tension pneumothorax (Fig. 10.3) impairs venous return by caval distortion from mediastinal shift and raised intrathoracic pressure with compression of the contralateral lung. Clinical features are shown in Table 10.1 and include weak pulse, low blood pressure and rapidly spreading emphysema. A sudden collapse after ventilation suggests tension pneumothorax, which may require immediate relief with a 16-gauge needle before confirmation by chest X-ray or formal drainage.

Haemothorax

A haemothorax occurs in 20–30% of chest injuries (Carrero & Wayne 1989). The hemithorax holds 2–3 l. On an erect chest X-ray, blunting of the costophrenic angle occurs with 250–400 ml but on a supine film opacification is not apparent with less than 1000 ml and is less obvious when bilateral (Fig. 10.4). Opacification is more obvious on lateral decubitus films. Haemothoraces should be drained to encourage full lung expansion which reduces bleeding and lessens the risk of empyema or cortex formation. Failure to obtain complete evacuation may be due to a blocked drain, poor tube position, clotted haemothorax or failure of lung expansion. Thoracotomy is required for immediate blood loss over 1500 ml, continued bleeding above 400 ml/h over four hours, suspicion of major intrathoracic injury, continued haemodynamic instability or a persistent haemothorax.

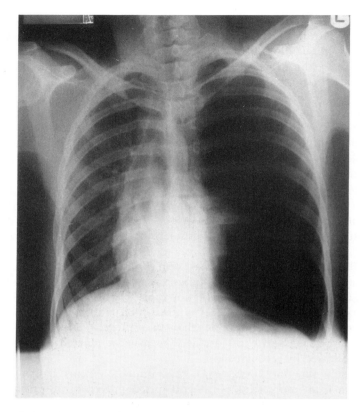

Fig. 10.3   Left tension pneumothorax. Large volume totally lucent (no lung at hilum) left hemithorax with spreading of the ribs and a low left hemidiaphragm, marked mediastinal shift.

Chylothorax

Thoracic duct rupture is rare and occurs with thoracic spinal hyper-extension, hydrostatic transmission of raised intra-abdominal pressure or penetrating injury. The effusion may not become opalescent until fat is ingested and its appearance may be delayed for up to six weeks after injury. Fluid loss should be replaced with plasma and the patient should be fed with parenteral nutrition. Oral medium-chain triglycerides, which are absorbed into portal blood, are less satisfactory. The localization of the site of leak by lymphangiography is rarely successful. About half of cases settle conservatively but surgery is required if drainage exceeds 1500 ml/day, continues for two weeks or is associated with metabolic complications. The thoracic duct is ligated via a right postero-lateral seventh interspace thoracotomy. The lower oesophagus is mobilized and retracted forwards to expose the duct which lies in front of the vertebral column between the

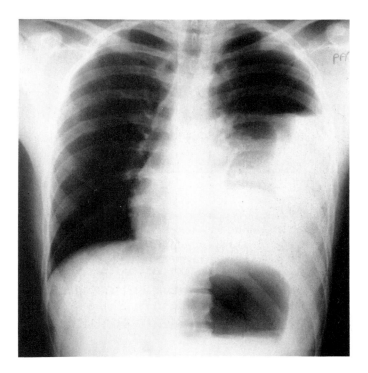

Fig. 10.4   Left traumatic haemopneumothorax. Left hemidiaphragm is intact and in normal position (shown by fundic gas shadow), apparent high diaphragm is a subpulmonary haemothorax with further lateral loculation and an air–fluid level.

aorta and azygos vein. The duct is made more obvious by intragastric cream given 30 min before exploration. Dyes should be avoided as these stain the tissues.

Intercostal drainage

Drains should be inserted between the anterior and mid-axillary lines above the fifth rib rather than anteriorly (see Table 10.2). A 28 French drain is used to prevent clotting. The arm is fully abducted to widen the chosen interspace which is widely infiltrated with 50 ml of 0.4% lignocaine. The skin incision is made one interspace lower and an oblique track is made with a blunt clip to pass over the top of the chosen rib. A finger is introduced and swept around the pleura to confirm intrathoracic position. A simple heavy suture is inserted where the drain will lie and tied when the drain is removed. Do not use a pursestring suture around the drain as this causes skin necrosis. The drain is inserted with the trocar pulled back from the tip and is guided to the desired position (apex for air, posteriorly for

Table 10.2 Comparison of axillary and anterior approach for chest drainage

	Axillary approach	Anterior approach
Interspace size	Large	Small
Chest wall muscles	Thin, intercostal + serratus anterior	Thick, intercostal + pectorals
Accessory respiratory muscles	No impairment	Impairs largest (pectoralis major)
Mediastinal structures	Away	Close
Internal mammary	Away	Close
Position	Usually goes to apex	Rarely goes to apex
Tube fixation	Easy without kinking	Difficult without kinking
Scar	Well hidden	Obvious

blood). It is fixed with a further heavy suture and the wound is closed. The drain is connected to an underwater seal bottle. High volume (up to 15 l/min) low pressure (3–5 kPa) suction (not a Roberts pump which is low volume low pressure) is applied to the bottle. The drain should not be clamped because of the risk of tension pneumothorax. The drain should be removed when there has been no air leak for 24 h with a fully expanded lung. If the patient is ventilated the drain should be left until after extubation or there has been no air leak for five days.

BLUNT INJURIES

Fractures

Rib fractures occur in 60–70% of patients following blunt chest trauma (Carrero & Wayne 1989) and 30% are missed on the initial chest X-ray. Oblique views are not helpful. Clinical signs of a rib fracture are crepitus, deformity and pain which limits chest wall movement and leads to atelectasis, sputum retention, hypoxia and hypercapnia. Forced Vital Capacity (FVC) indicates respiratory status (15–25 ml/kg poor, below 15 ml/kg requires ventilation). Ten percent of first rib fractures are associated with major vascular or brachial plexus injury (Dhasmana 1989). With more than six ribs fractured, 50% of patients have intrathoracic and 15% intra-abdominal injury (Jones 1980). Abdominal injuries are more common with fractures below the seventh rib. With multiple rib fractures respiratory function will deteriorate over the initial 48 h and requires analgesia sufficient for adequate coughing. With multiple fractures an intercostal drain should be inserted before ventilation.

Sternal fractures occur in 10% of significant impact injuries (Trinca & Dooley 1975) and are more common in those wearing seat belts. With the upper fragment displaced posteriorly there are often significant intrathoracic injuries. Local pain, bruising, swelling and sternal deformity occur. Treatment is usually conservative with adequate analgesia, although operative fixation may be performed during surgery for other injuries.

Posterior displacement of the upper fragment may need urgent reduction to prevent vascular or tracheal compression.

Scapular fracture is an unusual isolated injury and suggests significant impact. A total of 40% are missed on the initial chest X-ray (Harris & Harris 1988) but nearly all have ipsilateral chest injuries.

Fragments from clavicular fractures may damage the subclavian vessels or brachial plexus. Posterior claviculosternal dislocation may injure the trachea and innominate vessels and requires immediate reduction.

Vertebral fractures can occur during blunt chest trauma, most commonly thoracic, and may widen the mediastinum.

Flail chest

Flail chest occurs in 10–20% of significant chest injuries but is rare in children who have pliable ribs. Initially muscle splinting may mask paradoxical movement which is never obvious posteriorly. Factors leading to respiratory failure are pulmonary contusion, pain and paradoxical movement which causes increased dead space and mediastinal shift and leads to hypoventilation of the contralateral lung. Early stabilization by local support is important and the patient should be turned onto the flail segment or a sandbag placed over it.

Mortality and morbidity have been reduced significantly (Trinkle et al 1975) with careful management of the pulmonary contusion by limitation of crystalloid infusion to 1000 ml during resuscitation and 50 ml/h over the next 24 h. Diuretics are given if the circulation is overloaded. Circulating volume is maintained with blood or plasma but not plasma substitutes. Adequate analgesia is required for effective physiotherapy and regular sputum cultures give a basis for antibiotic therapy. Half of the patients can be managed without ventilation, particularly those without lung contusion. Features suggesting that mechanical ventilation is required are unsatisfactory respiratory function (Pao_2 below 8 kPa, $Paco_2$ above 8 kPa, tachypnoea above 35/min, FVC below 15 ml/kg), more than eight unilateral or four bilateral rib fractures, other significant injuries, severe shock, need for general anaesthetic, age over 65 years and pre-existing lung disease. Anterior flail segments can be effectively stabilized but others should only be fixed during thoracotomy for other injuries. Mortality depends on pre-existing respiratory state and other injuries and is 10% in those with an isolated flail segment. A third of survivors will have complications such as chest wall pain and respiratory dysfunction.

Pain control

Pain results in sleep deprivation, muscle splinting, hypoventilation, poor cough, retained secretions, hypertension and tachycardia. Adequate pain control should be achieved using systemic analgesics or nerve blockade (continuous infusion thoracic epidural gives excellent analgesia).

Aspiration pneumonitis

Aspiration of material below pH 3 causes severe bronchorrhoea and alveolar damage. Large fragments may lead to asphyxia. Surfactant is decreased and this causes alveolar collapse leading to hypoxaemia. Treatment is by oxygen, bronchodilators, high dose penicillin and early ventilatory support with PEEP. Steroids are contraindicated. Bronchoscopy is required only for removal of foreign bodies, lavage is unnecessary due to rapid spontaneous neutralization.

Traumatic asphyxia

This is a marker of severe compression of the upper body. There may be swelling, violaceous skin discolouration, subcutaneous and subconjunctival petechiae, retinal haemorrhage, epistaxis, haemoptysis, haematemesis, fits, confusion, coma, papilloedema and hyperthermia. Mortality is 10%, largely from associated injuries.

Adult Respiratory Distress Syndrome (ARDS)

ARDS usually occurs 12–48 h after injury and is unlikely to develop after 72 h unless further precipitating factors occur. There is a functional disruption of the alveolar-capillary membrane produced by the release of toxic products from neutrophils. This results in patchy atelectasis and interstitial oedema which lowers compliance and increases shunting. Diagnostic criteria are; Pao_2 below 10 kPa with FIo_2 above 0.5, which is resistant to increasing FIo_2, widespread infiltrates on chest X-ray, and a pulmonary wedge pressure below 18 mmHg. Clinically there is dyspnoea, tachypnoea and tachycardia. Radiographic changes appear 12–24 h after the initiating event and also after the physiological changes but do not correlate with them. There are patchy ill-defined bilateral pulmonary densities without evidence of left ventricular failure. Later these extend and coalesce. Quantification of the volume of damaged lung by computed tomography (CT) (Wagner 1989) relates to the need for ventilation: over 28% damage requires ventilation. The best predictor of ARDS is Pao_2 below 13.3 kPa with FIo_2 0.4 and below 46.7 kPa with FIo_2 1.0, when there is a 95% probability of ARDS (Weigelt 1981).

Risk factors include sepsis, 22 unit transfusion in less than 12 h, pulmonary contusion, multiple major fractures, aspiration, head injury and prolonged hypotension with factors acting cumulatively (Norwood & Civetta 1985). The likelihood of ARDS with two factors is 42% and with three factors 85%.

Treatment involves ventilation with PEEP, the maintenance of an effective circulation without fluid overload and the control of triggering factors. There is no evidence that steroids, PEEP or dehydration can prevent or curtail ARDS. Despite treatment there may be progressive hypoxaemia and hypercapnia. Average mortality is 50–65%, rising to 80–90% when sepsis is present. High airway pressure, which is necessary to ventilate undamaged lung to remove CO_2, leads to further damage. Early experience with extracorporeal membrane oxygenation (ECMO) showed no survival benefit (Zapol et al 1979). Extracorporeal CO_2 removal ($ECco_2R$) with veno-venous perfusion through a membrane removes all metabolic CO_2 with oxygenation by low frequency ventilation with ECMO during $ECco_2R$. In ARDS when Pao_2 is below 6.7 kPa with FIo_2 above 0.6 and PEEP above 5 cmH_2O, survival is 10%. $ECco_2R$ can increase this to 47% (Pesenti et al 1988). This technique requires heparinization, so bleeding is a major problem.

Lung injury

Pulmonary contusions are lacerations produced by direct trauma, shock waves or deceleration, with interstitial bleeding and alveolar collapse. Radiographic signs are an indistinct density, visible by one hour in 70% of cases and in the remainder by six hours, which becomes an irregular linear infiltrate. Treatment is conservative, as for flail chest, and the contusion resolves in 2–6 days. In half of the cases infection develops, and this may take 2–3 weeks to clear. Abscess formation is rare.

A pulmonary haematoma is a discrete mass, usually 2–5 cm in diameter, which resolves over six weeks. If it becomes infected or fails to resolve resection is indicated.

A pulmonary pseudocyst is a non-epithelialized intrapulmonary air space. It causes chest pain, cough, dyspnoea and haemoptysis and is visible on chest X-ray within 12 h of injury adjacent to a contusion. It may contain a fluid level and changes in shape and size rapidly. It is well demonstrated by CT. Air usually reabsorbs over 2–4 months but resection is indicated for enlargement or infection.

Diaphragmatic injury

This occurs in 3–5% of major trunk injuries (Johnson 1988). Considerable deceleration is required and the rupture is caused by increased intra-abdominal pressure or by laceration from rib fractures. Post mortem studies show equal frequency on both sides but more right-sided injuries are immediately fatal so clinical series show a ratio of one right- to three left-sided injuries. Three percent are bilateral, associated with other severe injuries. Injury usually occurs in the dome or postero-lateral area as a radial tear with about a third involving the oesophageal hiatus. Associated injuries such as lower rib fractures, splenic and hepatic injury occur in 70–90% of patients. Undoubtedly diagnosis requires a high index of suspicion. Presentation may be early (within hours), delayed (within days) or late (on average three years). Clinical features include hypotension (bleeding is usually from intra-abdominal injury) and shoulder, chest or upper abdominal pain (Table 10.1). Approximately 50–70% are missed on the initial chest X-ray (Table 10.3). Both clinical and radiological features (Figs. 10.5–10.8) may be masked by mechanical ventilation and deterioration after cessation of ventilation or a persistent haemothorax are both suspicious of a diaphragmatic rupture. There is no infallible test to exclude rupture. One can perform contrast gastrointestinal studies and peritoneal lavage (negative in 30–60% of cases). The appearance of lavage fluid in the chest drain is diagnostic. Other investigations include thoracoscopy within 24 h, laparoscopy after 24 h, ultrasound, isotope hepatosplenogram or angiography. Rupture is commonly missed, and a quarter of patients present late with epigastric discomfort, dysphagia, intestinal obstruction, recurrent chest infections or dyspnoea.

Table 10.3   Possible radiological features of a ruptured diaphragm

Incomplete visualization of the hemidiaphragm
Elevation of the hemidiaphragm
Blunting of the costophrenic angle
Multiple lower rib fractures
Persistent lower lobe collapse
Persistent haemothorax
Mediastinal shift in the absence of a pneumothorax
Aberrant course of a nasogastric tube
Gas filled viscera in chest which is distinguished from a
   haemopneumothorax by apex containing compressed lung not air, and fluid level not
   across the whole hemithorax

Respiratory distress may be relieved by a nasogastric tube. Most acute ruptures are repaired via laparotomy with thoracotomy used for isolated left injury, right-sided injury for control of hepatic veins with laparotomy if required, and delayed repair because of adhesions. The diaphragm is repaired with strong absorbable interrupted single layer sutures. Mortality depends upon associated injuries and is low for isolated rupture.

Phrenic nerve injury is rare and occurs from cervical hyperextension. There is paradoxical movement of the hemidiaphragm. The paralysis recovers over six months and is only a problem when there is pre-existing respiratory disease.

Laryngeal and tracheo-bronchial injury

Laryngeal injury occurs in 1% (Gussack & Jurkovich 1988) and tracheobronchial injury in 1–3% (Dhasmana 1989) of major chest injuries. They are produced by direct compression from a blow to the neck with vertical fracture of the thyroid cartilage or laryngo-tracheal separation, by backwards displacement of the sternum, by raised intrabronchial pressure, by shear with forward movement of the main bronchi against the fixed carina during deceleration, or widening during antero-posterior chest compression with lateral shear or longitudinal shear from hyperextension. Incomplete tears are more common than circumferential disruption. Pulmonary vessels are rarely injured. Tracheo-bronchial injury is seen more commonly in children and young adults, within 2.5 cm of the carina and more often in the right main bronchus. Half have other injuries. Clinical features include dyspnoea, mediastinal or cervical emphysema which is severe and spreads rapidly with pneumothorax if the pleura is torn, haemoptysis, stridor, cough, neck pain, dysphonia and loss of laryngeal outline. The chest X-ray may show emphysema, pneumothorax, lung collapse or the lung 'falling away' from the hilum. Tracheo-oesophageal fistula can occur 3–5 days after blunt cervical trauma. Over the first few weeks there may be persistent collapse or a continuing air leak. Delayed presentation with dyspnoea and recurrent infection from obstruction is more common with more distal injuries.

The greatest danger is complete loss of the airway, so when this injury is suspected bronchoscopy and intubation are required before paralysis. With laryngo-tracheal separation it is normally possible to intubate with direct visualization, but failing this the neck is explored to intubate the distal airway. Tears involving less than a third of the circumference or sited more distal than secondary lobar bronchi settle with conservative management, but there may be late obstruction. The upper trachea is approached by a cervical incision, the lower trachea, carina, right and proximal left main bronchus through a right postero-lateral thoracotomy and the distal left main bronchi through a left thoracotomy. It is important to avoid extensive mobilization as this impairs the blood supply. On the right side, divide the azygos vein and ventilate the opposite lung by selective intubation through the wound. After debridement repair the bronchus with fine absorbable sutures, knots on the outside, and extubate as soon as possible. With major haemorrhage, oxygenate by selective intubation of the uninjured lung, control the bleeding and then repair.

Cardiac injury

Myocardial contusion occurs in 20–30% of chest injuries but is clinically significant in less than 2% (Pevec et al 1989). It is caused by compression between the sternum and vertebrae or by impaction against the sternum from deceleration. Decreased contractility occurs leading to unexpected deterioration or failure to respond to treatment, dysrhythmias or angina. ECG shows non-specific ST and T wave changes in one-third of patients with significant trauma. New Q waves and conduction defects are

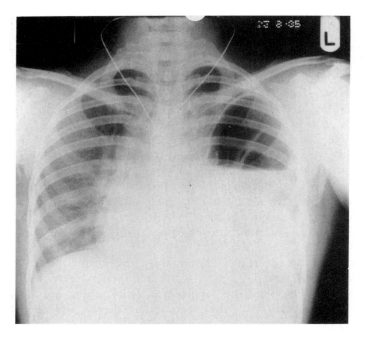

Fig. 10.5 Ruptured left hemidiaphragm. Stomach containing a fluid level within the left hemithorax, compressed lung lying above and medial to the top of the intrathoracic stomach, shift of mediastinum to the right.

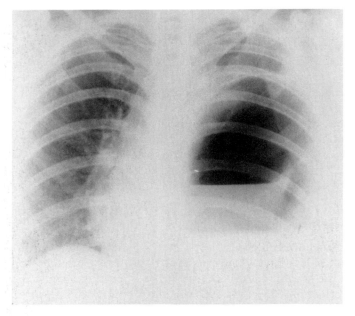

Fig. 10.6 Ruptured left hemidiaphragm. Fluid level in intrathoracic stomach not completely across the hemithorax, compressed lung above and medial to the intrathoracic stomach, with mediastinum shifted to the right.

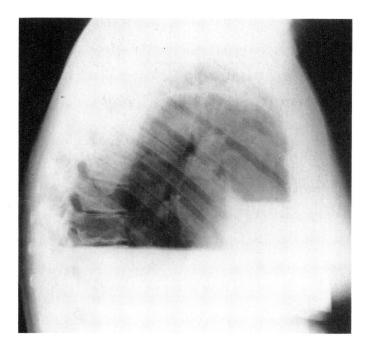

Fig. 10.7 Ruptured left hemidiaphragm. Lateral view showing double fluid level from intrathoracic gastric volvulus which distinguishes it from a haemopneumothorax.

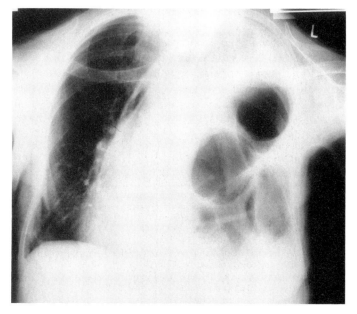

Fig. 10.8 Ruptured left hemidiaphragm. Gas shadows are from intrathoracic colon with an effusion obscuring the lung at the apex.

significant. Myocardial creatinekinase is neither specific nor sensitive in trauma: up to half of patients have raised levels but few have significant myocardial injury. Abnormal ventricular wall motion is seen in 20–30% by two-dimensional echocardiography or isotope imaging. If the ECG is normal on admission, repeat it at 24 h; if it is abnormal perform an echocardiogram and monitor for 24 h; with abnormal wall motion close observation is required for 48 h. Changes usually resolve within a few weeks. Low output and dysrhythmias are treated conventionally. All new murmurs must be fully investigated.

Other injuries such as myocardial infarction or rupture, mural thrombus formation, coronary artery damage, conducting system damage, valve injury and pericarditis are rare.

Great vessel injury

Fewer than 20% of patients with traumatic aortic ruptures (TAR) reach hospital alive. TAR are caused by severe deceleration producing shear at the junction of the mobile arch and fixed descending aorta, by impact between the ascending aorta and sternum or from hyperextension of the thoracic spine injuring the descending aorta. The intima and media tear. Survival depends on adventitial and pleural integrity. The commonest site for TAR is just distal to the left subclavian artery: 60% occur here but they account for 90% in surgical series (Bryan & Angelini 1989). Other sites are the ascending (15%) or distal descending (15%) aorta or multiple sites (10%).

When TAR is suspected, systolic pressure is kept below 100 mmHg by vasodilators and beta-blockade until surgical repair. Clinial signs include unexplained hypotension, upper body hypertension, variation of major pulses, arm/leg pressure discrepancy, chest pain, external chest injury, haemothorax, systolic murmur, dyspnoea, anuria, paraplegia and coma. About 60% of patients with TAR have pulmonary contusions and may develop ARDS. Radiological signs are shown in Table 10.4 and Figure

Table 10.4   Possible radiological features of traumatic aortic rupture

Mediastinal widening from peri-aortic haematoma
Mediastinum at the aortic knuckle above 10 cm (normal below 8 cm)
Mediastinal thoracic width ratio above 0.30 (normal below 0.27)
Right paratracheal stripe width above 1 cm
Loss of contour of the aortic knuckle
Separation of intimal calcification from adventitia at aortic knuckle
Obliteration of the aortopulmonary window
Oesophageal, tracheal or CVP line deviation to the right at T4
Apical pleural cap, usually on the left
Depression of the left main bronchus more than 40° from the horizontal
Fractured first and second rib particularly with sternal fracture
Multiple upper rib fractures

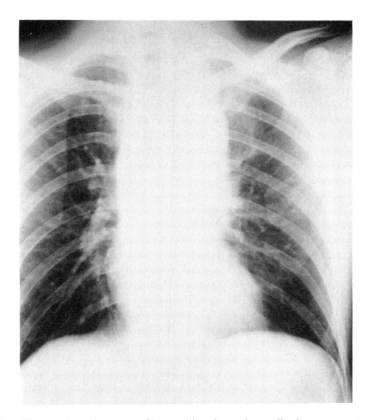

Fig. 10.9 Traumatic aortic rupture. Shows widened superior mediastinum.

10.9. The likelihood of TAR increases with the number of signs present. Spinal fractures are present in 10% (Woodring et al 1988). CT will confirm a mediastinal haematoma which is an absolute indication for angiography to localize the site. Contrast enhanced CT, digital subtraction angiography and two-dimensional echo are not reliable.

Without intervention mortality is 70% by two days and 90% by seven days. Immediate repair is required except in the presence of injuries likely to significantly worsen prognosis (severe head injury, sepsis, severe respiratory insufficiency, paraplegia) when controlled hypotension can be maintained, with surgery delayed until the patient's condition improves. The ascending aorta is repaired via a median sternotomy on cardiopulmonary bypass and all other TAR's through a left postero-lateral thoracotomy. It is necessary to clamp distal to the left carotid artery and below the rupture with pharmacological control of proximal hypertension. A heparin-bonded shunt from the left ventricle or ascending aorta to the femoral artery can be used. Pumped extracorporeal circuits require heparinization with risk of intracranial bleeding. Repair is by direct suture or interposition graft if mobilization will damage intercostal vessels. Operative survival is 70–90%. Post-operative paraplegia (5–7%) and renal failure (about 25%) occur irrespective of the method used. Unoperated survivors form saccular aneurysms which may cause compression resulting in dysphagia, dyspnoea, stridor, cough and back pain.

The innominate artery may be avulsed at its origin producing a widened upper mediastinum on chest X-ray. Bypass graft via a median sternotomy extended into the neck, separated from oesophageal or tracheal repair by muscle graft results in 90% survival.

Oesophageal injury

The oesophagus is injured in 0.01% cases of blunt trauma with 80% of these involving the upper two-thirds (Beal et al 1988). Causes include direct compression of the upper oesophagus from posterior sternal displacement, increased intraluminal pressure or damage to the blood supply by deceleration, which causes distraction of the aorta from the oesophagus and leads to delayed perforation up to five days later. Half of the patients with blunt injuries to the cervical oesophagus have laryngo-tracheal trauma. Oesophageal rupture results in dysphagia, odynophagia, mediastinal or cervical emphysema, neck or chest pain, hydropneumo-thorax, fever, severe systemic toxicity or an acute abdomen.

When oesophageal rupture is suspected the patient should have nil orally and antibiotics should be given. A water soluble contrast study is performed, followed, if negative, by a barium study as thin contrast will miss 25% of ruptures (Carrero & Wayne 1989). Endoscopy shows a haematoma rather than the perforation. Management depends on the time since rupture and the general condition of the patient. Repair should occur within 18 h of rupture. The cervical oesophagus is exposed by an incision along the anterior border of the left sternomastoid with division of the inferior belly of omohyoid, retraction of the thyroid medially and carotid sheath laterally to expose the oesophagus behind the trachea. The upper two-thirds of the intrathoracic oesophagus is explored via a right thoracotomy and the lower third from the left. In order to preserve the blood supply, mobilization is restricted to the ipsilateral and posterior aspect in the neck or the ipsilateral and anterior aspect in the chest. If the rupture is difficult to locate the oesophagus is insufflated with CO_2 through a nasogastric tube. Debride the rupture and repair it with single full thickness interrupted fine absorbable sutures with the knots outside. The repair is separated from any tracheal or vascular repair by pleural or muscle flaps. The mediastinum is drained and the patient is given nil orally for five days until a contrast study confirms healing. With extensive damage or delayed operation the oesophagus should be resected and the stomach advanced to the neck. When the patient is unfit for resection it is wise to defunction the oesophagus and plan a later replacement or to drain via a limited thoracotomy and irrigate with antibiotic solution via the nasogastric tube. Mortality is up to 80% because of delay in treatment.

PENETRATING INJURIES

Approximately 10% of penetrating chest injuries require thoracotomy (Carrero & Wayne 1989). It is important not to probe the wound or fill it with contrast since this is misleading and invites infection. The entry and exit wounds should be marked before a chest X-ray to assess the track. The penetrating object should not be removed until operation unless the surgeon is in a position to perform an immediate thoracotomy if severe haemorrhage occurs.

Pulmonary injury

The initial management of a penetrating pulmonary injury is tube drainage, as 90% of stab wounds (Mandal & Oparah 1989) and 70% of low velocity missile injuries (Robison et al 1988) settle with this alone. High velocity wounds (above $500\,\mathrm{ms}^{-1}$) cause extensive tissue damage and all require exploration (Robison et al 1988). Anterior thoracotomy is required for patients in an unstable condition as passage of a double lumen tube takes time and the lateral position worsens the haemodynamic state. Other patients require a postero-lateral thoracotomy. When possible, undertake vascular repair rather than pulmonary resection which is only required with complete maceration. A total of 2% of stab wounds involve the hilum and immediate vascular control is required by application of a Satinsky clamp across the hilum. If the site of injury is close to the clamp the vessels are controlled intrapericardially and then repaired.

Air embolism is rare but occurs with injury producing tracheo-bronchial-pulmonary vein communication. This causes focal neurological signs without head injury or cardiovascular collapse, especially with mechanical ventilation. The patient is tipped head down and an immediate anterior thoracotomy performed for hilar control.

Diaphragmatic injury

Ten percent of diaphragmatic injuries in the UK are penetrating (Johnson 1988). The diaphragm is injured in 15–25% of wounds below the fourth interspace anteriorly, sixth space laterally and eighth space posteriorly. A total of 75–95% of these require laparotomy. The chest X-ray may be normal or may show a haemo- or pneumothorax, or an obscured or elevated hemidiaphragm. Peritoneal lavage is negative in 10–40% of cases unless there is obvious abdominal injury. Defects are unlikely to heal but may seal with omentum. There is a risk of late herniation but surgical exploration is not justified in the presence of a normal chest X-ray and in the absence of abdominal signs.

Laryngeal and tracheo-bronchial injury

In this type of injury, 75% involve the cervical trachea (Pate 1989). They present the same clinical features as blunt injury and also frothy bleeding from the wound. Conventional intubation (not through the wound) and exploration are required. Small anterior defects are sutured, large anterior and all posterior defects must be debrided and repaired. Intrathoracic tracheal injury is usually discovered during thoracotomy for other injuries and is treated by debridement and repair.

Cardiac injury

Immediate mortality is 20% with stabbings and 60–80% with low velocity missiles. Survival depends on tamponade as free bleeding causes exsanguination. There is a 60% risk of cardiac injury if the wound overlies the cardiac silhouette on chest X-ray (Siemens et al 1977). Myocardial stab wounds may seal temporarily with tamponade and as little as 100 ml of blood can cause tamponade. Beck's triad of elevated JVP (which may be masked by hypovolaemia or caused by tension pneumothorax), diminished heart sounds and pulse paradox (15 mmHg fall on inspiration) is only present in 40%. Seventy per cent of patients will be hypotensive. Absence of fluid on echocardiogram does not exclude tamponade. Systemic blood pressure may improve transiently after an increase in the CVP. Pericardiocentesis gives a 30% error rate and should be avoided except in experienced hands. When tamponade is present, drape the operative field before induction of general anaesthetic as this may cause severe hypotension secondary to vasodilatation. Tamponade is relieved through a left anterior fifth interspace thoracotomy without lung isolation (right thoracotomy with right-sided wounds). The incision extends from the sternal edge to the axilla. A rib retractor is inserted and the pericardium is opened longitudinally anterior to the phrenic nerve. Bleeding is controlled by digital pressure whilst the laceration is repaired with interrupted horizontal mattress buttressed 2/0 Prolene sutures, tied to just appose the edges, as myocardium is friable. With a laceration near a coronary vessel the sutures are passed deep to the vessel. Divided coronary vessels are controlled by passing a suture under them and snugging this whilst obtaining specialized advice.

Retained intracardiac foreign bodies are rare. Those in the left heart or systemic arteries must be removed immediately whereas those in the right heart or systemic veins are removed electively (Van Way 1989).

Careful follow up is mandatory as 5–30% of survivors will have an intrapericardial defect (septal defect, intracardiac fistula, valve injury) which may require elective repair.

Great vessel injury

Extrapericardial penetrating injuries of the aorta usually exsanguinate. Penetrating injury to the innominate artery usually occurs near its bifurcation and this is repaired via a median sternotomy. Venous injuries are repaired when possible, otherwise they are ligated, except below the level of the azygos vein when the SVC must be repaired. This requires an intracaval shunt.

Oesophageal injury

Five percent of penetrating neck wounds injure the oesophagus and most have associated vascular or laryngo-tracheal injury. Thoracic oesophageal injuries are rare and usually present because of the associated aortic injury. The presentation is as for blunt injury. The mortality depends on associated injuries and on any delay in treatment.

THORACOTOMY FOR THORACIC TRAUMA

Thoracotomy is required in 10% of major injuries. Indications are listed in Table 10.5. When vital signs have been absent for more than five minutes there will be no survivors but if absent less than five minutes, 30% of stab wounds but no blunt injuries survive.

Table 10.5   Indications for thoracotomy following thoracic trauma

Absent vital signs
Agonal
Great vessel injury
Persistent bleeding
Haemothorax—massive, recurrent or undrained
Tracheo-bronchial rupture
Persistent air leak or recurrent pneumothorax
Cardiac injury—significant likelihood, tamponade, intracardiac damage
High velocity missile injuries
Injuries traversing the mediastinum
Some diaphragmatic ruptures
Air embolism
Oesophageal injury
Major loss of chest wall
Removal of some foreign bodies
Some thoracic duct injury
Non-resolving intrapulmonary pseudocysts and haematomas

Thoracotomy with actual or incipient circulatory arrest should be performed via a left anterior approach. Coronary and cerebral perfusion is improved during internal massage by occlusion of the descending aorta which also limits intra-abdominal bleeding. It is safest to compress the aorta against the vertebrae near the diaphragm as cross-clamping runs the risk of tearing intercostal vessels. To find the aorta sweep the hand across the diaphragm postero-medially to reach the vertebral bodies then the aorta is the first structure anteriorly. Immediate venous access can be achieved by cannulation of the atrium or pulmonary artery. Ensure that air does not enter the circulation. Internal defibrillation (10–30 J) will fail if the heart is empty and acidotic. Abandon resuscitation with irreparable cardiac injury, when there is no sign of cardiac activity after 15 min or the systolic pressure remains below 60 mmHg on maximal support after 30 min. Possible cerebral damage is never an indication to discontinue resuscitation. Complications of immediate thoracotomy include pulmonary or pericardial infection, re-exploration for bleeding, injury to breast, lung or heart during incision and anoxic damage.

Chronic complications

Chronic complications of chest trauma are listed in Table 10.6.

Table 10.6   Chronic complications of chest trauma

Pleural space	Empyema, residual haemothorax, chylothorax, fibrothorax
Chest wall	Chronic pain, non-union of fractures, infection, discharging sinus, AV fistula
Lung	Impaired respiratory function, traumatic pseudocysts, retained foreign bodies, AV fistula, pulmonary artery aneurysm
Oesophagus	Stricture, fistula
Diaphragm	Delayed effects of missed rupture
Heart	Pericarditis (traumatic, suppurative, constrictive), coronary damage, valve damage, intrapericardial fistula, intracardiac shunts (septal defects, fistula), retained intracardiac foreign body, myocardial damage
Great vessels	Aneurysm and fistula formation

KEY POINTS FOR CLINICAL PRACTICE

The major immediate aims of treatment are the control of hypoxia and haemorrhage. The greater the impact/deceleration force the higher the risk of significant injury. A high degree of suspicion is necessary to avoid missing significant injuries. When in doubt seek expert advice or transfer the patient to a specialist centre.

REFERENCES

Anderson I D, Woodford M, de Dombal F T, Irving M 1988 Retrospective study of 1000 deaths from injury in England and Wales. Br Med J 296: 1305–1308

Beal S L, Pottmeyer E W, Spisso J M 1988 Oesophageal perforation following external blunt trauma. J Trauma 28: 1425–1432

Bryan A J, Angelini G D 1989 Traumatic rupture of the thoracic aorta. Br J Hosp Med 41: 320–326

Carrero R C, Wayne M 1989 Chest trauma. Emerg Med Clin North Am 7: 389–418

Dhasmana J P 1989 Management of severe chest injuries. Br J Hosp Med 41: 554–562

Gussack G S, Jurkovich G J 1988 Treatment dilemmas in laryngotracheal trauma. J Trauma 28: 1439–1444

Harris R D, Harris J H 1988 The prevalence and significance of missed scapular fractures in blunt chest trauma. AJR 151: 747–750

Johnson C D 1988 Blunt injuries to the diaphragm. Br J Surg 75: 226–230

Jones K W 1980 Thoracic trauma. Surg Clin North Am 60: 957–981

Mandal A K, Oparah S S 1989 Unusually low mortality of penetrating wounds of the chest. Twelve year's experience. J Thorac Cardiovasc Surg 97: 119–125

Mattox K L 1989 Prehospital care of the patient with an injured chest. Surg Clin North Am 69: 21–30

Norwood S H, Civetta J M 1985 Ventilatory support in patients with ARDS. Surg Clin North Am 65: 895–916

Pate J W 1989 Tracheobronchial and oesophageal injuries. Surg Clin North Am 69: 111–124

Pepe P E 1989 Acute post-traumatic respiratory physiology and insufficiency. Surg Clin North Am 69: 157–174

Pesenti A, Kolobow T, Gaitinoni L 1988 Extracorporeal respiratory support in the adult. Trans Am Soc Artif Intern Organs 34: 1006–1008

Pevec W C, Udekwu A O, Peitzman A B 1989 Blunt rupture of the myocardium. Ann Thorac Surg 48: 139–142

Robison P D, Harman P K, Trinkle J K, Grover F L 1988 Management of penetrating lung injuries in civilian practice. J Thorac Cardiovasc Surg 95: 184–190

Siemens R, Polk H C, Gray L A, Folton R L 1977 Indications for thoracotomy following penetrating thoracic injury. J Trauma 17: 493–500

Trinca G W, Dooley B J 1975 The effects of mandatory seat belt wearing on the mortality and pattern of injury of car occupants involved in motor vehicle crashes in Victoria. Med J Aust 1: 675–678

Trinkle J K, Richardson J D, Franz J L 1975 Management of flail chest without mechanical ventilation. Ann Thorac Surg 19: 355–363

Van Way C W 1989 Intrathoracic and intravascular migratory foreign bodies. Surg Clin North Am 69: 125–134

Wagner R B 1989 Pulmonary contusions: evaluation and classification by computed tomography. Surg Clin North Am 69: 31–40

Weigelt J A 1981 Early identification of patients prone to develop adult respiratory distress syndrome. Am J Surg 142: 687–691

Woodring J H, Lee C, Jenkins K 1988 Spinal fractures in blunt chest trauma. J Trauma 28: 789–793

Zapol W M, Snider M T, Hill J D et al 1979 Extracorporeal membrane oxygenation in severe acute respiratory failure: a randomised prospective study. JAMA 242: 2193–2196

11

Pathophysiology and management of rectal prolapse

G. S. Duthie   D. C. C. Bartolo

Full thickness rectal prolapse is an uncommon condition and the clinical features make the diagnosis relatively easy to make. The fact that there are a large variety of operative treatment options suggests that many of the questions of both pathophysiology and management of this condition are unanswered.

AETIOLOGY AND PATHOPHYSIOLOGY

Despite intense investigation over many years our understanding of the pathophysiology of complete rectal prolapse remains incomplete.

Moschcowitz (1912) suggested that rectal prolapse represented a sliding type of hernia. Indeed most patients have deep rectovesical or rectovaginal extensions of the pouch of Douglas and it is accepted that with continued progression the rectum herniates through the pelvic floor. It is also recognized that the mobility of the mesorectum is an important aetiological factor which allows the rectum to straighten with loss of the normal rectal curvature (Ripstein & Lanter 1963).

An elegant study on the pathogenesis of prolapse using radio-opaque markers confirmed the theory that rectal prolapse represents a rectal intussusception (Theuerkauf et al 1970). It seems likely that prolapse is a progressive condition through stages of mucosal prolapse and perhaps the Solitary Rectal Ulcer Syndrome, to rectorectal and rectoanal intussusception and thence to full thickness rectal prolapse, and moreover, that these three conditions share a common pathogenesis (Sun et al 1989).

There is however little understanding of the underlying patho-physiological events although it has been shown that prolapse is associated with pelvic floor denervation (Parks et al 1977, Neill et al 1981). Since many patients are female some of this deterioration may be attributable to childbirth, but a significant minority of patients are nulliparous. Chronic neurophysiological damage may also result from chronic straining at defaecation (Bartolo et al 1983) and this may explain many of the remaining cases. Another factor in the pathogenesis of prolapse may be failure of rectal support by the levators and pelvic fascia due to defective collagen maturation in the pelvic floor. Extensive stretching of these supporting structures and partial pelvic floor denervation during parturition would explain the association of prolapse with childbirth.

Porter (1962) reported the physiological findings in this condition. He found that the sphincters were lax and contracted poorly in reflex response to raised intra-abdominal pressure. A significant association was seen between rectal prolapse and spinal cord injury (Porter 1962), but Fry et al (1966) considered the majority had no underlying neurological disorder. The prolapse almost certainly initiates a persistent recto-anal inhibitory reflex which means that the internal anal sphincter remains chronicly relaxed. Indeed following repair pressures improve (see below). The intus-susception theory is now widely accepted and since this usually progresses from above the pelvic floor it seems full thickness rectal prolapse is due to a combination of rectal and pelvic floor abnormalities.

PHYSIOLOGICAL INVESTIGATION

Routine anorectal assessment of rectal prolapse involves anal canal and rectal manometric studies together with measurement of anal and rectal sensibility and proctography. We believe that all patients should undergo pre-operative colonic transit studies since constipation is a common association and may contribute to post-operative recurrence (Boulos et al 1984).

Patients with rectal prolapse can usefully be divided into two groups: those with prolapse, and those with prolapse and faecal incontinence. In our unit 73 patients have been physiologically assessed, and 65 have undergone postoperative followup studies. Table 11.1 shows details for 73 patients with prolapse compared with a control group of 30 patients with no anorectal complaints.

Table 11.1 Anorectal physiology in prolapse [median (range)]

	Controls	Prolapse continent	Prolapse incontinent
Numbers	30	22	51
Manometry			
Sphincter length (cm)	3 (2–4)	2 (0–3)*	1 (0–3)*
MRP (cmH$_2$O)	90 (55–180)	60 (20–160)*	35 (10–85)*†
MVC (cmH$_2$O)	225 (140–465)	120 (30–265)*	90 (15–135)*
Anal sensation			
Lower (mA)	4.5 (2–9)	8.5 (3–21)*	10 (3–26)*
Middle (mA)	5 (2–10)	12 (5–24)*	15 (3–26)*†
Upper (mA)	5 (2–11)	18 (3–22)*	23 (3–26)*†

MRP = maximum resting pressure; MVC = maximum voluntary contraction; mA = milliamps.
*$P < 0.05$ compared with controls; †$P < 0.05$ compared with prolapse continent.

Sphincter function

Both continent and incontinent patients with prolapse have significantly shorter sphincters compared with normal subjects and in addition have very poor resting anal canal pressures. Incontinent patients are significantly worse than continent patients in this respect. It seems likely that this is due to internal anal sphincter inhibition induced by the advancing prolapse, which acts like a faecal bolus to activate the rectoanal inhibitory reflex. This was supported by the fact that sphincter inhibition in incontinent patients was induced by smaller volumes of rectal distension than in normal controls. They did, however, require much larger volumes to produce prolonged inhibition but this most probably reflects the fact that they already have near maximal inhibition. It would seem that since incontinent patients have the worst sphincter function overall, there is indeed progression of anal sphincter dysfunction from normals through patients with intussusception without overt prolapse to patients with prolapse and incontinence.

Voluntary sphincter function is also significantly impaired compared with controls and shows the same trend towards progressive failure seen in the internal sphincter, when one considers the patients with intussusception. This may reflect pelvic floor trauma in the post-partum females, and in males and nulliparous females may be the result of neuropathy associated with excessive defecatory straining.

Anal and rectal sensation

Anal sensation

Continence and normal defecation depend on both motor and sensory components. A perceived threat to continence will normally elicit either a voluntary or involuntary reflex response from the anal sphincters. However, if sensation is defective then threats to continence will not be appreciated and leakage will involuntarily ensue. The rectoanal inhibitory reflex allows contact between rectal contents and the sensitive anal canal epithelium. This is an unconscious event in response to rectal filling. Any threat to continence should normally be coped with by reflex somatic muscle recruitment which maintains pressure in the distal anal canal. All this depends on the ability of the sphincters to sense the threat and respond appropriately. We see from the results of electrosensitivity testing that anal canal sensation is impaired in the upper, mid, and lower anal canal in rectal prolapse. The incontinent patients had significantly higher thresholds (greater impairment) than the continent patients. We believe that this sensory defect is an important component of the pathogenesis of incontinence and prolapse.

Rectal sensation

The volume of first rectal sensation was lower in rectal prolapse compared with normal subjects. We found that patients with incontinence and prolapse appreciated lower volumes than continent patients or controls. The same pattern was seen in intussusception where the continent patients appeared less sensitive to rectal filling. This was somewhat surprising since biofeedback training for incontinence aims to teach the patients with incontinence to sense smaller volumes within the rectum. Rectal sensation is considered to depend on the muscle spindles of the pelvic floor and is almost certainly modified by rectal autonomic afferents (Oresland et al 1990).

Proctography

In our hands proctographic assessment of rectal prolapse has been generally unhelpful. Evacuation studies confirmed the full thickness rectal prolapse in all cases. The main usefulness of proctography is to confirm the presence of intussusception in incontinent patients without overt prolapse.

Parks' flap valve theory of continence has not been supported by recent studies (Bartolo et al 1986). We believe that continence depends mainly on the ability of the sphincters to respond to raised intra-abdominal or rectal pressures. It is therefore not surprising that there is no correlation between obliquity of the anorectal angle and continence. There was however a trend to increased perineal descent at rest in the prolapse patients and during straining there was significantly more descent seen in patients compared with controls.

Overall there seems good evidence for sensory and motor pelvic floor dysfunction. The poor anal resting pressures are the result of rectoanal inhibition induced by the rectal intussusception. Pelvic floor nerve damage is responsible for the somatic weakness of the external anal sphincters. The underlying pathophysiology that allows the initiation of the prolapse still remains unclear but there is good evidence that this is a progressive phenomenon. Certainly, internal rectal prolapse appears to show the early physiological changes that are found to a greater extent in full thickness rectal prolapse. There is good corroboration from other investigators that mucosal prolapse and solitary rectal ulcer syndrome should also be included in this group of diseases (Sun et al 1989).

MANAGEMENT

Non-operative

Conservative management has nothing to offer the adult with full thickness rectal prolapse. Correction of associated constipation is very important as a number of these constipated patients will actually have impaired colonic transit. The operative strategy can then be planned appropriately and modified to deal with the constipation and prolapse.

Only in the poorest risk patients can conservative management be justified and even then local perineal procedures under regional anaesthesia should be possible. Injection of sclerosant is only useful in an attempt to fix the mucosa to the underlying rectal musculature in mucosal prolapse. Whenever possible we advocate an abdominal approach for full thickness rectal prolapse because the results of this approach are superior to other techniques.

Local operative procedures

Thiersch first described anal encirclage using silver wire in 1912 and since then many modifications using nylon, silastic and other materials have been reported. These procedures are designed simply to increase anal basal pressure by a local effect and thus retain the prolapse. They have no effect on the underlying pathophysiology. In addition, the encircling material restricts anal relaxation during defecation and so constipation and faecal impaction are common complications.

The Delorme procedure (Christiansen & Kirkegaard 1981) is a relatively non-invasive operation in which the prolapse is everted to its fullest extent following which the rectum is denuded of its mucosa for the length of the prolapse. The underlying rectal musculature is then plicated. The mucosal defect is subsequently repaired by suturing the proximal and distal resection margins over the plicated rectal wall. The results of this procedure are reasonably good but inferior to abdominal procedures. It does not attempt to repair the main anatomical or physiological defects. Moreover, there is a significant long term relapse rate (Aminev & Malyshev 1964). This procedure should be held in reserve for very old or infirm patients.

A more logical perineal approach is that popularized by Altmeir et al (1971) although this procedure remains more common in the USA than in the UK. Instead of a mucosal excision, the full thickness of the rectum is resected starting at the upper end of the anal canal. This allows the prolapsing rectum and sigmoid colon to be dissected in stages through the anal orifice. After the redundant bowel has been resected the colon is anastomosed to the top of the anal canal. In addition, the levator ani and puborectalis muscles can be plicated to improve continence. While this approach has the advantage of allowing surplus bowel to be resected the resultant anatomy is abnormal in that the compliant rectum is removed and replaced by sigmoid colon which is often diverticular and relatively non-distensible. Thus the patient will experience urgency and in the presence of sphincter weakness will be unable to defer defecation. This may exacerbate the patient's incontinence. Altmeir et al (1971) reported very good results although his experience involved a considerable number of patients with either a psychiatric or a neurological history. He does however claim that there is a good recovery of external sphincter function in patients without neuropathy but the mechanism for this is unclear. Watts et al (1985) offered this operation only to the elderly and infirm because of their anxiety about recurrence. In fact there were no recurrences in their series of 33 patients. Unfortunately only 6% (2 patients) considered their continence was improved and 22% were worse. Certainly resting pressures might be expected to recover with removal of the prolapse although resection and anastomosis close to the dentate line may damage the rectoanal inhibitory reflex. Despite some reports of excellent results there are some series (Hughes 1949) where there has been a high failure rate and overall it is probably superior to the Delorme procedure but inferior to abdominal procedures.

Abdominal operative procedures

Many different abdominal procedures have been reported over the years. Various sling operations, colpopexy, colonic plication, and reversed intus-susception procedures have been described, but the current modern management in most centres is an abdominal rectopexy, with or without resection of the redundant bowel.

One of the most popular procedures in North America is the Ripstein operation (Ripstein 1972). After full mobilization, the rectum is fixed to the sacral promontory with an encircling sling of teflon mesh. Ripstein's own series reports only 1.5% recurrence but there are a significant number of complications, most notably constipation which is probably due to a combination of the sling and the redundant sigmoid colon (Jurgeleit et al 1975). If the sling is too tight it obstructs the proximal bowel, while the sigmoid is commonly partially obstructed where it is angulated at the point of attachment to the mesh. The bowel above this prolapses down into the pouch of Douglas.

There are four rectopexy procedures used in the UK today: simple suture rectopexy, posterior Ivalon sponge rectopexy, anterior and posterior Marlex rectopexy, and resection and rectopexy. We have experience of all.

Mobilization of the bowel for rectopexy

Figure 11.1a depicts the mobilization of the rectum and distal sigmoid colon for all but the resection and rectopexy. We now routinely approach these operations using a transverse lower abdominal muscle cutting incision.

After mobilization of the distal sigmoid and upper rectum the peritoneal reflection is incised and the dissection carried distally to the level of the levators. Care is taken to avoid damaging the autonomic nerves in this region since sacrifice of these can cause considerable urinary, faecal and

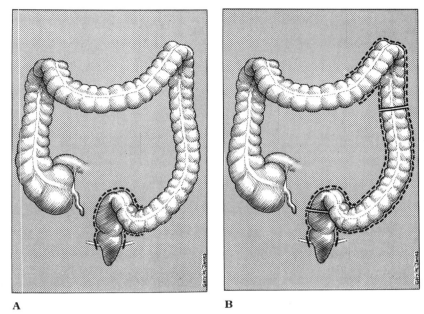

A   **B**

Fig. 11.1   Colorectal mobilization for rectopexy. **A** For non-resectional procedures. Lateral ligaments divided; **B** for resection and rectopexy. Lateral ligaments divided.

sexual morbidity which is unacceptable during operations for benign disease. The lateral ligaments of the rectum are usually divided to obtain maximal mobilization.

The distal dissection for resection and rectopexy is similar to that described by Frykman & Goldberg (Watts et al 1985) but we always mobilize the splenic flexure because we consider this provides a healthy descending colon for anastomosis without tension (Fig. 11.1b). We do not believe that low anterior resection is justified since this removes most of the important rectal reservoir and, furthermore, low anastomoses are more liable to leak.

Simple suture rectopexy

This is the easiest of the abdominal procedures and we have tended to reserve it for elderly patients because of its relative simplicity. After mobilization the lower rectum is fixed to the pelvic floor and presacral fascia by four prolene sutures (Fig. 11.2a), two of which are placed distally and two more proximally. It is important that the proximal fixation is high enough onto the presacral fascia to prevent rectal intussusception which will lead to incontinence and recurrence, but not so high as to cause the angulation of the rectosigmoid seen following the Ripstein operation. We

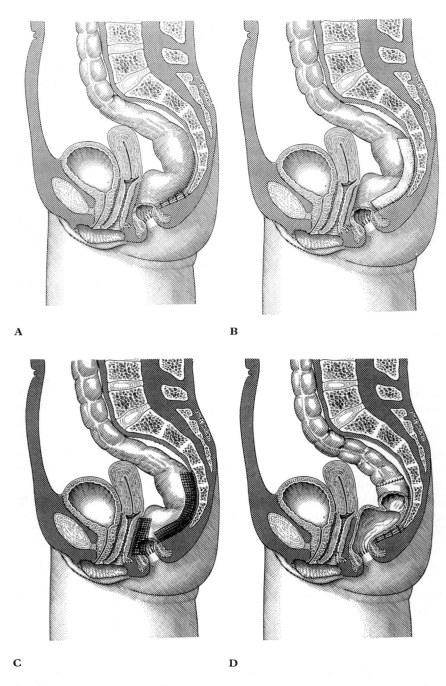

A   B

C   D

Fig. 11.2 **A** Simple suture rectopexy; **B** posterior Ivalon sponge rectopexy; **C** anterior and posterior Marlex rectopexy; **D** resection and rectopexy.

have had one recurrence in an elderly patient, who declined pre-operative physiological assessment, in whom we have no manometric data, and she could not therefore be included in the subsequent physiological analysis. We believe the fixation sutures were placed too low and consequently the rectum was still able to intussuscept and therefore partially prolapse above the point of fixation.

Posterior Ivalon sponge rectopexy

We have followed the procedure described by Wells in 1959. Polyvinyl alcohol sponge (Ivalon) is secured by non-absorbable sutures to the presacral fascia posteriorly and to the back of the rectum (Fig. 11.2b). The rationale for the use of prosthetic material is the dense fibrous reaction that it produces which fixes the rectum into the sacral curvature thereby preventing recurrence. Unlike other materials, Ivalon is thought to be absorbed over a number of years so for this reason and to avoid the recognized septic complications seen with non-absorbable material, some authors have advocated the use of absorbable prosthetic material (Arndt & Pircher 1988).

Anterior and posterior Marlex rectopexy

The rationale for this approach is that in addition to the mobility of the posterior rectum the anterior rectum, particularly in women, is poorly supported. Furthermore, prolapse may be initiated by anterior rectal wall descent. The deep pouch of Douglas and the rectovesical pouch in males is considered to be an important component of prolapse, and it seems logical to add support in this area as well. In addition, many elderly female patients have rectoceles which are the end result of pelvic floor weakness and obstetric trauma. We have used a procedure similar to that described by Nicholls & Simson (1986) in a number of the patients in this series.

A sheet of Marlex was sutured posteriorly as in the Ivalon sponge procedure, but in addition the anterior rectal wall was separated from the vagina in females. In male patients, to avoid injury to the nervae errigentes, Denonvillier's fascia was incised above the seminal vesicles and the dis- section was continued distally on the rectal muscle tube. Following this mobilization, a strip of Marlex was fixed in place on the distal anterior wall of the rectum in the rectovaginal septum to give additional anterior support (Fig. 11.2c).

Resection rectopexy

Our technique has been modified from that described by Frykman & Goldberg (1969). The mobilization has been described above. We aim to construct an anastomosis without tension 12 cm from the anal verge. This

Table 11.2 Functional outcome

	Number of patients	Continence to solid and liquids Number of patients (%)		Bowel frequency (per day)		Straining at stool Number of patients (%)		Incomplete emptying Number of patients (%)	
		Pre-op	Post-op	Pre-op	Post-op	Pre-op	Post-op	Pre-op	Post-op
Suture rectopexy	10	2 (20)	9 (90)*	2.5 (0.5–5)	1.5 (1–3)	5 (50)	4 (40)	5 (50)	2 (20)
Ivalon rectopexy	9	4 (44)	6 (66)*	1 (0.5–3)	1.7 (1–5)	7 (77)	4 (44)	6 (66)	5 (55)
Marlex rectopexy	20	5 (25)	15 (75)*	3 (0.2–5)	2.3 (1–5)	13 (65)	11 (55)	13 (65)	7 (35)
Resection rectopexy	26	6 (23)	23 (88)*	1.5 (0.1–5)	1 (0.5–5)	23 (88)	17 (65)	16 (61)	9 (26)

Bowel frequencies are medians (range).
*$0.01 < P < 0.05$.

procedure provides the opportunity to resect the redundant sigmoid and distal descending colon. We believe splenic flexure mobilization allows healthy well vascularized descending colon to be used for the anastomosis rather than the sigmoid which may have a compromised blood supply especially in the elderly. In addition to the resection the distal rectal remnant is fixed to the pelvic floor and presacral fascia in a similar manner to that described for simple suture rectopexy (Fig. 11.2d).

Results of abdominal rectopexy

We have assessed our results for these four types of abdominal rectopexy. There are no significant differences in the ages of the patient groups although there is a trend to perform simple suture rectopexy on older patients. We offer a non-resectional procedure to patients with intestinal hurry and diarrhoea. Apart from the previously mentioned failure of one suture rectopexy there have been no recurrences. There has been no operative mortality and no serious morbidity. We believe that the extensive dissection in the resection cases has proved worthwhile in that there has been no anastomotic complication. Furthermore, contrary to our initial anxieties about resection in patients with incontinence, diarrhoea has not proved to be a consequence. We have not seen to date any infective complications following the insertion of prosthetic material.

Table 11.2 shows the paired pre- and post-operative data relating to bowel function. Post-operatively there was no significant alteration in bowel function nor in the presence of a normal call to stool. This is especially rewarding since operations involving an implant are frequently complicated by post-operative constipation. Overall neither constipation nor diarrhoea proved to be significant problems. Furthermore, straining at stool and a feeling of incomplete emptying after defecation did not increase after rectopexy. In fact there has been a tendency to reduced constipation after surgery.

Simple suture and resection rectopexy were the most successful at restoring continence in incontinent patients (Fig. 11.3). While there was still a significant improvement in the implant groups it was less marked and we wonder whether the presence of prosthetic material may interfere with sphincter recovery due to the inflammatory response that ensues. We believe the implant makes the rectum less compliant and this may contribute towards the lack of improvement in sphincter function in these patients. We have no experience of the use of absorbable implants such as Dexon or Vicryl mesh. It is possible that the inflammatory response and the risks of sepsis due to the prosthetic material could be reduced by using these absorbable materials. In our opinion, their use runs counter to the rationale for the use of an implant whose purpose is to provide prolonged support to prevent the well-known problem of late recurrence.

The argument for the use of synthetic implants to fix the rectum has been

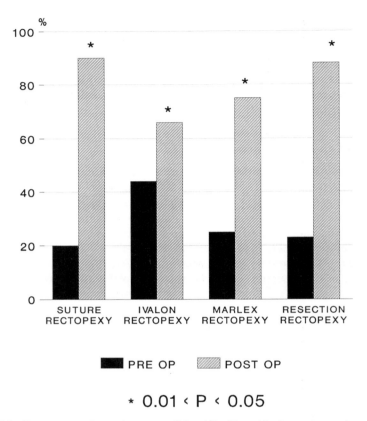

* 0.01 < P < 0.05

Fig. 11.3   Improvement in continence to solid and liquid stool in the post-operative period.

their low recurrence rates, but many series using simple suture fixation or resection and rectopexy have shown similar results (Watts et al 1985). Most of the available options achieve their primary objective, namely, to control the rectal prolapse. It is perhaps in the secondary objective, restoration of continence, that comparison between the functional results is important. On the basis of our own functional results we question whether insertion of prosthetic material, with its inherent risk of infective complications, is justified. The objective physiological measurements post-operatively in these patients were inferior to those in whom no implant was employed, and brings into question the mechanism of restoration of continence following Marlex and Ivalon rectopexy.

It can be argued that resection carries an unacceptable risk of anastomotic dehiscence. We consider that this risk should be low with careful attention to detail. Resection deals with the presence of redundant loops of sigmoid, and in theory should reduce any tendency to constipation. We assiduously avoid low anastomoses with their higher risk of complications, and because

Table 11.3 Pre- and post-operative physiology [median (range)]

	Suture rectopexy		Ivalon rectopexy		Marlex rectopexy		Resection rectopexy	
	Pre-op	Post-op	Pre-op	Post-op	Pre-op	Post-op	Pre-op	Post-op
Manometry								
Sphincter length (cm)	3 (1–4)	3 (2–3.5)	3 (2–4)	3 (2.5–4)	3 (2–4)	3 (2–4)	3 (0–4)	3 (2–4)
MRP (cmH$_2$O)	25 (10–100)	45 (20–60)	53 (35–85)	55 (30–125)	65 (20–160)	50 (20–125)	43 (12–145)	60 (25–185)*
MVC (cmH$_2$O)	90 (40–200)	70 (40–175)	175 (70–265)	135 (85–315)	170 (45–265)	190 (30–225)	120 (30–215)	130 (50–230)
1st rectal sensation (ml)	ND	ND	ND	ND	77 (30–415)	50 (25–301)	57 (20–250)	40 (15–95)
Anal sensation								
Lower (mA)	8.5 (3–26)	7.5 (3–26)	8 (3–19)	6.2 (2–10)	6.5 (3–20)	8 (1–14)	10 (4–26)	7 (4–14)
Middle (mA)	9 (6–26)	7.5 (3–15)*	9 (3–26)	6.7 (3–12)	8 (3–26)	9 (3–17)	10 (4–25)	7.5 (3–15)
Upper (mA)	23 (5–26)	12.5 (9–23)*	15 (3–26)	11 (4–23)*	18 (3–26)	13 (3–26)*	20 (5–26)	13 (1–20)†

MRP = Maximum resting pressure; MVC = Maximum voluntary contraction; ND = Not Done.
*p < 0.05, †p < 0.01, Wilcoxon signed ranked pairs test.

a low resection would remove the compliant rectal reservoir. In favouring resection and rectopexy over simple suture rectopexy we believe that dealing with the redundant colon will improve the outcome and in addition will overcome the denervation of the left colon that may result from the rectal and sigmoid dissection.

Physiological analysis

In an attempt to evaluate the physiological alterations associated with the different procedures and to determine which changes, if any, were responsible for restoration of continence we have evaluated our patients post-operatively using the same physiological parameters as in the pre-operative assessment. Table 11.3 shows the changes in pre- and post-operative physiology.

Anal manometry

None of the operative procedures significantly increased sphincter length. In the resection group we demonstrated a significant rise in resting anal canal pressure and there was a similar trend in the sutured group. The implant groups show no such sphincter recovery with a small tendency for pressures to fall. It has been suggested that recovery of internal anal sphincter function is a major factor in the restoration of continence. It seems logical to assume that this improvement is due to removal of the sphincter inhibition caused by the presence of the prolapsed rectum. This recovery has been reported by other authors (Broden et al 1988). Keighley et al (1983) on the other hand presented a series of patients treated by Marlex rectopexy following which there was no evidence of significant recovery of sphincter function. Their data is in agreement with our own findings following implant surgery. The reason for the trend towards lower post-operative resting pressures in our implant patients is unclear and warrants further study if implant procedures are to be continued. Despite this unimpressive physiological data, implant procedures do restore continence and other factors must also be important or we would have much poorer results for these groups.

As expected, there was no improvement in somatic muscle function overall following any procedure. There is good evidence of partial denervation of the external anal sphincter and puborectalis in these patients, both on electromyography (Neill et al 1981) and histology (Parks et al 1977) and clearly rectopexy could not be expected to improve this damage.

Anal and rectal sensation

The improved function of our implant group may be the result of improved sensory awareness in the post-operative patients. Spencer (1984) suggested that the presence of recto-anal inhibition and a failure to appreciate the descent of either the prolapse or bowel contents were the important aetiological factors in incontinence. Our patients certainly did not demonstrate reduced rectal awareness pre-operatively, which, as discussed above, was an unexpected finding. After surgery there was a trend towards a reduction in the volume of first rectal sensation in the post-operative period. This would allow a perceived threat to continence to be appreciated at a smaller volume of rectal distension. The importance of this finding is uncertain and would require larger numbers to resolve the issue.

The physiological reduction in anal sensation has been discussed but in the post-operative period we noted significant improvements in sensory awareness in the upper anal canal, and in some cases the mid anal canal. If we consider those patients in whom continence was restored and compare them to the failures, the same pattern emerges in that improved mid anal canal sensation was seen in those in whom continence was restored. We believe that this improved sensation comes about because of the restoration of normal upper anal canal and lower rectal anatomy. The prolapsing insensitive rectal mucosa has been lifted out of the anal canal to a more normal anatomic position.

When rectal contents come into contact with the anal lining the patient will perceive a threat to continence and can take steps to avoid leakage using remaining sphincter function. Before surgery the anal epithelium lies below the sphincter so the subject will be unaware of faecal leakage. It is reasonable to conclude from our data that recovery of sensation and internal anal sphincter function are both important in the restoration of continence. Moreover, other, as yet unexplained factors, are probably involved in a multifactorial restoration of continence.

Radiology

In contrast to the findings of Yoshioka et al (1989), we have demonstrated no significant alterations in either the anorectal angle or in the degree of perineal descent. Certainly there are no predictive values in these parameters, after rectopexy. This is perhaps not surprising, as we found no systematic disturbance of these measurements pre-operatively. The lack of correlation between operative success and radiological changes is well documented (Miller et al 1989).

CONCLUSIONS

Complete rectal prolapse can be a distressing condition for the patient. Some are elderly and infirm, others are otherwise fit and in reasonable health. There should be two primary objectives in treating these patients. The first is to carry out a procedure that safely corrects the prolapse with minimal morbidity and without mortality. The second is to cure or significantly improve the associated incontinence and the underlying defecatory disorder.

If the patient is frail and unfit for a major procedure, one of the perineal procedures should be chosen as these can be carried out under regional anaesthesia. In our experience this rarely proves to be the case and the majority, with modern safe anaesthesia can withstand an abdominal operation. The advantages of the abdominal approaches are the high probability that the patient can be rendered continent and that recurrence rates are kept to a minimum. Recurrence following surgery is a major problem and although further surgery may be successful, the probability of restoring continence following a secondary procedure is much lower. The various sphincter-tightening procedures can be tried as backup operations, but the overall success rates are relatively low (Keighley et al 1983, Miller et al 1989). As is so often the case in surgery, the first procedure provides the ideal opportunity for a successful outcome.

In our hands, resection rectopexy appears to be the procedure of choice. The continence rates are high and to date we have seen no recurrences. This is in agreement with the series reported by Watts et al (1985). Most published work concentrates on correcting the prolapse with little attention given to incontinence, yet this is a humiliating experience for both patients and their supporting relatives. Clearly every effort should be made to deal with both aspects of this condition.

Constipation is a common association. Resection theoretically helps, but the limited sigmoid exision would not be expected to cure severe slow transit constipation. Although when surgery proves necessary in slow transit constipation, we normally advocate a radical colonic resection with an ileorectal anastomosis, we do not pursue this approach in prolapse patients. In patients with weak sphincters we would expect severe incontinence to ensue if so radical a colonic resection were undertaken. The primary purpose of the resection is to reduce recurrence and prevent obstruction which may result from distortion at the rectosigmoid junction following high fixation of the rectum with redundant sigmoid colon.

The management of prolapse remains a challenging condition. There is still a great deal to learn. It is only by studying the patients we treat, and carefully auditing the results, that we will be in a position to refine decision-making and select the procedure that will correct the prolapse and associated defecatory disorders.

REFERENCES

Altmeir W A, Cuthbertson W R, Schowengerdt C, Hunt J 1971 Nineteen years experience with the one stage perineal repair of rectal prolapse. Ann Surg 173: 993–1006
Aminev A M, Malyshev J U I 1964 Rectal prolapse. Am J Proctol Gastroenterol Colon Rectal Surg 15: 355–360

Arndt M, Pircher W 1988 Absorbable mesh in the treatment of rectal prolapse. Int J Colorect Dis 3: 141–143

Bartolo D C C, Read N W, Jarret J A, Read M G, Donnely T C, Johnson A G 1983 Differences in anal sphincter function and clinical presentation in patients with pelvic floor descent. Gastroenterology 85: 68–75

Bartolo D C C, Roe A M, Locke-Edmunds J C, Virjee J, Mortensen N J Mc C 1986 Flap valve theory of anorectal continence. Br J Surg 73: 1012–1014

Boulos P B, Stryker S J, Nicholls R J 1984 The long term results of polyvinyl alcohol (Ivalon) sponge for rectal prolapse in young patients. Br J Surg 71: 213–214

Broden G, Dolk A, Holmstrom B 1988 Recovery of the internal anal sphincter following rectopexy: a possible explanation for continence improvement. Int J Colorect Dis 3: 23–28

Christiansen J, Kirkegaard P 1981 Delormes operation for complete rectal prolapse. Br J Surg 68: 537–538

Fry I K, Griffiths J D, Smart P J G 1966 Some observations on the movement of the pelvic floor and rectum with special reference to rectal prolapse. Br J Surg 53: 784–787

Frykman H M, Goldberg S M 1969 The surgical treatment of rectal procidentia. Surg Gynecol Obstet 129: 1225–1230

Hughes E S R 1949 In discussion on rectal prolapse. Proc R Soc Med 42: 1007–1011

Jurgeleit H C, Corman M L, Coller J A, Veidenheimer M C 1975 Procidentia of the rectum: Teflon sling repair of rectal prolapse, Lahey clinic experience. Dis Colon Rectum 18: 464–467

Keighley M R B, Fielding J W L, Alexander-Williams J 1983 Results of Marlex mesh rectopexy for rectal prolapse in 11 consecutive patients. Br J Surg 70: 229–232

Miller R, Orrom W J, Cornes H, Duthie G S, Bartolo D C C 1989 Anterior sphincter plication and levatorplasty in the treatment of faecal incontinence. Br J Surg 76: 1059–1060

Moschcowitz A V 1912 The pathogenesis anatomy and cure of prolapse of the rectum. Surg Gynecol Obstet 15: 7–21

Neill M E, Parks A G, Swash M 1981 Physiological studies of the anal musculature in faecal incontinence and rectal prolapse. Br J Surg 68: 531–536

Nicholls R J, Simson J N L 1986 Anteroposterior rectopexy in the treatment of solitary rectal ulcer syndrome without overt rectal prolapse. Br J Surg 73: 222–224

Oresland T, Fasth S, Akervall S, Nordgren S, Hulten L 1990 Manovolumetric and sensory characteristics of the ileoanal J pouch compared with healthy rectum. Br J Surg 77: 803–806

Parks A G, Swash M, Urich H 1977 Sphincter denervation in anorectal incontinence and rectal prolapse. Gut 18: 656–665

Porter N H 1962 A physiological study of the pelvic floor in rectal prolapse. Ann R Coll Surg Engl 31: 379–404

Ripstein C B 1972 Procidentia: definitive corrective surgery. Dis Colon Rectum 15: 334–336

Ripstein C B, Lanter B 1963 Etiology and surgical therapy of massive prolapse of the rectum. Ann Surg 157: 259–264

Spencer R J 1984 Manometric studies in rectal prolapse. Dis Colon Rectum 27: 523–525

Sun W M, Read N W, Donnely T C, Bannister J J, Shorthouse A J 1989 A common pathophysiology for full thickness rectal prolapse, anterior mucosal prolapse and solitary rectal ulcer. Br J Surg 76: 290–295

Theuerkauf F J, Beahrs O H, Hill J R 1970 Rectal prolapse: causation and surgical treatment. Ann Surg 171: 819–835

Watts J D, Rothenberger D A, Buls J G, Goldberg S M, Nivatvongs S 1985 The management of procidentia: 30 years experience. Dis Colon Rectum 28: 96–102

Wells C 1959 New operation for rectal prolapse. Proc R Soc Med 52: 602–603

Yoshioka K, Hyland G, Keighley M R B 1989 Anorectal function after abdominal rectopexy: parameters of predictive value in identifying return of continence. Br J Surg 76: 64–68

12

Liver resection

I. S. Benjamin

Major hepatic resection remains a procedure which is mainly carried out in specialist centres where there is the investigative and post-operative backup required for the most complex cases. However, the last decade has seen liver surgery emerge from the darkness and as both understanding and the results of liver resection have improved, more surgeons not only now refer patients to specialist centres, but even undertake the more straightforward resections themselves. The aim of this review is to define current indications for liver resection and to outline the techniques commonly used, with particular emphasis on new approaches which have brought about this change in perception.

INDICATIONS FOR LIVER RESECTION

Malignant tumours

Primary

Primary hepatocellular carcinoma (HCC) remains the commonest cancer in men worldwide, largely because of the high prevalence of hepatoma in cirrhosis due to hepatitis B virus in Eastern populations. HCC is relatively uncommon in the West and Western surgeons have mostly been brought up with the view that resection of the cirrhotic liver is an almost uniformly fatal procedure. It remains true that major liver resection in cirrhosis commonly results in liver failure and death, but encouraging results have been obtained in patients with small tumours detected as the result of ultrasound or tumour marker screening. Resection of multiple tumours under 5 cm in size has been shown to be feasible in Japanese series, and there has been some interest in this also in France. These efforts have been further stimulated by the disappointing results of transplantation for HCC, with the exception of those patients who undergo transplant for cirrhosis and are found to have small incidental tumours. Nonetheless, Western experience remains small.

A variant of primary liver cell cancer, the fibrolamellar hepatoma (FLH), has been recognized increasingly in the last decade. This tumour contrasts in almost every possible respect with the commoner variants of HCC. It occurs in the non-cirrhotic liver, predominantly in young females, and may reach a very large size within the liver in a 'pushing' rather than invasive manner. It metastasizes late. It rarely expresses the tumour marker alpha-fetoprotein, but has been found to carry its own markers, plasma neurotensin and vitamin B12 binding capacity. Although some have disputed that FLH has an inherently better prognosis than HCC, these tumours are nevertheless more often resected (or transplanted) than the other varieties, and it may be that long-term survival is better (Soreide et al 1986).

Secondary

Secondary tumours are the commonest hepatic malignancy in Western practice. They are very common from colorectal primaries, and perhaps as many as 40% of patients have occult or overt metastases at the time of colectomy. Surprisingly, it is still unknown how many of these tumours are truly resectable. Moreover, not all surgeons agree that resection, even of solitary metastases, significantly affects the natural history of the disease. This question will be discussed later in this chapter, but it must be said that this remains the commonest indication for liver resection in the UK. Secondaries from other primary tumours are much less often resected. The exception to this may be metastases from functioning endocrine tumours, which are often slow growing and exercise their main effects by their secretory products. Rather special criteria may therefore be adopted for resection of these liver secondaries, since palliation of endocrine syndromes (such as severe carcinoid syndrome or Verner–Morrison syndrome) may be most effective. Resection of other secondaries cannot be universally recommended, although in individual cases it may be justified: the author has resected secondaries from breast, leiomyosarcomas and teratomas, in specific cases. Hilar cholangiocarcinoma is another controversial indication for liver resection. Only approximately 20% of all hilar cancers are amenable to resection, and half of these require liver resection to obtain tumour clearance. It remains uncertain whether this major procedure, with its attendant high morbidity and mortality, will find a permanent place in the management of this condition.

Benign lesions

Liver cell adenoma is seen increasingly, both because of its association with the oral contraceptive pill and because of the increasing use of abdominal ultrasound. The indications for resection hinge on the risk of complications such as rupture (very rare), and of malignant transformation (probably equally rare, and some would doubt its occurrence at all), or on the uncertainty of the diagnosis. The consensus would now be that large or symptomatic adenomas should be resected if this can be done safely, while smaller or asymptomatic lesions should be observed intermittently with ultrasound. Focal nodular hyperplasia may be treated in the same way, and although there is no evidence of malignant transformation in this lesion, there remains a small risk of traumatic rupture. Spontaneous rupture is exceedingly rare. Haemangiomas are very common and are now often seen on routine ultrasound. Improvements in radiological imaging frequently allow a confident diagnosis by a combination of dynamic contrast CT scanning, angiography and magnetic resonance imaging. There is no risk of malignant change and in fact few increase in size during a period of observation. It is therefore only necessary to resect the few 'giant' haemangiomas which are judged to be truly symptomatic. Some may respond to embolization, but experience in this Unit with resection for symptomatic tumours has been good (Lancet 1988). Cysts of the liver rarely warrant resection, with the exception of large and complicated hydatid cysts, which will not be considered further in this chapter. Simple cysts and some symptomatic polycystic livers may require resection or marsupialization, but it is often worth a trial of radiologically guided aspiration and alcohol instillation before considering this.

Occasionally liver resection is required for patients with benign biliary disease, particularly when biliary strictures are associated with lobar atrophy and intrahepatic stones. This situation is more common in Asiatic cholangiohepatitis, but is rarely indicated in Western practice.

ANATOMY

Improvements in anatomical understanding are the key to modern liver surgery. While early anatomists recognized the branching lobular pattern of the liver, terminology remained confusing until the work of the French anatomists and surgeons in the 1950s gained recognition outside Europe. No surgical text on the liver is now complete without a version of the diagram showing the nomenclature of the eight liver segments defined by Hepp & Couinaud (Fig. 12.1). The hepatic veins are the true key to the anatomy of the liver (Ger 1989). Three in number, they run in vertically disposed fissures which divide the liver, working from right to left, into segments VI/VII, V/VIII, IV, and II/III.

The nomenclature of liver resection is still confusing in much of the literature, not least because American authors remain reluctant to accept the segmental descriptions. The 'classical' liver resections should really be named as follows:

1. Right hepatectomy—segments V, VI, VII, VIII.
2. Extended right hepatectomy—segments IV, V, VI, VII, VIII (sometimes including I).
3. Left hepatectomy—segments II, III, IV (sometimes including I).
4. Left lateral segmentectomy—segments II and III.
5. Extended left hepatectomy—segments I (usually), II, III, IV, V, VIII.

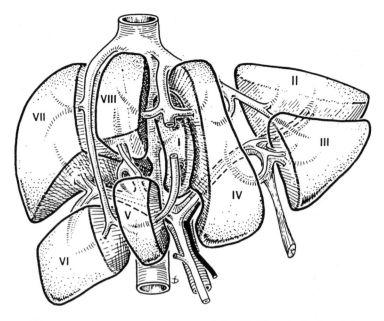

Fig. 12.1   The segmental anatomy of the liver, as defined by Hepp & Couinaud, shown in exploded form. Reproduced with permission from Blumgart (1987).

For some purposes it may be useful to divide segment IV (the quadrate lobe) by a horizontal line into IVa and IVb. Resection of segment IVb may sometimes be undertaken alone or with segment V in resection of hilar cholangiocarcinomas or gallbladder tumours. Note that the so-called 'trisegmentectomy' resects not three but five (or sometimes six) segments and this terminology should be avoided. This emphasis on nomenclature of segmental anatomy should not be dismissed as mere pedantry. It is from this systematic approach that advances in surgical resection techniques such as single or multiple segmentectomies and cranial hepatic resections have sprung.

   Turning attention to the inflow tracts of the liver, each segment is provided with a branch of the hepatic artery and portal vein, and drains into a single hepatic duct. Variants in the arterial anatomy are well recognized. It must be emphasized that very rarely are these variants 'accessory' arteries, but *replaced* arteries, supplying well-defined and often large territories of the liver. The commonest such variant is the origin of the right hepatic artery from the superior mesenteric artery, which is seen in some 20% of angiograms. This aberrant vessel runs behind the head of the pancreas and lies posteriorly in the free edge of the lesser omentum. Here it can generally be palpated, but it is useful to have advance knowledge of its presence either from pre-operative angiography or from good quality ultrasound studies.

In up to 10% of patients the left hepatic artery arises from the left gastric artery, or directly from the coeliac axis. At operation this artery runs in the ligamentum venosum, which joins the cleft between segments I and II/III of the liver to the lesser curve of the stomach, where it can be usually readily palpated. Prior knowledge of these aberrant vessels from angiography may save some time in dissection.

In contrast to the hepatic arteries, the portal veins have few variants. The left portal vein is more accessible than the right and runs horizontally at the base of segment IV, below and behind the left hepatic duct. The left hepatic

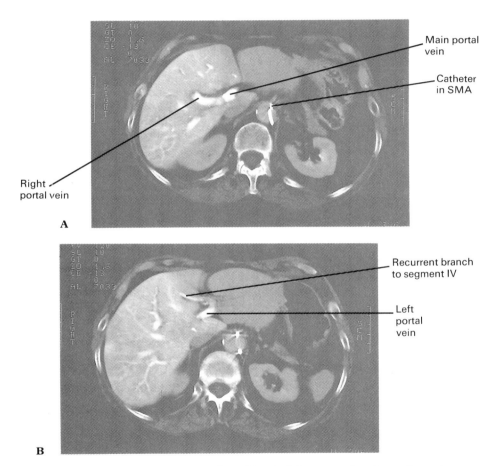

Fig. 12.2 CT scans of the liver in a patient with a single large secondary from colorectal cancer. Contrast has been delivered via a catheter in the superior mesenteric artery, and the portal veins are clearly seen. In **A** contrast fills the right liver and portal vein radicles, but the tumour has occluded the portal supply to segments II and III. In **B** a lower cut of this examination shows clearly the main left portal vein, and the recurrent branch to segment IV while no contrast enters segments II and III. This tumour was resected by a left lateral segmentectomy, with 5 mm of tumour clearance.

artery may also run in this plane, but quite commonly enters the liver more vertically at the umbilical fissure. Crossing the umbilical fissure the left portal vein divides to segments II and III, and in the fissure it gives off the recurrent branches to segment IV. It is important to be aware of this structure when resecting segments II and III, since inadvertent dissection too far to the right of the umbilical fissure may deprive segment IV of its portal venous supply. These recurrent vessels can be seen clearly in the CT scan in Figure 12.2; a secondary tumour has occluded the portal supply to segments II and III but the recurring branch to segment IV is spared. It is worthwhile but not essential to preserve this branch, but this certainly should not be allowed to prejudice radical tumour clearance.

Note that the right portal vein frequently divides very early into its anterior and posterior sectoral branches at the hilus, and the posterior branch is in danger of injury if blind dissection is undertaken behind the portal vein in this region.

The biliary anatomy is of great importance, and the numerous variants of the hilar ducts have been well described. Probably the most important points to make are that the left hepatic duct is *always* an extrahepatic structure, and can be separated from the base of segment IV by division of the peritoneum which overlies the portal vein and left duct in this region and fuses with Glisson's capsule. This manoeuvre is described by the French as 'lowering the hilar plate'. The right hepatic duct is not so obligingly constant and is subject to considerable variation, particularly in the mode of junction of the right anterior (V/VIII) and posterior (VI/VII) sectoral ducts.

Finally, to return to the hepatic veins, it is worth reiterating that these are the absolute key to the anatomy of liver resection (Ger 1989). The middle hepatic vein runs in the principal plane of the liver, usually from the left side of the vena cava towards the fundus of the gallbladder. It is in this plane that right or left hepatectomy will be performed, usually ligating tributaries from the side to be resected, but leaving the vein itself intact. The left hepatic vein commonly joins the middle hepatic vein before its entry into the vena cava, although this is variable and it may be helpful to define the junction by intra-operative ultrasound. Sometimes the left hepatic vein enters the cava separately from the middle hepatic vein, which is a convenient arrangement when it is necessary to carry out resections of segments II and III (Fig. 12.3).

The right hepatic vein enters the right side of the vena cava just below the diaphragm, and a phrenic vein (which may be quite large) is often the anatomical clue to the location of this vein. The vein is usually accessible outside the liver, and it is the author's practice to attempt to control and divide this whenever possible during a right hepatectomy (see below). There are a variable number of small hepatic veins running from the posterior surface of the right liver and the right half of the caudate lobe (segment I) into the vena cava. These may be very short and are easily

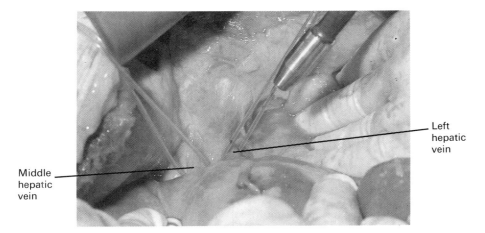

Left hepatic vein

Middle hepatic vein

Fig. 12.3 This operative photograph, from the same case as Figure 12.2, shows slings around the left and middle hepatic veins which in this case enter the inferior vena cava separately. The tumour was resected with formal ligation and division of the left hepatic vein, preserving the middle hepatic vein and ligating only tributaries from segment II.

damaged during mobilization of the right liver. A vein commonly present but infrequently described in texts is the inferior right hepatic vein. This vein drains from segment VI directly into the vena cava and may be encountered during mobilization of the right liver from the vena cava posteriorly. It is generally very short but may be as long as 1 cm in its cranio-caudal axis, and its ligation may require the use of a vascular clamp on the vena cava. It is important to be aware of the possibility of this vein, since its inadvertent division may give rise to catastrophic haemorrhage.

The inferior vena cava runs in a groove behind the whole length of liver. It is not frequently appreciated that the vena cava can if necessary be separated from the liver by careful dissection and ligation of small venous branches throughout its length.

NEW TECHNOLOGY

It must be emphasized that liver surgery depends not upon the availability of special instruments but upon understanding of the anatomy and careful technique. However, a number of significant technological advances have contributed to the development of liver resection.

Intra-operative ultrasound

This has been valuable in three distinct areas. First, ultrasound may be used to define the hepatic anatomy, and in particular to show the position and relation of tumours to the hepatic veins and portal venous branches. The extent of resection judged to be required may be either increased or reduced by use of the ultrasound probe. While it is useful to have a radiologist experienced in ultrasound in theatre to help in the early stages, there is no substitute for the surgeon learning to use the ultrasound as an extension of his hands and eyes.

Secondly, ultrasound may be more sensitive than pre-operative imaging in detecting small lesions in the liver which would render resection of a known liver tumour futile. This is most important since experience has shown that in about a quarter of all patients who undergo liver resection for colorectal secondaries the only site of recurrent tumour is in the liver itself. However, one must also be aware of the false positive diagnosis of additional liver tumours, since the highly sensitive contact ultrasound probe may show small haemangiomas and granulomas in the liver, and results must be interpreted with caution.

The third application has been little used outside highly specialized units (Shimamura et al 1986), particularly in Japan and France. In cirrhotic patients, in whom major liver resection for a primary HCC may be contra-indicated, ultrasound may be used to guide placement of a catheter with an occlusion balloon into a portal venous radicle. Dye is then injected to mark the extent of the tumour bearing segment. This can then be safely and radically resected, without major parenchymal loss. This elegant technique has yet to find a major place but is applicable in a few situations.

Hepatotomy devices

It is the highly vascular nature of the liver parenchyma which (rightly) holds most fear for the majority of surgeons. The liver is generally divided by a 'tissue fracture' technique, crushing small amounts of liver tissue between the finger and thumb, or more commonly with a haemostat, leaving the vessels and ducts intact to be individually ligated and divided. A major technological advance was the use of ultrasonic energy to divide the liver (Hodgson & Del Guercio 1984). There are now a variety of such instruments, but the first one to be used was the Cavitron ultrasonic surgical aspirator (CUSA). This sophisticated device has a hand piece with a tip which vibrates in its longitudinal axis at ultrasonic frequency. At the appropriate power setting these oscillations shatter the hepatocytes but leave fibrous tissue undamaged, allowing precise dissection around medium and large biliary and vascular structures and accurate, controlled precise placement of ligatures or clips. The device has continuous saline irrigation and suction to remove fluid and debris, and use of this instrument has come close to allowing virtually 'bloodless' hepatic resection.

An alternative to the CUSA for parenchymal division is the waterjet knife, which directs a fine high powered jet of water at the liver tissue, allowing the same sort of dissection to be performed. This has not yet been widely reported, but may in fact prove to have many of the benefits of the CUSA.

The use of lasers to divide the liver is not new, but although many people have experimented with this technology it has not been widely applied. One comparison between the CUSA and the laser in experimental animals showed that the laser produced more tissue damage at the cut edge of the liver than the CUSA device.

A cheap and effective alternative to all of these devices is the 'suction knife' (Almersjo & Hafstrom 1974). This can be made by squeezing the end of a plastic sucker with a heavy haemostat and cutting it off at an oblique angle. This sucker is then used to tease apart the tissue mechanically. It is the author's practice to use a fine metal sucker for hepatotomy, and as long as care is taken not to disrupt small vessels before they can be coagulated, or larger ones before they are ligated or clipped, then blood loss during the division of the liver should not be significantly more than that achieved with the CUSA (Sugarbaker & Leighton 1986, Schroder et al 1987). The CUSA and other devices really come into their own when carrying out segmental and non-anatomical resections, but lack of such a device should not in itself deter a well-trained and experienced surgeon from undertaking liver resection.

Haemostatic aids

Following a right hepatectomy there may be a raw surface some 10 cm in diameter, which may continue to ooze slowly post-operatively. A variety of materials are available to assist haemostasis including collagen matting or fleece. A more recent approach used widely in Europe has been to spray the surface of the liver with a rapid setting fibrin glue (Tisseel®, Immuno, Austria). Separate solutions of human lyophilized fibrinogen and thrombin are mixed directly on the liver surface. As the components mix, the fibrinogen is activated and forms an instant clot of fibrin which very effectively seals small bleeding points and even small bile leaks. This may be used alone or in combination with collagen matting, and is very effective as a final stage in haemostasis. Electrical devices such as the infra-red coagulator may be used, but all have the disadvantage of inducing a degree of tissue damage.

Haemostasis can also be assisted by suturing of the cut liver surface. This is made easier by the use of absorbable ox fibrin liver buffers (Biethium®, Ethicon, Scotland) which allow the tying of catgut sutures without cutting through the liver capsule (Wood et al 1976). In practice with careful haemostasis during the hepatotomy and the use of fibrin glue, these buffers are rarely necessary and are best avoided if possible because of the inevitable production of a small cuff of ischaemic liver.

Liver clamps

Various clamps have been devised to apply an even pressure around the liver. The Longmire clamp is a large spring loaded device which is too

A

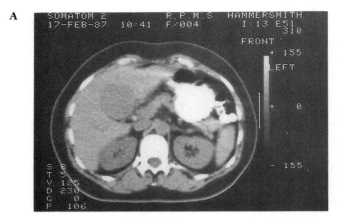

B

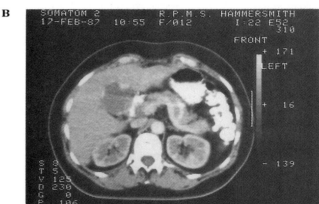

Fig. 12.4   A–D A sequence of scans taken between 10 and 30 min after injection of an intravenous bolus of contrast. In this case a large haemangioma can be seen in segment VII which fills in progressively during the delayed scans until it is almost completely opacified.

ungainly for general use although it may be useful for some pedunculated tumours and occasionally for left lateral segmentectomies. Lim has described the use of a tourniquet around the liver for the same purpose, but there is no wide experience of this.

Retractors

Exposure is of paramount importance during major liver resection and is greatly aided by a fixed retractor system such as the Omnitract (CLS Medical, UK) or Bookwalter systems. These give excellent exposure of the subphrenic spaces, allowing safer dissection of the hepatic veins and vena cava, and freeing the assistants' hands to help with dislocating and supporting the liver during the dissection.

C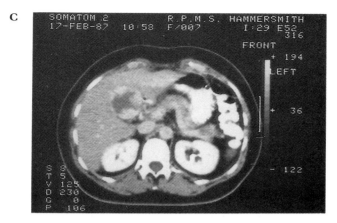

D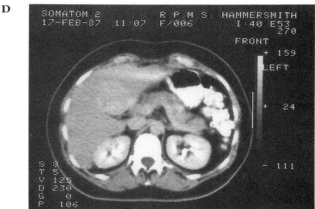

Fig. 12.4 Continued.

Hepatic vascular isolation

This can be a useful technique, and although many methods have been described using intracaval shunts, particularly for trauma, these are rarely necessary. As will be discussed below, most patients, especially the young, can tolerate a period of total caval clamping without venous bypass for a long enough period to enable the surgeon to carry out most complex liver resections.

PRE-OPERATIVE PREPARATION

Laboratory tests

As well as routine haematology and biochemistry, laboratory tests must include a full investigation of clotting, especially in jaundiced patients. The need for vitamin K, fresh frozen plasma or platelets pre-operatively should be considered. Even though blood losses are now very small with most elective resections, it is the author's practice to crossmatch 10 units of blood for a major hepatectomy. Baseline liver function tests are important to be able to interpret post-operative changes. Careful attention must be paid to renal function and full hydration. In the case of known or suspected liver tumours, appropriate serum markers should be examined, including alpha-fetoprotein, CEA, neurotensin, vitamin B12, binding capacity, and other gastrointestinal hormones in the case of secondary tumours of unknown origin. These tests are not only of diagnostic value, but may allow early diagnosis of recurrent tumour after resection.

Radiology

Radiological imaging is aimed at defining the anatomical location and extent of hepatic lesions, and may also give valuable information about resectability (Mukai et al 1987).

Isotope scanning is now of limited usefulness and has largely been superseded by other scanning modalities. Ultrasound is the simplest test and is extremely accurate in defining the size and location of tumours and their relationship to the hepatic and portal veins. A careful search of the whole liver must be made for other tumours. In jaundiced patients the level of ductal obstruction can be defined, and precise diagnostic information may be obtained about vascular anatomy and invasion.

CT scanning is probably the current gold standard for pre-operative investigation, and will show the size and location of tumours, even for lesions less than 1 cm in size. Excellent delineation of the vessels can be obtained following intravenous contrast. If a haemangioma is suspected then delayed centripetal enhancement of the tumour following a bolus of intravenous contrast may be observed, but scans up to 15 or 30 min after injection must be performed (Fig. 12.4). CT clearly detects atrophy in the right or left liver in the case of bile duct cancers. Portal venous anatomy can sometimes be seen in great detail, as can the relation of tumours to the hepatic veins (Fig. 12.5). Greater definition for very small lesions may be seen as negative areas in the portogram phase, and this may be assisted by bolus injection into a visceral artery through a catheter left in place following an angiogram. This technique (CT arterioportography) has achieved popularity in the United States. Apparent diaphragmatic involvement on CT scanning is usually inflammatory rather than invasive, and does not contraindicate resection (Weinbren et al 1987).

Visceral angiography is performed for all but the most minor and peripheral liver lesions. An angiogram will give not only a 'roadmap' of arterial anatomy, but may reveal small vascular deposits in the liver, especially from endocrine secondaries. It is in fact rare for such lesions to be found on angiography alone, and not on CT scans with intravenous contrast. It has been observed that lipiodol injected into the hepatic arterial

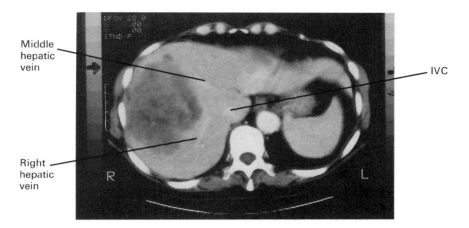

Middle hepatic vein

IVC

Right hepatic vein

R

L

Fig. 12.5 An intravenous contrast CT scan showing clear filling of the right, middle and left hepatic vein close to their entry to the inferior vena cava. The relation to these veins of a tumour in the right liver can be seen clearly.

tree is initially taken up diffusely throughout the liver (probably by Kupffer cells), but clears from the normal liver more rapidly than from tumour circulation. A CT scan one week after lipiodol injection may show an abnormal pattern of tumour uptake (Bruneton et al 1988). Although this procedure has a number of false positives, it is occasionally useful in revealing the site of an occult tumour (Fig. 12.6).

Embolization of tumours in order to shrink them before resection is an appealing concept, but has not proved valuable in practice. Many tumours do not shrink significantly after embolization, and timing is critical to avoid increased difficulty at operation due to formation of large collateral vessels. However, some workers have used forms of therapeutic chemoembolization or radioactive labelled embolization and have apparently brought irresectable tumours within the range of surgical management (Sasaki et al 1987).

Cholangiography, either retrograde or percutaneous transhepatic, is essential only for patients with suspected bile duct cancer.

General radiological screening must not be ignored, particularly for patients with secondary disease. A chest X-ray must of course be examined, and it is now the author's practice to carry out CT scanning of the chest at the same time as the liver to avoid missing small metastases, particularly at the lung bases.

Assessment of liver function

Routine biochemical liver function tests have already been mentioned. Nutritional assessment should be carried out in patients who have lost weight, and a period of pre-operative nutritional support should be

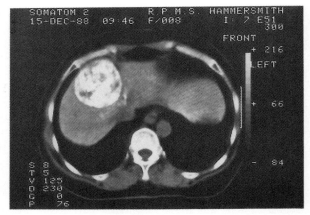

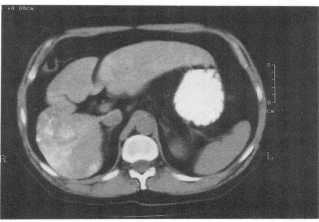

Fig. 12.6   Lipiodol angiograms. **A** Shows very bright imaging of a well localized primary HCC in segment VIII of the liver, one week after lipiodol angiography; **B** shows patchy retention of lipiodol in segment V in a patient with haemochromatosis and a rising alpha-fetoprotein, in whom other attempts at tumour localization had failed. This patient underwent a segmental resection for this tumour with good clearance and no complications.

considered. Dynamic liver function tests aimed at assessing the functional hepatic mass or estimating the amount of liver which can safely be removed have been reported, but have not been widely used (Matsumata et al 1987). Risk scoring systems have been applied to liver resection, for example the well-known Child/Pugh classification used for patients with portal hypertension. It is not yet clear if any such classification has a sufficient predictive value to be of use.

Pre-operative preparation

Apart from general nutritional support and chest physiotherapy, the need for pre-operative transfusion should be assessed. It is the author's practice to administer prophylactic antibiotics (currently piperacillin and gentamicin) as a single intravenous dose before operation and 6 h thereafter. There is no need to continue antibiotic therapy beyond this period, unless there is a specific therapeutic indication. The question of pre-operative drainage of the biliary tree for patients presenting with jaundice remains unresolved despite a number of trials, mostly showing no effect. Nevertheless, deeply jaundiced patients undergoing complex hepatic resection and hilar reconstruction for bile duct tumour are at a very high risk of post-operative complications and if jaundice has been very prolonged (six weeks or more) then a period of stenting to achieve internal drainage as a temporary measure should be considered.

OPERATIVE TECHNIQUE

Anaesthesia

An experienced anaesthetist is essential for major hepatic resection. Good venous access must be secured, and full relaxation and endotracheal intubation are used, in preparation for what may be a long operation. We frequently use epidural analgesia for the first 24 h after operation, followed by patient controlled analgesia with automatic boluses of intravenous opiates. The anaesthetist must watch for changes in central venous pressure during operation. Major changes in haemodynamic parameters may be due to compression of the IVC during mobilization, but are sometimes due to release of vasoactive substances into the circulation consequent on handling of the tumours. This may occur not only with endocrine tumours but with apparently non-secreting HCCs. Volume replacement during surgery should be adequate but on no account should the circulation be over-filled 'prophylactically'. This simply increases bleeding from the cut surface of the liver because of the increased venous pressure. Similarly, positive end-expiratory pressure should be avoided, particularly during the hepatotomy phase of the operation.

Position

The patient is positioned supine and the abdomen and entire chest should be prepared up to the sternal notch and over the lateral chest wall, in case there is a need for a thoracotomy or sternotomy.

Incision

A bilateral subcostal incision is sufficient for almost every liver resection. Right thoracotomy is now extremely rare in the author's practice, although it may sometimes be required in cases of atrophy and hyperplasia with rotation of the liver. If it is necessary to gain access to the inferior vena cava above the liver, especially in trauma cases, it is best to split the sternum and divide the diaphragmatic fibres down to the cava, controlling the IVC from within the pericardium.

Assessment

Full laparotomy must be performed. If operation is for secondary disease following resection of a primary colorectal cancer, the region of the previous colectomy must be examined carefully. Any nodes along the aorta should be sampled and frozen section carried out. Unless a deliberately palliative resection is being performed, positive nodes on frozen section should preclude major liver resection. Following full bimanual palpation of the whole liver, intra-operative ultrasound is used if available, to search for small occult tumours, to define the extent of the known tumour, and to establish the anatomy, particularly of the hepatic veins. Coeliac axis nodes may also be sampled for frozen section if appropriate.

Mobilization

Most of the manoeuvres to be described relate to resections of the right liver, and separate comment will be made on matters relating to left hepatectomy. It is often helpful to mobilize the hepatic flexure fully and to Kocherize the duodenum, in order to gain access to the inferior vena cava below the liver. The ligamentum teres is divided between ligatures, and the falciform ligament is divided all the way up to the dome of the diaphragm above the liver. Mobilization of the right liver can now commence by division of the right coronary ligament. Once this has begun an assistant on the opposite side of the table lifts the liver upwards and forwards, while strong retraction is applied to the right costal margin, using a fixed retractor system. Great care must be taken at this point because small veins entering the vena cava can be torn if excessive traction is applied. It is sometimes necessary to divide the right adrenal vein, particularly if a posteriorly placed tumour restricts access at this point. As a precaution, once there is a sufficient length of inferior vena cava exposed between the right renal vein and the liver, the cava should be mobilized at this point and a sling placed around it above the renal veins. Mobilization of the right liver continues with division of the caval ligament, which becomes a stout fibrous structure as the dome of the diaphragm and right hepatic vein are approached. At this point great care must be taken as substantial hepatic veins may run close to the caval ligament. It is usually necessary to divide several small hepatic veins between fine silk ligatures. Metal clips can be used here, but there is a danger that these may become displaced by a gauze swab at a later point, and the author avoids their use in this setting.

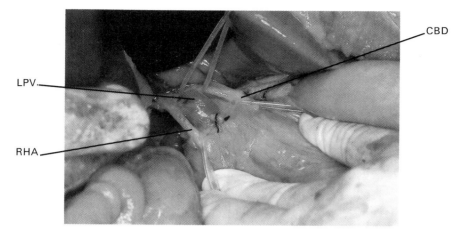

Fig. 12.7   Slings are shown in place around the common bile duct, the left branch of the portal vein, and an anomalous right hepatic artery arising from the superior mesenteric artery.

It is not necessary to complete the mobilization of the right liver at this stage, and attention can now be turned to dissection of the hilar structures. These should be dissected carefully and their anatomy precisely defined. It is useful to place slings around the bile duct, arteries and main portal veins (Fig. 12.7). If possible and safe, it is best to divide the vessels which supply the area to be resected out with the liver. The artery can be doubly ligated and divided, but the portal vein should be controlled with a vascular clamp and the splanchnic end formally closed with a vascular stitch. Ligation and division of these vessels is the first irreversible step in the operation, and should not be performed until resectability has been fully assessed. Once this is done a line of demarcation will appear (in the case of a right hepatectomy) which marks the principal plane of the liver dividing segment IV from segments V and VIII.

Final mobilization of the right liver can now be continued. Dissection above and below the level of the right hepatic vein will usually allow its isolation outside the liver. If its course is long enough to apply clamps and to divide the vessel, this can be done at this stage. If not, then a suture can usually be placed and the vein doubly ligated in continuity. At this point it is usually also possible, although not always necessary, to dissect behind the IVC above the liver, and to place another sling at this point. It should be emphasized that every step of this procedure should be aimed at total control and safety, and if there is a sling around the IVC above and below the liver and another around the free edge of the lesser omentum, then almost any mishap can be dealt with under complete vascular control.

The liver surface can now be marked in preparation for the final hepatotomy. The liver capsule is incised along the resection line using the

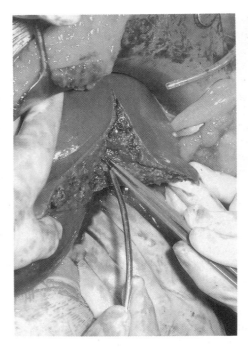

Fig. 12.8   Hepatotomy for a right hepatectomy. A metal sucker is being used to tease apart the tissues, while an assistant uses the diathermy forceps to coagulate small vessels. By progressing slowly using this technique very little blood loss is encountered during the hepatotomy phase.

diathermy. If the tumour is peripheral, it is safest to swing the line of resection well clear of the hilar structures, particularly if these have not been ligated outside the liver. It is often safest to avoid dissection of the right branches of the biliary tree if the anatomy is at all unclear at the hilus. These sectoral ducts can then be ligated within the liver substance at a safe distance, avoiding any possible damage to the main hepatic duct or left hepatic duct. Division of the liver is now commenced at the free edge, in the centre of the gallbladder bed. This is done with an instrument crushing or gentle finger fracture technique, or using the CUSA if available. The use of a fine sucker to tease the tissues apart is an equally effective technique (Fig. 12.8). A soft bowel clamp may be applied to the free edge of the lesser omentum as a Pringle manoeuvre, or bulldog clamps may be applied to the portal vein and hepatic artery to the liver remnant. This reduces troublesome oozing from the cut surface of the residual liver during the hepatotomy. The time of total hepatic vascular occlusion is recorded. Although it has been shown that up to at least one hour of hepatic ischaemia is quite safe, it is the author's practice to release such clamps after 15 min, pressing on the cut surface liver with a gauze pack. The clamps can be reapplied after allowing liver perfusion for one or two minutes. This manoeuvre is carried out not so much to minimize hepatic ischaemic damage as to prevent a large bolus of stagnant blood being released into the circulation at one time. Even during the most complex liver resection it is rarely necessary to apply the clamps for more than 30 min.

During the hepatotomy phase small vessels can be coagulated; medium size vessels are ligated with fine silk ligatures or controlled with metal clips. More substantial vessels and bile ducts should be suture-ligated as they are encountered, particularly main portal and hepatic venous pedicles. The major difficulty for the occasional liver surgeon is losing orientation within the liver. It helps to place the left hand behind the right liver, with the fingers between the hepatotomy and the vena cava, so that the correct direction can be determined at all times. If the dissection strays to the left, the middle hepatic vein will be encountered in the depths of the wound. The ideal resection plane is immediately to the right of this vein, and only tributaries of the vein from segment IV need to be ligated. Frequent review of the resection line is needed, both to avoid entering the wrong plane and to ensure that the cut surface is at least 1 cm away from a large or central liver tumour. Paradoxically, extended right hepatectomy (segments IV to VIII) may be easier at this point than right hepatectomy, since the amount of liver divided is less. In this case, it is especially important for the surgeon to have the fingers of the left hand in front of the inferior vena cava, as the hepatotomy proceeds just to the right of the umbilical fissure. The middle hepatic vein in this case will be encountered at the top of the resection, and should be suture ligated, taking care not to damage the confluence with the left hepatic vein.

Conclusion

The hepatotomy proceeds postero-superiorly through the liver, and finally the specimen can be removed. At this point a pack is placed over the cut surface and gentle pressure is applied, as the clamps are released from the inflow vessels. After a few minutes the pack is carefully removed and any further bleeding points are treated appropriately, with diathermy to small vessels and suturing of larger or more persistent bleeding points. There should be very few of these if the hepatotomy has proceeded carefully and all vessels have been ligated and divided as they are encountered. Other haemostatic aids (such as Tisseel or collagen fibre—see above) may now be applied. It is important to search for bile leaks, especially if the resection has been close to or involving the hepatic ducts. In the special case of extended right hepatectomy with the confluence of the hepatic ducts in continuity for a hilar tumour, it will now be necessary to perform a hepaticojejunostomy between the residual left hepatic duct at the umbilical fissure and a Roux loop of jejunum. These procedures will not be discussed here in detail, but have been described elsewhere recently (Blumgart & Benjamin 1989).

All other areas must be inspected carefully for bleeding. Particular attention is paid to the divided ligaments and any area of denuded diaphragm. The abdomen is then closed with drainage of the deadspace. It is the author's preference to use a closed tube drain of silicone, without suction. While it is accepted that if persistent oozing occurs then no drain is guaranteed to be effective in preventing a subphrenic collection, it is the author's practice to drain every case except for minor wedge excisions. There is absolutely no need to place a T-tube into a normal bile duct following an uncomplicated liver resection. However, if there has been doubt about involvement of bile ducts, it is reasonable to insert a catheter into the cystic duct and to inject dilute methylene blue in order to identify any bile leaks on the cut surface. This may be a particularly valuable manoeuvre following complex resections for bile duct cancers or for hydatid disease.

Different techniques are applicable to some cases. Palliative metastasectomy for carcinoid secondaries is a remarkably straightforward procedure. The liver is incised around the tumour, and blunt dissection with a finger or a haemostat readily allows the tumour to be shelled out (Fig. 12.9). Multiple metastases may be removed in this way. Careful haemostasis is required in the residual cavities, and this may require several deep sutures to be placed because substantial veins may have been stretched around the metastases in such cases.

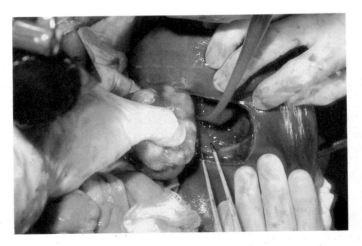

Fig. 12.9   Local resection in a patient with multiple carcinoid metastases and severe carcinoid syndrome. A 5 cm tumour is being shelled out of the liver. A total of 600 g of tumour was removed from this patient by multiple metastasectomies and two segmentectomies. A bile fistula resulted from one of the cavities, but closed spontaneously, and chemotherapy for the carcinoid syndrome could be discontinued. Reproduced with permission of the Medical Illustration Department, Royal Postgraduate Medical School and Hammersmith Hospital.

Resection of segments II and III of the liver is generally a straight-forward procedure. If this is for a tumour situated well away from the umbilical fissure then there is no need to dissect closely into the fissure. This avoids damage to the recurring portal branch to segment IV. However, if the tumour encroaches into the fissure, the portal supply should be deliberately dissected within the fissure, or else consideration should be given to extending resection into a formal left hepatectomy (segments II, III and IV). Resection of segment I (caudate lobe) can be tedious, because numerous small hepatic veins have to be carefully ligated and divided as they enter the IVC. This mobilization is often best done from the right and from below, even if a left hepatectomy is being performed. Partial resection of segment I may be appropriate in some instances, in which case a careful search must be made in the cut surface of this segment for small biliary radicles which will otherwise give rise to a troublesome post-operative biliary fistula. Occasionally large tumours of the right or left liver have a very pedunculated configuration, and in these cases one of the specially designed liver clamps may make the operation very straightforward.

Finally, it must be noted that whatever technique is adopted the most important determinant of long-term survival after resection is radical clearance of the tumour. It is absolutely essential therefore that the resection should be tailored to the position of the tumour, and if radical clearance cannot be achieved, a change of strategy should be considered.

POST-OPERATIVE COURSE

Most of our patients spend one night in an intensive care or high dependency unit, although assisted ventilation can usually be discontinued shortly after operation. The use of epidural or patient controlled analgesia has already been mentioned. It is uncommon to have large quantities of blood loss through the drains post-operatively, but there may be a considerable ooze of serous fluid because of the opened peritoneal spaces. Occasionally a chylous leak occurs, especially when there has been a major hilar dissection. Bile leaks are uncommon unless there has been biliary reconstruction, but when this occurs it is essential to leave the tube to drain until the fistula is closing spontaneously. In other cases the drains are removed when the volume has fallen to under 30 ml per day and this may take 3–4 days.

The remarkable process of regenerative hyperplasia can restore the liver of a rat to its normal size within three weeks of a two-thirds hepatectomy. The time course of regeneration is unclear in man, but may nevertheless be very rapid (Nagasue et al 1987). Even following extended right hepatectomy, the liver mass may be restored to normal within three months (Fig. 12.10). However, during this time synthetic liver function may be impaired, resulting in the need for administration of exogenous albumin and clotting factors. One unit of human albumin solution or fresh frozen

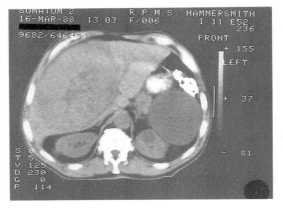

Fig. 12.10 CT scans. **A** CT scan of a patient with a large primary HCC in a non-cirrhotic liver. Extended right hepatectomy was performed; **B** CT scan three months after resection showing enormous regeneration of segments II and III of the liver.

plasma as appropriate should be given each day. Careful monitoring of blood glucose should be carried out, although hypoglycaemia is seldom a problem if a continuous infusion of 5% dextrose is maintained. If the hourly blood glucose measurements should fall below normal, then a bolus of 50% dextrose should be given intravenously. Following major liver resection patients may develop mild jaundice. This can generally be shown to be due to unconjugated hyperbilirubinaemia because of impaired hepatocyte function during regeneration. However, if the bilirubin continues to rise an ultrasound scan should be performed to exclude biliary obstruction or a major intra-abdominal bile collection. If present, such a collection can be drained percutaneously under ultrasound guidance. Re-operation is seldom indicated.

Follow-up will depend upon the indication for and nature of the resection. It is our practice to carry out a repeat CT scan approximately three months after the operation, by which time the liver will probably have reached its final regenerated size. This serves as a useful baseline from which to assess possible recurrent disease. A second scan is carried out at six months and annually thereafter. In cases of recurrent primary liver tumour, re-resection may be considered if necessary, or even transplantation. Unfortunately, even a five-year survival apparently free from disease is not a guarantee of cure, and we have seen one patient in whom recurrent liver tumour first appeared six years after resection. It is therefore a question of philosophy how long one should continue to follow up a patient who has undergone liver resection for tumour.

RESULTS

Operative mortality

This has become much lower in recent years and should now be 5% or less for elective hepatic resection in uncomplicated cases. The mortality may rise to 10% in more complex situations, especially when a large tumour requires an extended resection with a risk of post-operative liver failure. The highest mortality is for large parenchymal resections in cirrhotic patients, and these are probably best avoided. Hilar cholangiocarcinoma with biliary reconstruction in jaundiced patients also carries a high mortality. While straightforward hepatectomy can reasonably be performed in most hospitals by an appropriately trained surgeon, more complex cases should be treated only in major centres.

Morbidity

The major problem following liver resection used to be haemorrhage, but this has now become a much less significant threat. The major post-operative morbidity now is from sepsis, and this relates to the difficulty of avoiding collections in the deadspace. These collections consist of haematoma and bile which may contain organisms. There is a clear indication that the mortality following drainage by laparotomy in such cases is considerably higher than that after percutaneous approaches. If a collection is suspected, early ultrasound and catheter drainage are recommended.

Survival

For primary liver tumours several series now report three- to five-year survival rates of 23–73% for non-cirrhotic patients (Adson 1988). Five-year survival without resection for primary HCC is negligible. Survival after resection for secondary disease, particularly from colorectal cancer, remains a most controversial issue. There have been no trials of resection versus conservative management with chemotherapy for solitary or multiple secondaries for colorectal cancer. Nevertheless, historical data would suggest that five-year survival is well under 5% for unresected liver metastases, while there are numerous studies showing five-year survivals between 25 and 50% following resection (Benjamin & Blumgart 1988). Several groups have examined factors which determine survival or recurrence following resection (Hughes et al 1988). Age and the size of the secondary tumour may affect operative mortality, but have no additional effect on survival. The Dukes' stage of the primary tumour has a significant effect on survival, but it seems that resection of a liver secondary returns the individual patient to the survival curve appropriate to the stage of the primary tumour. The presence of extrahepatic metastases, including lymph nodes, at the time of resection has a major adverse effect on survival, and resection in the presence of extrahepatic disease is seldom indicated. It has already been mentioned that tumour clearance is of major importance and at least 1 cm should be aimed at. It is a matter of considerable debate whether the number of metastases has an important effect on survival. Some groups have suggested that patients with four or more metastases have significantly impaired survival, and that this is a contraindication to resection. Others would differ from this view, and this may be the one area in which there is considerable need for controlled trials. Our own data for resection of both primary and secondary liver tumours are shown in Figure 12.11.

Liver resection for bile duct cancer remains controversial. The problem is how to ensure complete tumour clearance for these very difficult slow-growing locally invasive tumours. In our experience, patients with radical resection have a significantly better survival rate than those with residual tumours. While results are often disappointing, palliation is good and a small group of patients may benefit from such resections.

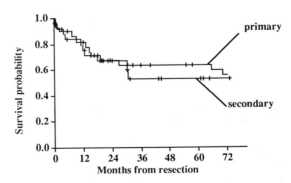

Fig. 12.11 Actuarial survival curves for patients undergoing liver resection for primary tumours (solid line) or colorectal secondaries. The curves are remarkably similar with predicted five-year survival rate of greater than 50%.

KEY POINTS FOR CLINICAL PRACTICE

Improvements in morbidity and mortality for liver resection have followed a better understanding of hepatic anatomy and physiology, accompanied by some technical innovations. More centres are now practising liver resection, for somewhat wider indications, including palliative resection in a small number of cases. Resection for secondary disease is gaining wider acceptance, although there remains considerable scepticism about its overall value. However, until better techniques of chemotherapy or novel approaches to liver cancer emerge, resection remains the only hope of cure for these patients. This author cannot do better than to end by quoting Adson: 'We cannot always act so that hope might triumph over judgement, but we cannot ignore the patient's need for hope when operative risk and morbidity are low, when there are no therapeutic alternatives, and when, at times, our palliative efforts may give rise to cure' (Adson 1987).

REFERENCES

Adson M A 1987 Resection of liver metastases—when is it worthwhile? World J Surg 11: 511–520

Adson M A 1988 Primary hepatocellular cancers—Western experience. In: Blumgart L H (ed) Surgery of the liver and biliary tract. Churchill Livingstone, London: 1153–1165

Almersjo O, Hafstrom L 1974 The "Suction Knife". A new device for dividing liver parenchyma. Acta Chir Scand 140: 581–583

Benjamin I S, Blumgart L H 1988 Hepatic resection for liver metastases. Dig Surg 6: 40–51

Blumgart L H (ed) 1987 Surgery of the liver and biliary tract. Churchill Livingstone, Edinburgh, p 5

Blumgart L H, Benjamin I S 1989 Liver resection for bile duct cancer. Surg Clin North Am 69: 323–337

Bruneton J N, Kerboul P, Grimaldi C et al 1988 Hepatic intra-arterial lipiodol: technique, semiologic patterns, and value for hepatic tumours. Gastroint Radiol 13: 45–51

Ger R 1989 Surgical anatomy of the liver. Surg Clin North Am 69: 179–192

Hodgson W J, Del-Guercio L R 1984 Preliminary experience in liver surgery using the ultrasonic scalpel. Surgery 95: 230–234

Hughes K S, Rosenstein R B, Songhorabodi S et al 1988 Resection of the liver for colorectal carcinoma metastases: a multi-institutional study of long-term survivors. Dis Colon Rectum 31: 1–4

Lancet leading article 1988 Hepatic haemangioma—a suitable case for treatment. Lancet ii: 882–884

Matsumata T, Kanematsu T, Yoshida Y et al 1987 The indocyanine green test enables prediction of postoperative complications after hepatic resection. World J Surg 11: 678–681

Mukai J K, Stack C M, Turner D A et al 1987 Imaging of surgically relevant hepatic vascular and segmental anatomy. Parts I and II. AJR 149: 287–292, 293–297

Nagasue N, Yukaya H, Ogawa Y et al 1987 Human liver regeneration after major hepatic resection. A study of normal liver and livers with chronic hepatitis and cirrhosis. Ann Surg 206: 30–39

Sasaki Y, Imaoka S, Kasugai H et al 1987 A new approach to chemoembolization therapy for hepatoma using ethiodized oil, cisplatin and gelatin sponge. Cancer 60: 1194–1203

Schroder T, Hasseigren P O, Bracket M et al 1987 Techniques of liver resection. Comparison of suction knife, ultrasonic dissector and contact neodymium-YAG laser. Arch Surg 122: 1166–1171

Shimamura Y, Gunven P, Takenaka Y et al 1986 Selective portal branch occlusion by balloon catheter during liver resection. Surgery 100: 938–941

Soreide O, Czerniak A, Bradpiece H A et al 1986 Characteristics of fibrolamellar
    hepatocellular carcinoma. A study of nine cases and a review of the literature. Am J Surg
    151: 518–523
Sugarbaker P H, Leighton S B 1986 Hepatic parenchymal suction dissector. SG&O 163:
    267–269
Weinbren K, Adam A, Blumgart L H et al 1987 Apparent extrahepatic invasion by metastatic
    tumours in the liver. Clin Radiol 38: 357–362
Wood C B, Capperauld I, Blumgart L H 1976 Bioplast fibrin buttons for liver biopsy and
    partial hepatic resection. Ann R Coll Surg Engl 58: 401–404

13

Quality assurance in surgical practice—audit, surveillance and decision analysis

Stephen Karran   Stuart Scott

'The joy of excellent performance' (Aristotle)

WHY?

The patient

When illness strikes, the priority is clear. With minimal delay the patient needs the help of the person who, above all, can determine and achieve optimal management of the illness. The degree to which this aim can be achieved is the fundamental determinant of quality assurance. Whilst the evaluation of many aspects of health care provision requires no medical input, e.g. waiting lists, outpatient clinic throughput, waiting room amenities, pharmacy budget, etc., these remain, essentially *secondary* to the core issue of quality assurance which requires consultant surgical peer review. Performance indicators in these other fields cannot, in themselves, provide *true* determinants of 'quality'.

Patient expectations

It is essential to consider the rightful expectations of the patient. Most patients will put up with significant inconvenience and discomfort, providing they can be secure in the knowledge that they will obtain from their physician an honest and informed assessment of their complaint, together with a recommendation of a course of action (or inaction!) best suited to *their own* individual situation. Confirmatory investigations should be ordered only when of direct benefit to management, with minimal risk and discomfort, and optimal treatment undertaken, which may need to be tailored *specifically* to their needs. Nonmedical assessment of such complex matters will invariably prove inappropriate as opinions and subsequent advice *within* the medical profession often differ greatly. To achieve these objectives we need ever more precise definitions of pathological processes, co-morbidity and other secondary factors, and of the relative chances of benefit or possible adverse events associated with the chosen therapy. In addition, knowledge of the extent by which the proposed management will drain the resources available is required.

The service

Every society worth its salt desires the best possible care for its members. One yardstick of society itself is the relative value it places on this welfare and the provision it is able to make to achieve that end, and the relative expenditure of the wealth of the society on vital areas such as defence, education and health is a continual source of debate.

Within the National Health Service there will always be need for an increase in resource. The gap between the reasonable expectations of the patient and the ability of the service to provide those expectations widens inexorably year by year (Thwaites 1987, 1988) (Fig. 13.1). The growing realization of this fundamental problem has produced a positive response through 'resource management'. How successful this strategy will prove however in coping with this gap remains to be seen.

Integral to optimal utilization of limited resources are meaningful costings of the many components of health care. This is clearly both an enormous and an extremely complex task. Health care provision for all, regardless of cost, is a recipe for disaster. At the inception of the NHS, some believed that the institution of a universally available health care service would make disease go away. They argued, as a result, that the relative cost of the service would gradually diminish! The folly of such a dream can be seen all too clearly today as the population lives longer to suffer ever more expensive incapacities with old age. These conditions are usually more expensive to treat and carry with them an ever diminishing chance of cure. Too little has, as yet, been done to define accurately just what *can* be achieved in this field, where palliation is the sole objective. It therefore becomes impossible realistically to inform the patient and relatives what any proposed management truly has to offer. In parallel with

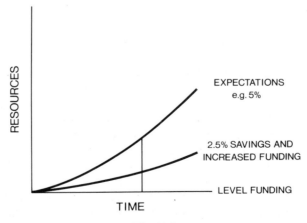

Fig. 13.1

this need to inform the patient meaningfully is the equally important need for realistic costings. The service can never otherwise be managed in an efficient or 'businesslike' way. Emotive and illogical responses abound to these problems. Objectors to the development of a cost-conscious, yet caring, service demand things of society which they do not expect of their own behaviour! In an eloquent demonstration of such ambivalence, Roberts (1982) demonstrated that the 'acceptable level of risk' relating to voluntary (and therefore presumably pleasurable) activities such as hazardous sporting activities, or indeed smoking, was an order of magnitude greater than that which was demanded from the health system. One example he quoted was the demand by patients for skull X-rays, over and above competent clinical examination, following head injury. This expectation is present even though the relative statistical benefit is minimal compared with the risks involved in the events which caused the head injury in the first place. It may well be 'right' that such different standards should exist, but surely not simply as a result of ignorance. In surgical practice, the reassessment of the need for routine preoperative chest X-rays in fit young adults is one sign of improved resource management based on knowledge of the actual, rather than imagined, risk. Progress in these areas can only be achieved by meaningful audit.

We therefore have a pressing need to quantify more precisely just what the service *can* provide, and *how much* each component of that care will cost. In this way alone can reasoned and reasonable decisions be made.

The agent—education and training

There are few who enter into a career in surgery without the desire to excel. The unique attraction of this specialty lies not, as in the biased, and possibly envious, opinion of many outside the specialty, merely in the fundamental 'craft' aspects. Equally as important and challenging are the decisions regarding the many differing options, both conservative and operative, and also the timing of any intervention. Indeed it is probably true that the most difficult decisions in surgery are related to the decision *not* to operate!

With the inevitable, and desirable, progression towards specialization, and nowadays even super-specialization, the surgeon may learn fewer operative procedures than his predecessors, though these include techniques that may be far more complex. The demise of 'general' surgery has been bemoaned for some time, yet is the 'speciality' less challenging than the generality? Surely the converse is true, as the most critical challenges within any specialty more often reside in areas of 'judgement' rather than technique alone. More than one famous teacher has emphasized the pre-eminent importance of this (J. Burke, 1990, personal communication). Rushing headlong into an inappropriate operation, with disastrous consequences for patient and relatives, remains too common a problem.

The value of experience, inevitably hard won, is usually underestimated by initiates full of their imagined technical prowess. Humility sits uncomfortably on some shoulders!

The recognition of the importance in certain areas of surgical practice of 'supratentorial' aspects of a patient's symptoms highlights particular problems within a hard pressed service. Too often it is heard that the clinician can only give so many minutes of his time to each patient in his clinic. Often twice as much time is allowed for similar patients in the more 'civilized' environment of private practice. Although some of this extra time is spent on 'courtesies' which may have little bearing on clinical outcome, it is nevertheless germane to examine the clinical and economic consequences, as well as the effects on both professional and patient satisfaction, of underallocation of time to each patient within the clinic.

There are few patients who are totally relaxed, and thus fully communicative, within the first few minutes of an interview with 'the man in the white coat'. A too cursory history, devoid of the educated, sensitive probing of the expert clinician, commonly leads to a totally undesirable sequence of events. Managerial ineptitude of this ilk usually escapes the attention of nursing staff and administrators. The educational disincentive to junior medical staff, however, is incalculable. Too often the interests of the latter are more attuned to self-preservation than to critical evaluation of management policies. Instead of patient, sensitive and detailed discourse with the patient and his relatives, giving due notice to their intelligence and sensibilities, a cursory history is taken and an inadequate examination is performed. Inexorably this leads to unnecessary, expensive and possibly hazardous investigations. This rushed and uncritical 'processing' of the patient may achieve a high 'throughput' within the clinic, but to what avail? In truth, it constitutes a potent waste of limited resources and imposes inconvenience and possible danger on the unfortunate patient. The prime function of the consultant is to consult! Why else his years of training and experience? It is at this level that the choice or appropriateness of possible management pathways must be made. When will it be fully appreciated by those responsible for the NHS that it is *highly cost-effective*, as well as professionally satisfying, to 'get it right' first time?

A typical example of the potential dangers of overemphasis on the commercial aspects of providing a 'market service' without requisite safeguards, lies in the apparently serious recent suggestion that varicose veins operations should be put out to competitive tender by competing hospitals or units. On the basis of such 'pricing' arrangements general practitioners would then be asked to choose where to send their patient. Not every family practitioner may wish to decide which of support stockings, bed rest, injection sclerotherapy, sapheno-femoral disconnection, avulsions, ligations or 'stripping' procedures, (or even no treatment at all), is the most appropriate management for an individual patient! If such be true of a common, 'simple' condition such as varicose veins, how much more of an intolerable burden would be placed on our general practitioner colleagues in more complex situations? Within the speciality of gastroenterology, the development of joint medical and surgical clinics during the last 20 years is fulsome testament to the *absolute* necessity of obtaining the greatest breadth, as well as depth, of expertise and experience at the *earliest* opportunity in the management of complex clinical problems.

It is clear, therefore, that it is in the interest of every practitioner to document, and then evaluate critically, each aspect of his practice in which, through thought and experience, he places credence. It is up to him to be able to defend these practices, not only in terms of clinical efficacy, but also

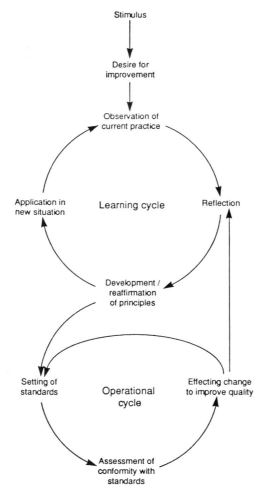

Fig. 13.2 Integration of learning and audit cycles. Reproduced with permission from Batstone 1990.

in the utilization of limited resources. He will prove an indifferent advocate at the best if he bases his case on 'emotive' arguments, potent though they often seem! At the end of the day, facts must be the substance of his case. Without them he deserves little sympathy, and will surely never reach the Aristotelian goal. This objective can only be achieved by peer review as described below.

In a recent review by Batstone (1990) the fundamental educational nature of audit has been forcibly re-emphasized. Figure 13.2 shows the complex inter-relationship between the components of audit, education and clinical performance.

HOW?

Audit, surveillance and decision analysis

The quality of decision making is proportional to the quality of the information available. Although lip service is often given to this fact, optimal data to enable value judgement are seldom obtained. In this section some of the common pitfalls are examined.

Many important items of information are readily available to hospital management. Staffing levels, bed availability and occupancy, operating theatre time and usage (National Audit Office 1987, HMSO 1989b, Wyatt et al 1990, Young 1990), patient throughput, outpatient clinic usage, and waiting lists are examples that are already at management's fingertips. However, as already stressed, the information that is required to assess how *good*, as opposed to how busy, a service is, is usually totally lacking. Without knowledge of the quality of clinical decision making, and the clinical outcome of such decision making, any assessment of the quality of the service is illusory. In the present financial climate within the NHS many vital decisions are taken in ignorance of this critical information. With the pressure to introduce 'market forces' into the NHS with the White Paper 'Working for Patients' (HMSO 1989) managers are being forced into taking 'best guess' decisions; often there can be very little of the 'best' about the guess! Who, if anyone, is to blame for this dangerous state of affairs? The medical profession itself, by and large, has failed to meet the requirements outlined above. Therefore many important battles are lost by default. It is too facile to blame 'management' for these problems, as, in most cases, they have not created them! Attempts to develop common strategies and programmes jointly between the profession and the management are vitally needed.

A common approach

The way forward must be for medical, nursing and, indeed, all health care professionals to work *with* management. In this way alone can we hope to achieve the common goal of 'optimal' utilization of limited resources. Simultaneously, every effort to increase resources must also be made to narrow the 'expectation gap'.

What, however, constitutes 'optimal' in this context? The age old dilemma of choice between reasonable standards of care for the majority, or high-cost intensive care for a few, has to be faced at many levels and in many situations. Controversies over what exactly constitute 'acceptable' levels of risk in different situations has been eloquently expounded by Roberts (1982). It is clear that in such matters professional statistical and economic advice is crucial to sensible decision-making.

When reasonable targets have been determined, it is then essential to establish means of obtaining data which are:

1. Relevant,
2. Accurate and standardized,
3. Complete (in so far as is possible),
4. Confidential.

If these criteria are agreed, how should they be obtained?

Audit or surveillance

The term 'audit' is nowadays used widely. However, 'audit' means different things to different people. Not only does it refer to matters economic, but is now increasingly used in clinical contexts. This is, of course, entirely welcome, provided the potential limitations of any system evolved for providing critical information are appreciated.

The term 'surveillance' is, in many situations we believe, a far more useful word, in that it conveys concepts of greater importance. High-quality surveillance programmes are capable of providing the best information base for decision-making (i.e. 'decision analysis').

Audit is an activity assessment within a given period of time. This can be as short or as long as desired. The purpose, generally, is to obtain the maximum amount of relevant information to aid decision-making processes. These may be relevant either to maintenance or improvement in the service under audit. Relevant information may relate to recruitment and/or throughput, i.e. 'process'. Further audits may assess the 'unit' cost of items such as the management of the 'average' patient or of particular procedures or services. Within broad guidelines these may be helpful in assessing and even comparing relative performances. Such aspects of audit are already well understood by management and need no further emphasis here.

However, in recent years, more attention has been paid to the *clinical* aspects of audit. Herein lie several problems which are still unfortunately often poorly perceived. Most audits of this type are *retrospective* and, as such they rely, firstly, on the availability of records. As all investigators know this is far from universally satisfactory! Secondly, contained within these records, it is vital that the *relevant* information is recorded accurately. Absence of information, or inaccuracy or incompleteness of that which is recorded, all vitiate the purpose of audit. The limited usefulness of most medical records for these purposes is well known, particularly to those with medico-legal experience!

However, one positive thing that can be said about such retrospective reviews is that the *minimum* level of any problem is usually established. Such information can prove extremely valuable. For example, approximately 80% of information regarding major events such as death and anastomotic complications can usually be retrieved. This information may be sufficient to change clinical practice. In a recent survey of major complications following re-anastomosis after emergency (Hartmann's) resection of the sigmoid colon undertaken over the previous 10 years in Southampton (Pearce & Karran 1989), it was conclusively demonstrated that delaying the second procedure for at least six months conferred a highly significant reduction of mortality and morbidity.

By contrast, a recent study undertaken by the Public Health Laboratory Services (H. Glennister, 1989, personal communication) to determine the incidence of wound and other complications showed that less than 30% of all such events were recorded in either the nursing or medical records. Such an incomplete data base makes nonsense of any attempts to evaluate the clinical outcome of, for example, patients undergoing 'short stay' surgery (i.e. hospitalized for less than two days) by performing 'audit' based on medical records alone. Our own surveillance programme, in which all 'clean' surgery has been followed up within the community by research nurses, has shown that over 70% of all wound complications occur *after* discharge from the surgical ward. These studies were undertaken in an attempt to extend the pioneering work of Cruse (1980), Birnbaum (1984) and others from North America. For many years such workers have recognized the crucial importance of a properly structured, relevant, sensitive and specific programme. Data produced by such programmes are accurate. As yet in the UK, hospital managements generally remain to be convinced of the necessity of establishing permanent programmes of this sort, which not only confer benefit to patients, but also avoid considerable wastage of limited resources. It is our belief that *no* surgical unit in future should be allowed to function *unless* it is capable of producing accurate and relevant data of the true clinical outcome of the patients for which it has been responsible. It is, surely, the right of every patient and his relatives to be given meaningful information regarding the various risks of proposed operative or other therapeutic strategies.

The essence of surveillance, therefore, is that of *continuous* prospective 'audit', with careful documentation of *all* relevant events. In this context, it is important to emphasize that successes, as well as failures, should be discussed, as these may prove to be every bit as educational. The same applies to 'near misses'! In this way the vital necessity of 'closing the feedback loop' (Smith 1990) can be achieved. In virtually all of our own 'audit' studies, the stimulus to critical self-examination itself has produced improvements in performance (the well known 'Hawthorne effect'). This is almost certainly the result of greater care and attention to detail, particularly in matters of technique such as prevention of haematoma formation. Dramatic benefits such as a threefold reduction in avoidable complications have been documented (Karran et al 1987, Royal College of Surgeons of England 1989, Shaw & Costain 1989). Indeed, in some clinical areas the establishment of critical surveillance by a dedicated team, such as the Southampton Nutrition Team, has achieved even more dramatic benefits within three months of its inception (Royce et al 1985), producing savings far greater than the cost of supporting the team.

The critical difference between audit, performed on a once and for all basis, and an effective ongoing surveillance programme, as so elegantly demonstrated by Birnbaum (1981, 1984) and others from North America, is that a surveillance programme is capable not only of detecting important improvements, but that these improvements invariably pay many times over for the investment in the programme itself (Haley et al 1981, 1986, Haley 1985, Beyt et al 1985, Mead et al 1986, Reimer et al 1987, Rosendorf et al 1983). Deterioration in the service is invariably detected at an *early* stage, the cause of the problem is usually readily identified and can therefore be rapidly corrected. Serious wastage of vital resources is thus avoided (de la Hunt et al 1986).

Data collection

There are important criteria for clinical data collection, not only for scientific validity, but in many clinical situations, for ethical and professional reasons also. Firstly, it is *essential* that the critical primary data must be collected by persons with the appropriate professional training. For example, wound assessment on our unit is made by trained audit nurses or members of the surgical team. Secondly, once collected, such data must be *verified* through the process of confidential peer review. Only then should they be submitted to analysis. Computerization is clearly of great value at this stage and with the institution of a system with the relevant safeguards of confidentiality, trends can be rapidly identified and appropriate action instituted at an early stage.

Decision analysis—expert systems

The prime function of any audit/surveillance programme must be *educational*, and as already stressed, the *quality* of data available to the primary health care team is of paramount importance. Decision analysis is a tool which has been 'borrowed' from industry to ensure optimal utilization of resources (Nettleman 1990). The key feature of this process is the determination of the quality of the data which is compared with the 'gold standard' of an 'expert system'. An example of the latter in our own experience is the community surveillance programme conducted by trained independent audit nurses who are responsible for feeding back accurate, complete data to the surgical team at the next morbidity/mortality meeting. An expert system is capable of high *sensitivity*, i.e. it 'misses' few, if any, events which are relevant. It must be appreciated, however, that some events, by their very nature (e.g. late complications) fall outwith of any 'one-off' audit programme. These events should eventually be detected by a permanent, carefully designed surveillance programme.

The 'expert system', by its very design, is also capable of achieving high *specificity*, that is it identifies problems which are *genuine* events, and are, therefore, not 'false positives'.

With the high sensitivity and also specificity that such systems can obtain, the consequent overall accuracy and positive predictive value provide the *only* valid means for ensuring reliable decision analysis.

Any audit system proposed *must* be validated against the appropriate current gold standard 'expert system'. It must also be revalidated if, subsequently, an improved 'gold standard' is developed. Audit systems which have not undergone such validation are a waste of valuable resource in themselves, and, more seriously, are highly likely to produce spurious results. The clinician, together with his managerial and professional colleagues, is misled, and the health care provided is thus endangered.

Setting up an audit/surveillance programme

Some of the major practicalities in developing programmes capable of producing meaningful decision analysis are described below (Karran 1988).

Responsibility for development and maintenance of the programme

This responsibility clearly must be that of the senior medical staff. If *they* fail to establish the correct attitudes, ethos and logistic support, any programme is doomed.

Regular surveillance/audit meetings

These must be held *within normal working hours* at fixed, regular times. Depending on the amount of information to be discussed, a meeting held every two weeks is reasonable, though many units have found weekly meetings useful. Meetings which are held less frequently lose value, partly as a result of difficulties of staff remembering important details.

Ethos of meeting

Again, this is the responsibility of the senior medical staff. The whole intention of any audit meeting must be *educational*, not punitive. Even a suspicion of 'witch hunting' inhibits truthfulness—and not only on the part of junior staff! The consequence of a lack of honesty can be disastrous, and obviates the educational intent and content of the meeting. Provision of coffee also helps!

Confidentiality

Every patient and topic discussed must be treated with *total* confidentiality by all present. It is essential to emphasize this to any students or occasional visitors invited to the meeting. Data must be 'depersonalized' as soon as possible before inclusion in any analysis or report. Care must be taken that after the meeting no confidential documents are left lying around but are gathered and kept in a secure place. Failure to preserve confidentiality has led to disastrous consequences especially in North America due to attempts at litigation. In most countries, however, the overriding need for collection of accurate confidential data is protected by statute. In this way the vital professional necessity of achieving meaningful audit can be ensured.

Attendance

This should be compulsory to *all* members of the surgical staff. In our experience the attendance of our ward and theatre nursing staff enhances the value of such meetings considerably, and confidentiality has not proved a problem to us, though serious breaches of confidence have been reported (Meeting on surgical audit, Royal College of Surgeons of England, London, December 1988).

Data collection

This clearly must be a *team effort* involving medical, nursing, and other professional staff where relevant. In our experience over the last six years, the completeness and objectivity of the data presented for discussion by the surgical team have been greatly enhanced since the appointment of dedicated audit nurses. Their task is simplified by the use of standard record forms (see Appendix at the end of the chapter). Medical staff, by and large, have considerable and genuine difficulties in recording all data which may prove relevant, even with the help of 'aids' such as 'complications books' kept on the ward or in theatre. In addition, they never, of course, actually see a large proportion of the significant postoperative events, particularly those occurring in 'short-stay' patients. The study by Bird (1988) showed convincingly that 'audit' nurses can prove highly cost-effective to the NHS by stimulating improved performance 'across the board' through rapid closing of the 'feed-back loop'. As stated above, it is our conviction that such a member of staff will become vitally necessary in the future to achieve the highest quality of surgical practice.

Computers and computer analysis

It is by deliberate intent that no more than a passing reference to computers or computer assistants has been made so far! Their merit in handling and analysing *verified* information is known too well. Many excellent computer systems have already been developed (Dunn 1988, Ellis et al 1987) to assist the audit/surveillance process. Yet the commonest, and possibly most serious, mistake of all who become interested in clinical audit, is the assumption that meaningful audit will automatically follow acquisition of computer assistance. The aphorism about the quality of 'data in and data out' is too well known to repeat, but how often is it actually heeded? One must beware of the assumption that the mere provision of computerized facilities means that satisfactory audit programmes are 'in situ'. Funds are now being widely released throughout the NHS to facilitate audit. What proportion of these vital resources, however, will actually end up being spent in fruitful ways remains to be seen! Or will the audit be audited effectively?

Funding

Meaningful clinical audit and surveillance programmes require *permanent* funding. Of particular importance for each unit is the salary for a trained professional member of staff (e.g. an audit sister) whose function is to collect and collate accurate and complete primary data and present them for peer group discussion and analysis. Such an appointment is not only highly beneficial to patient welfare, and thus to professional morale, but is also *highly cost-effective.*

Secondary to this basic vital requirement must be the provision of appropriate secretarial and computer assistance. Investment in these latter components, however, *without* securing the former will almost certainly result in acquisition of false or incomplete data. False judgements will follow, resulting in an impoverished health service.

CRITICAL QUESTIONS

1. In the light of current knowledge and technology what is the optimum that can be achieved for each individual patient?
2. What are the inevitable, or at least the probable, costs (e.g. inconvenience, risk and financial) of both investigations and treatment to the patient and his relatives?
3. Can we achieve, or closely approximate, optimal benefits and costs in *this* unit? If not, are there alternatives, e.g. further specialist referral?
4. Do we know, with any degree of accuracy, the chances of achieving, or not achieving, optimal results. Conversely, what are the actual chances of an adverse outcome? i.e. do we have *accurate* local 'audit' data?

5. Do we know how much the proposed course of action will cost our health care service—or, indeed, in the new market approach, how much funding might it attract?

CRITICAL CRITERIA FOR 'AUDIT'

1. Honesty!
2. Education not punishment
3. Relevance
4. Objectivity
5. Reproducibility
6. Completeness
7. Confidentiality
8. Appropriate professional qualifications essential for primary data collection

REFERENCES

Batstone G F 1990 Educational aspects of medical audit. Br Med J 301: 326–328

Bird S 1988 Surgical surveillance—clinical and financial implications. IVth Year Study in Depth, University of Southampton

Birnbaum D 1981 Risk management vs infection control committees. Dimensions 58 (12): 16–19

Birnbaum D 1984 Analysis of hospital infection surveillance data. Infect Control 5 (7): 332–338

Beyt B E, Troxler S, Cavaness J 1985 Prospective payment and infection control. Infect Control 6 (4): 161–164

Cruse P J E 1980 Surgical infection surveillance. In Karran S J (ed) Controversies in surgical sepsis. Praeger, Eastbourne, pp 327–332

de la Hunt M N, Chan Y C, Karran S J 1986 Postoperative complications: how much do they cost? Ann R Coll Surg 68: 199–202

Dunn D C 1988 Audit of a surgical firm by microcomputer: five years' experience. Br Med J 296: 687–691

Ellis B W, Michie H R, Esufali S T et al 1987 Development of a microcomputer-based system for surgical audit and patient administration: a review. J R Soc Med 80: 157–161

Haley R 1985 Infection control strategies save $250,000. Hospitals 59 (22): 63–65

Haley R W, Schaberg D R, Crossley K B et al 1981 Extra charges due to prolongation of stay attributable to nosocomial infections: a prospective interhospital comparison. Am J Med 70: 51–58

Haley R W, Culver D H, White J W et al 1986 The efficiency of infection surveillance and control programmes in preventing nosocomial infections in US hospitals. Am J Epidemiol 12 (2): 182–205

HMSO 1989 Working for patients. Medical Audit Working Paper 6. London (CMND 55)

HMSO 1989a Working for patients: The Health Service, caring for the 1990s. London

HMSO 1989b The management and utilisation of operating departments. NHS Management Executive. London

Karran S J 1988 Recommendations of the Wessex Working Party for Quality Assurance and Audit in Surgical Practice

Karran S J, Toyn K, Karran S E 1987 Community surveillance—should we in future operate without it? Paper presented at International Symposium on Sepsis in Surgery, Postgraduate Medical Federation, Vienna, October 1987

Mead P B, Porles S E, Hall P et al 1986 Decreasing the incidence of surgical wound infections. Validation of a surveillance notification programme. Arch Surg 121 (4): 458–461

National Audit Office 1987 The use of operating theatres in the National Health Service. HMSO, London

Nettleman M 1990 Use of decision analysis in preventing nosocomial infections. Proceedings of the 1st International Conference on the Prevention of Infection. Nice, May 1990, p 53

Pearce N, Karran S J 1989 Hartmann's reversal—when and how? Gut 30 (10): A1470

Reimer K, Gleed C, Nicolle L E 1987 The impact of postdischarge infection on surgical wound infection rates. Infect Control 8 (6): 237–240

Roberts C J 1982 Medical care as a risk-avoidance procedure: underwriting the cost of care in the UK. Br Med J 285: 751–755

Rosendorf L F, Octavio J, Estes J P 1983 Effects of methods of post discharge wound infection surveillance on reported infection rates. Am J Infect Control 11 (6): 226–229

Royal College of Surgeons of England 1989 Guidelines to clinical audit in surgical practice. Royal College of Surgeons of England, London

Royce C, de la Hunt M, Taylor M, Walker E, Karran S J 1985 Central venous access for nutritional support—initial experience of a nutrition team. Ann R Coll Surg Engl 67: 197

Shaw C D, Costain D W 1989 Guidelines for medical audit: seven principles. Br Med J 299: 498–499

Smith A 1990 Medical audit—closing the feedback loop is vital. Br Med J 300: 65

Thwaites B 1987 The N.H.S.: the end of the rainbow. Foundation Lecture, University of Southampton, 27th May. Institute of Health Policy Studies, 1987

Thwaites B 1988 The grand dilemmas of a National Health Service. Keynote Lecture, University of Leeds. Nuffield Institute for Health Service Studies, Leeds

Wyatt M G, Houghton P W J, Brodribb A M J 1990 Theatre delay for emergency general surgical patients: a cause for concern? Ann R Coll Surg Engl 72: 236–238

Young A 1990 The empty theatre. Br Med J 300: 1289–1290

FURTHER READING

Pollock A, Evans M 1989 Surgical audit. Butterworths, Guildford

APPENDIX

POSTOPERATIVE ASSESSMENT

Patient	*Date of assessment:*
Name	Consultant...
DOB	Hospital..
Address	Surgeon..
....	Date of operation ....
GP	Operation ....

Date of removal of sutures:

(A) WOUND   Please tick
(1) No problems   ☐

(2) Minor problems

    1) Inflamed
                a) at one point only.. ☐
                b) at suture points .... ☐
                c) along length of wound .... ☐
                d) area around wound .... ☐

    2) Discharge
       (clear or haemoserous)   a) at one point only or small volume (< 2 ml) ☐
                           b) extensive, prolonged or large volume (> 2 ml) ☐

    3) Bruising   mild or moderate ☐

    4) Suture problems   e.g. difficult removal (please specify) ☐

    5) Other
       (please specify).. ☐

(3) Major problems

    1) Extensive cellulitis   ☐
    2) Extensive bruising   ☐
    3) Pus   a) one area only, small vol (> 2 ml) ☐
                       b) extensive, prolonged or large volume (> 2 ml) ☐

    4) Deep or severe infection
       or wound breakdown   ☐

    5) Other..
       (please specify)..

(4) Drugs (e.g. antibiotics) prescribed   ☐
    (please specify)..

Contd over ...

235

(B) OTHER POSTOPERATIVE COMPLICATIONS (please specify)

(1)

(2)

(3)

(4)

(5)

14

A review of recent advances in general surgery

I. Taylor

In this selected review of General Surgery during 1989 topics of general interest related to gastroenterology (both upper and lower), pancreatico-biliary, hepatic and breast surgery will be discussed. Emphasis is placed on those aspects which are likely to have direct significance in patient management.

UPPER GASTROINTESTINAL SURGERY

Oesophagus

The treatment of reflux oesophagitis is initially medical. In a trial of 162 patients with endoscopically proven reflux oesophagitis, omeprazole was more effective than ranitidine in the relief of major symptoms such as heartburn, regurgitation and dysphagia (Hoffman & Rasmussen 1989).

When medical measures fail then surgery may be required. Several procedures have been described and subjected to prospective study. Deakin et al (1989) found similar results at 2 years with Nissen fundoplication and the Angelchik prosthesis. Taylor et al (1989) report favourable results with the new technique of vertical gastric plication but further assessment is required.

The management of peptic oesophageal stricture has always been controversial. The combination of endoscopic dilatation and anti-reflux medication is advocated by Hands et al (1989) and excellent results are reported. Alternative methods of dealing with stricture include dilatation with balloons (Grundy & Belli 1988) and for achalasia, forceful pneumatic dilatation using the Mosher bag (Csendes et al 1989).

Resection offers the only hope of cure for patients with oesophageal cancer. In order to achieve good results careful surgical technique is essential. In two studies from Hong Kong the cause of leakage was analysed (Paterson & Wong 1989, Lorentz T et al 1989) and appeared to be chiefly related to ischaemia of the oesophageal substitute. Gastric reconstruction was regarded as the procedure of choice. There is also increasing interest in the use of stapling instruments for construction of the anastomosis. Walther et al (1989) have utilized linear stapling techniques and Brough &

Tweedle (1989) described a new technique with a curved circular stapler with detachable head.

Gastro-duodenal surgery

In England and Wales, bleeding and perforation account for 4500 deaths annually. Taylor (1989) recommends ulcer surgery for those patients who frequently relapse on maintenance therapy, those who relapse early after three or more two-monthly courses of these drugs and for those who have relapsed after three or more courses of the drug at or about the age of 50.

Certainly elective ulcer surgery is safe with a mortality of 0.15–0.3%. Recently anterior lesser curvature seromyotomy has been advocated as a simple and effective procedure. In an animal study Hunter et al (1989) have used an Argon laser to perform the technique with significant acid reduction.

The prognosis associated with massive upper gastrointestinal haemorrhage from peptic ulceration is still poor with mortality rates of over 20%. Several attempts have been made to produce prognostic scores for the recognition of 'high-risk' patients. One such study utilized the APACHE II scoring system in 96 patients undergoing surgery for gastric ulcers and 58 for duodenal ulcers (Schein & Gecelter 1989). None of the patients with a score less than 11 died whereas the mortality rate for those who scored greater than 10 was 22%. It is probable, however, that most surgeons will rely more upon their own experience and expertise than being confined by a prognostic score.

Surgeons should be aware of the increasing availability of non-operative procedures for the management of bleeding peptic ulcer. Two randomized trials deserve comment. Rutgeerts et al (1989) randomized 140 patients with bleeding peptic ulceration into three endoscopic treatments; adrenalin alone, adrenalin plus 1% polidocanol, and adrenalin followed by YAG photocoagulation. The efficacy of all three treatments was enhanced by repeated application.

Injection with adrenalin and polidocanol was as effective as and cheaper than laser treatment and easier to use. It should be noted that seven patients required emergency surgery despite endoscopic treatment. The overall mortality was 8.6% including two deaths due to bleeding. Lin et al (1988) have found that heat probe thermocoagulation was more effective than local injection of pure alcohol whereas Nakagawa et al (1989) favour the latter. Clearly all these techniques depend very much upon the expertise and enthusiasm of the individual but nevertheless provide an important alternative to major surgery in patients with actively bleeding ulceration.

Despite the advent of H_2 receptor antagonists the incidence of perforated duodenal ulcer has not significantly reduced and is still associated with a high post-operative mortality, particularly in patients over 70 years old

(Ball et al 1989). Irvin has reported a 34% mortality in this group and particular risk factors include delayed presentation and concurrent medical illness. These figures would suggest that non-operative treatment should be considered in selected patients. Berne & Donovan (1989) have, once again, advocated such a policy providing a gastroduodenogram suggests self-sealing. In their selected series of 35 patients, mortality was 3% and only one patient developed an intra-abdominal abscess. Conservative treatment consists of antibiotics, nasogastric aspiration, intravenous fluids and H_2 blockers.

Gastric cancer still remains a most depressing disease to treat. Allum et al (1989a) have reviewed the results of gastric cancer treatment in the West Midlands between 1957 and 1981. It is particularly sad that the stage at diagnosis has remained constant with 79% of patients having Stage IV disease whereas less than 1% had Stage I disease. The curative resection rate remains at 21% and operative mortality rates for partial and total gastrectomy are 13% and 29%, respectively. Overall 5 year survival was 5% at 5 years although 72% survived 5 years with Stage I disease. This emphasizes once again the importance of early diagnosis and treatment in this condition. For example, Percivale et al (1989) have reported a long term follow-up study of 54 patients with early gastric cancer treated by sub-total gastrectomy and report age-corrected 5- and 10-year survival rates of 95.7% and 84.3%, respectively. The authors stress the need for accurate lymph node dissection. It should also be noted that adjuvant chemotherapy has not demonstrated a survival advantage in operable gastric cancer. In one recent study (Allum et al 1989b) of 5FU and mitomycin C in 411 patients no benefit was demonstrated and toxicity was significant.

LOWER GASTROINTESTINAL SURGERY

Inflammatory bowel disease

Restorative proctocolectomy with ileo-anal anastomosis is becoming increasingly popular for ulcerative colitis (and familial polyposis coli). Technical advances have meant that it is becoming a less demanding technical procedure. The pouch-anal anastomosis can now be completed entirely with the ingenious use of staples—both linear and circular (Williams 1989, Brough & Schofield 1989, Kmiot & Keighley 1989). This ensures that the median operating time in experienced hands is about two and a half hours. Nevertheless, it still remains a procedure where selection is most important and even in the most experienced hands post-operative complications can be serious.

Long-term clinical and functional results of this procedure are now becoming available. Oresland et al (1989) have published results in a hundred consecutive patients treated by ileo-anal anastomosis and a J- or

S-shaped reservoir. There was a re-laparotomy rate of 14% for complications (sepsis, fistula and obstruction). Stool frequency stabilized at about 5 evacuations per 24 hours at 1 year, although 40% had night evacuations. Other problems included mucous leakage, sexual disturbances (8%) and dyspareunia. Patient satisfaction was reported as high and only three patients preferred conversion to an ileostomy. In addition, the cumulative risk of pouchitis was 30% at 2 years.

The problem of pouchitis or non-specific ileitis is clearly a serious accompaniment of restorative surgery in ulcerative colitis. There have been many suggestions as to its aetiology but it clearly results in a good deal of morbidity. It is most likely to be the result of an abnormal host response to the underlying pathogenesis of ulcerative colitis.

The epidemiology of inflammatory bowel disease is of great interest in our understanding of the aetiology of these conditions and particularly their relationship to subsequent malignancy. Two excellent review articles have addressed this latter problem (Cola 1989, Fozard & Dixon 1989). The conclusions of both are similar. In patients with long-standing total colitis, colonoscopic surveillance is necessary and the appearance of severe dysplasia is an indication for surgery. It should also be noted that as a result of asymptomatic population screening for colorectal cancer, the prevalence of inflammatory bowel disease has been found to be about 56 per 100 000. This figure suggests that traditional studies have underestimated the true prevalence by about 30% (Mayberry et al 1989).

Crohn's disease is characterized by a high incidence of recurrence. The risk of recurrence and re-operation has been investigated in a careful study from Holland (Shivananda et al 1989). Two-hundred and ten patients were followed up after surgical resection. Life table analysis showed that after 10 years 17% required further resection for recurrence and 8% for relapse. By 20 years the rate of recurrence had risen to 56%. An intriguing study from Cardiff (Williams & Hughes 1989) has suggested, albeit on retrospective data, that the incidence of recurrence in Crohn's disease may be reduced in patients who received a peri-operative blood transfusion. Five years after bowel resection the cumulative recurrence rate in transfused patients was 19% compared with 59% in controls.

In Crohn's disease those patients with short fibrous strictures may benefit from strictureplasty. However, the lesions are often multiple and the procedure may need to be repeated. Dehn et al (1989) from Oxford and Sayfan et al (1989) from Birmingham have discussed their experiences with this technique. In selected patients it is of value and can be carried out safely. It is an alternative to wide or multiple resections and should be considered.

Other complications of Crohn's disease require surgical intervention but the timing and type of procedure may be difficult to determine. Enterovesical fistulas can occasionally be managed conservatively but Heyen et al (1989) in reporting the experience from Birmingham favour resection of symptomatic fistulas with primary anastomosis if possible. Most would agree that the bladder defect should be closed over an indwelling catheter which should not be removed until there is radiological confirmation of satisfactory healing. Greenstein (1988) in reviewing the indications for repeated surgery in Crohn's disease observed that operations for perforation were followed by re-operation approximately twice as quickly as operations for non-perforating indications.

Two final therapeutic points require comment in the management of Crohn's disease. In patients with painful anal Crohn's in which there is no evidence of sepsis but deep cavitating ulceration, local depot methyl prednisolone injection may be beneficial and is worth trying (Hughes 1988). The benefit of pre-operative total parenteral nutrition in patients with severe Crohn's disease has been evaluated in 67 patients with serious complications, such as fistulas or obstruction (Gouma 1989). Spontaneous closure of fistulas was achieved in 75% of patients and mean body weights improved. Although it is expensive, such a regimen may provide significant advantage to patients with active Crohn's.

Cancer

Diagnosis

Increasing interest surrounds the concept of screening. Hardcastle et al (1989) and Pye et al (1989) have reviewed critically the present position of colorectal cancer screening and indicate most of the difficulties and pitfalls. Haemoccult has a positive predictive value for invasive cancer of 11–17% and for adenomas 36–41%. This specificity is achieved, however, at a loss of sensitivity, the interval cancer rate reported in screening studies being over 20%. In the Nottingham study (Hardcastle et al 1989) of 107 346 asymptomatic individuals, 2.3% of test subjects were positive and 63 cancers were detected (52% Stage A) as well as 367 adenomas. Only 10.6% of cancers in the control group were Dukes A. These are promising data but it is still too early to show any effect of screening on mortality in colorectal cancer. It is unlikely that a more specific test, such as an immunological one, will be more effective since Pye et al (1989) have shown that an increase in specificity is associated with a fall in sensitivity with a resulting enormous increase in laboratory work load. Other screening tests which have been evaluated include self-administration ('DIY') tests (Tate et al 1989). However, these are most unreliable with an unacceptable specificity.

Factors affecting prognosis and the accurate prediction of prognosis in colorectal cancer have attracted a good deal of attention in the last year. The influence of age on survival after curative resection has been investigated by Svendsen et al (1989). In a multivariate analysis of 1623 consecutive patients, Dukes C stage, poor differentiation and age between 40–60 years reached independent prognostic significance. This age group had a poorer prognosis than other groups despite the fact that younger patients had more advanced tumours. Other groups have utilized similar multivariate analyses to identify specific prognostic features. Domergue et al (1989) in 208 patients with rectal cancer identified lymph node status, tumour infiltration, histological type and pre-operative radiotherapy. Barillari et al (1989) in 571 patients with colorectal cancer looked specifically at symptom duration and survival but did not find any relationship between the duration of intestinal symptoms and stage or prognosis of colorectal cancer.

Peri-operative blood transfusion has also been investigated to determine whether it does indeed represent an independent prognostic factor. Vente et al (1989) in a study of 212 patients were unable to demonstrate such an effect but Stephenson et al (1988) found an adverse relationship between transfusion and survival in patients who had undergone resection of colorectal liver metastases. This is still a controversial topic and as yet the relationship between survival and transfusion is not proven. Prospective studies are required to resolve the dilemma. In an animal model, however, Carty et al (1989) were unable to determine a deleterious effect of syngeneic blood transfusion.

Two novel diagnostic techniques in colorectal cancer deserve mention. Rectal endosonography in rectal cancer is becoming increasingly widespread. It appears to be more accurate in staging local invasion pre-operatively than either digital examination or CT scans (Benyon 1989). In experienced hands it has an accuracy of over 80% in predicting mesorectal lymph node involvement (Benyon et al 1989) as well as definitive evidence of local extrarectal recurrence.

Radioimmunoscintigraphy has also attracted some recent attention. Anti-CEA monoclonal antibodies are most popular for this technique and Granowska et al (1989) have reported a prospective study using [III]In-labelled CEA in 23 patients with colorectal cancer. A sensitivity of 95% was found with an overall accuracy of 91%. Well and moderately-well differentiated tumours took up about four times more antibody than poorly differentiated tumours. This technique has yet to be of widespread value in the diagnosis of recurrent disease but the impetus is present for further studies.

The present status of tumour markers in large bowel cancer has been reviewed by Moore et al (1989). There is little doubt that with the progress in molecular analysis of colorectal cancer (Leading article 1989) constitutional genotypic markers are now being identified which may shortly be available as tumour specific markers and are likely to be far more useful than existing ones such as CEA and Ca 19-9.

Colonoscopic examination of the colon in patients with established colorectal cancer has been investigated in a study by Tate et al (1988). It would appear that early post-operative colonoscopy is likely to be most helpful in revealing small polyps.

Treatment

Treatment for colorectal cancer is predominantly surgical. The results of surgery alone, however, have not significantly improved the prognosis for this disease for many years. Nevertheless, surgery is now much safer and post-operative morbidity and mortality are reducing. Canivet et al (1989) have reviewed mortality in 476 patients operated on between 1973–1986. Operative mortality overall was 13.4%. However, this fell from 20.1% in 1973–1979 to 7.8% in 1980–1986. Specific risk factors were chronic obstructive airways disease, and previous myocardial infarction although age and emergency procedures were both important. The specific problem of obstruction has been investigated by Serpell et al (1989). There is no doubt that survival in patients presenting with obstruction is significantly worse than in non-obstructed patients. In this series, 5-year survival was 59.1% compared to 31.8% in obstructed patients (p < 0.001). This is probably in part related to the higher incidence of more advanced disease with far fewer Dukes' A lesions. Nevertheless, it would appear that completely obstructing colonic cancers are more aggressive than others. Malignant cells 'spilled' at surgery or in close proximity to a healing anastomosis or laparotomy scar have enhanced growth potential (Skipper et al 1989). This observation confirmed in an animal model has implications in emphasizing the need for surgeons to wash out the lumen of the bowel and the tumour bed, after surgical excision, with cytotoxic agents.

The question of adjuvant therapy of colorectal cancer is still under investigation and we still do not know whether it is beneficial. As Buyse et al (1988) point out, this is probably related in part to inadequate trials and insufficient patient numbers. Trials much larger than those published are required if adjuvant chemo- or radiotherapy are to be confirmed as being significantly beneficial. A meta-analysis of radiotherapy trials indicates that the incidence of local recurrence is reduced but this is not translated into unequivocal survival benefit. An example of this is the recent EORTC study (Gerard et al 1988) of 466 patients receiving pre-operative radiotherapy. Local recurrence rates at 5 years were 30% and 15% (p = 0.003), respectively, for control and radiotherapy. The effect was most marked in patients with locally advanced disease. However, 5-year survival rates were 59.1% and 69.1%, respectively, (p = 0.08). Levamisole, an immune stimulator has also been assessed as an adjuvant in colorectal cancer. Arnaud et al (1989) have reported the use of levamisole in 297 patients with Dukes' C colon cancer. The drug is well tolerated but no significant survival differences, or number of relapses were found in patients receiving levamisole compared to placebo. A most promising study reported by Moertel et al (1990) has demonstrated a survival benefit for patients with Dukes' C disease randomized to both 5FU and levamisole compared to surgery only or levamisole alone. Amazingly, the overall death rate was reduced by 33% (p = 0.006). They suggest that adjuvant therapy with levamisole and 5FU should be standard treatment for Dukes C carcinoma.

This year has seen an explosion of interest in the use of laser therapy in the management of colorectal cancer. In patients with advanced local disease who require palliation but are inoperable, Nd-YAG laser treatment has a role. Several studies have indicated a benefit (Krasner 1989, Mellow 1989, Brunetaud et al 1989) even for benign polypoid lesions. Laser combined with photodynamic therapy may enhance the response and has been suggested in addition for small tumours in the colon and rectum, anastomotic recurrences as well as dysplastic field changes (Barr et al 1989). One study, however, has suggested that although initial palliation can be achieved in over 80% of patients this is maintained in only 51% and 41% of patients surviving 6 months and 12 months, respectively (Van Cutsen et al 1989).

The management of patients with established liver metastases continues to attract a good deal of interest. Resection of solitary lesions (or certainly less than four) in one lobe can be carried out with a low morbidity and mortality and offers a realistic therapeutic option with 50–60% 2-year survivals (Holm et al 1989, Pinna Pintor et al 1989). However, such patients represent only approximately 5% of all patients with multiple colorectal liver metastases. New loco-regional approaches to this problem have been advocated but few are carefully assessed. Hunt & Taylor (1989) have critically reviewed the role of chemotherapy for both prophylaxis and treatment of liver metastases. In selected patients with less than 50% involvement, hepatic arterial chemotherapy with starch degradable microspheres may have a role. Such treatment has been advocated using either 5FU or mitomycin and promising results have emerged (Lorentz et al 1989). Nevertheless, further clinical trials to assess the optimal sequence and dosages are required. It is increasingly important to select specific treatments for individual patients and this should be based on, amongst other parameters, the percentage hepatic replacement with tumour.

Finally, anal carcinoma appears to be increasing in incidence and the management of this condition at St Marks Hospital between 1948–1984 has been reviewed (Pinna Pintor et al 1989). Prognosis depends on depth of invasion and the benefit of radiotherapy and particularly for locally invasive disease, is becoming increasingly established. As far as Bowen's disease of the anus is concerned local excision, often without skin grafting, is a reasonable approach if associated with a policy of careful follow-up.

Miscellaneous

The management of colorectal trauma is extremely difficult and continues to challenge surgeons. Trauma is either penetrating or blunt and always associated with severe peritoneal contamination and septic complications.

Two studies from the USA claim good results from contradictory policies. Orsay et al (1989) advocate 'no anastomosis' whereas George et al (1989) conclude that the majority of penetrating colon wounds can be repaired primarily or by resection and anastomosis regardless of risk factors. Many surgeons in the UK would favour measures which include, where possible, exteriorization of a segment.

Therapeutic colonoscopy is widening its horizons quite significantly. Novel uses include the balloon dilatation of colonic anastomotic strictures (Aston et al 1989), colonoscopic decompression in pseudo-obstruction (Martin et al 1988), and Nd-YAG laser photocoagulation for bleeding intestinal vascular abnormalities (Mathus-Vleigen 1989). Satisfactory results have been claimed for each of these innovations and surgeons should be aware of these therapeutic options in difficult selected patients.

Finally, major abdominal surgery (including colonic surgery) in the over-80s has been assessed in a prospective study (Palmer et al 1989). There is no doubt that this is associated with an increased mortality and increased post-operative dependency compared to similar surgery in 40–80-year-olds. This factor must be taken into account when deciding on treatment options in the elderly.

Colorectal haemorrhage

Rossini et al (1989) have reviewed their extensive experience of emergency colonoscopy in patients with active lower gastrointestinal bleeding. They were able to identify the site of bleeding in 80% of cases with a very low complication rate and treat the source of haemorrhage either by polypectomy (in 18 patients) or electrocoagulation (1 patient with angioma, 9 patients with angiodysplasia). They make a strong case, which many would agree with, for emergency colonoscopy being the first-choice examination in any patient with massive lower gastrointestinal bleeding. Trudel et al (1988) described very similar results in their series in which a diagnosis was established in 50% of patients and in 28 patients treated by endoscopic coagulation, 68% were controlled.

Another technique worthy of consideration in the difficult case is Technetium-99m red blood cell scintigraphy. Nicolson et al (1989) have described its use in 41 patients with major rectal bleeding. The red cells are labelled in vivo and serial scans taken with a large field gamma camera. A definite bleeding site was identified in 30 cases and red cell scintigraphy correctly localized 29 of these (sensitivity 97%). In the remaining 13 cases a bleeding site was not identified and there was 2 false positive scans (specificity 85%). Scintigraphy can detect bleeding rates of $0.05–0.1 \, \text{ml min}^{-1}$ and is particularly valuable for lesions which bleed either slowly or intermittently, e.g. colonic angiodysplasia.

Such techniques should reduce the need for 'blind' right hemicolectomy in colonic bleeding as recently advocated by Milewski & Schofield (1989).

Nevertheless, in their series of 14 patients, right hemicolectomy including the right half of the transverse colon resulted in a satisfactory outcome, although one patient re-bled at 11 months.

PANCREATICO-BILIARY DISEASE

Acute pancreatitis

Acute pancreatitis remains a major clinical problem even now associated with significant morbidity and mortality. Several studies have attempted to predict those patients most likely to develop severe pancreatitis.

The value of contrast enhanced abdominal CT scanning used prospectively in acute pancreatitis has been described in two studies by London et al (1989a, b). Highly significant differences were noted in pancreatic enhancement, peripancreatic tissue planes and indeed in pancreatic size between clinically severe and mild cases but these criteria did not add anything to standard prognostic indices (e.g. Glasgow criteria) for prediction of disease severity. The aetiology of the pancreatitis was inferred from 27% of admission scans. It is surely not justified to encourage serial CT scanning on all patients with acute pancreatitis. In selected cases—particularly if pancreatic necrosis or pseudocyst is suspected, and ultrasound is unhelpful, then CT scanning may be a valuable asset to management.

A number of biochemical tests have been investigated for prognostic value to predict and recognize disease severity. For example, serum phospholipase A2 activity has been performed during the first 6 days of admission (Bird et al 1989). Elevated initial activity correlated with clinical outcome and demonstrated a good agreement with the multiple prognostic criteria used to predict severe disease. Ten of 11 patients with raised activity had clinically severe disease.

Wilson et al (1989) have measured complement factors, antiproteases (α_2-macroglobulin and α_1-antiprotease), and C-reactive protein to determine the value of sequential measurement in prediction of outcome relative to clinical prognostic scoring systems. C-reactive protein was the best discriminator between mild and complicated attacks. It is also the simplest and quickest to perform. In effect a C-reactive protein of greater than $300\,\mathrm{mg\,l^{-1}}$ and which remains persistently elevated at the end of the first week provides a useful warning of the development of local pancreatic complications. It would appear reasonable to select out such patients for contrast-enhanced computed tomography and perhaps monitor such patients in an intensive care unit.

Finally, the APACHE-11 score has been assessed in acute pancreatitis. Larvin & McMahon (1989) demonstrated in 290 attacks of acute pancreatitis that outcome can be correctly predicted in 77% of attacks and identified 63% as severe compared to 44% achieved by clinical assessment.

The timing of surgical intervention in severe pancreatitis and deciding on the most effective procedure to perform have always been highly controversial issues. Kune & Brough (1989) reviewed the results of surgical intervention in a group of 476 consecutive patients with severe acute pancreatitis. The indications were laparotomy for diagnosis (77), excision of necrotic pancreas (7) and complications (18 pseudocysts, 53 pancreatic abscesses, 17 persistent obstructive jaundice and large bowel problems). There are several suggestions put forward from this experience but the main cause of mortality was pancreatic abscess formation and haemorrhage associated with them. All patients with pancreatic abscesses underwent laparotomy, necrosectomy, debridement of peripancreatic and retro-pancreatic slough and drainage of pus. Re-operation was required in 13% of patients and 19% of patients with a pancreatic abscess died.

Can such major complications of acute pancreatitis be avoided? Choi et al (1989) have reported a randomized prospective trial on the value of somatostatin. There were 36 patients randomized to receive somatostatin ($100\,\mu g\,hr^{-1}$ after a $250\,\mu g$ bolus for the first 2 days) and 35 randomized to control. Mortality in both groups was low but there was a tendency to fewer local complications in the somatostatin group (6 v 2 pancreatic inflammatory swellings).

The biliary tract

There are changing trends in surgery for benign gallbladder disease. Gutman et al (1988) has reported on 2181 consecutive cholecystectomies performed between 1969 and 1984. Over the years the population has become older, the proportion of males is increasing and there is an increasing incidence of diabetes. Periods of hospitalization have been reduced perhaps due to prophylactic antibiotics and anticoagulants.

Extracorporeal shock-wave lithotripsy may in due course alter the recommendations for cholecystectomy. Sackmann et al (1988) and Darzi et al (1989) have discussed their experience and indications for this form of treatment. Generally selection is limited to patients with symptomatic gallstone disease, with radiolucent stones of any size or number or radio-opaque stones less than 3 cm and a functioning gallbladder on oral cholecystography. Patients also receive a combination dissolution treatment comprising chenodeoxycholic and ursodeoxycholic acid. There are usually a maximum of six treatments at intervals of 2–3 weeks. Darzi et al (1989) reported a median time to clearance of stones of 7 months. The influence of subsequent oral dissolution therapy is probably critical and Sackmann et al (1988) noted that stones were completely cleared in only 30% of patients 2 months after lithotripsy compared with 93% at 18 months.

Ascending cholangitis is associated with significant morbidity. Treatment has altered in recent years but endoscopic drainage of the biliary system is a satisfactory approach. Leung et al (1989) have described results in 105 patients with acute calculous cholangitis who underwent urgent endoscopic drainage. Treatment was satisfactory in 102 (97%). Three of the patients in whom drainage was not successful underwent emergency surgery with one death. Despite successful endoscopic drainage three patients died of uncontrolled sepsis. It has been estimated that approximately 50% of patients with cholangitis develop septicaemia. In a randomized prospective study (Gerecht et al 1989) mezlocillin cured 83% of patients compared to 41% given gentamicin and ampicillin. There is a strong case for selecting mezlocillin or piperacillin in acute cholangitis.

Prophylactic antibiotics are still regarded as somewhat controversial by many surgeons. A study by Wells et al (1989) has demonstrated that a selective policy of prophylactic antibiotics solely to high-risk patients cannot be justified. Many studies have confirmed that prophylactic antibiotics should be given peri-operatively in all patients undergoing gallbladder surgery.

There are two other interesting topics which deserve mention. Ede et al (1989) report a useful technique in patients with inoperable cholangiocarcinoma. Fourteen patients were treated by the insertion of iridium-192 into a previously inserted endoscopic prosthesis and 9 have survived for a median period of 16.4 months.

The diagnosis of bile duct carcinoma can be extremely difficult. Okuda et al (1988) have compared and reviewed the available ongoing techniques in a series of 37 patients. Ultrasound and CT scan were most valuable. Percutaneous transhepatic cholangiography is more valuable than ERCP if the lesion is in the hilum or above. Magnetic Resonance Imaging is similar to CT but its value in the diagnosis of bile duct cancer was rather limited.

Finally, the management of patients with traumatic injury to the extrahepatic tract has been reviewed by Bade et al (1989). In essence, gallbladder stab wounds should be repaired if possible. Partial ductal transections can be managed by primary repair but complete transections should be dealt with by primary duct jejunal anastomosis. These recommendations are made on the basis of extensive experience of stab wounds in Durban.

LIVER DISEASE

The only real hope for long-term survival in patients with liver tumours is surgical resection. In patients with either localized primary hepatocellular carcinoma or solitary metastases (usually from primary colorectal cancer) resection should be considered. Brower et al (1989) have demonstrated the value of intra-operative ultrasound in both selection and assessment of resectability—especially in large tumours. The results of surgical resection of both primary and secondary tumours have been presented in a number of recent publications. Steele & Ravikumar (1989) have reviewed the literature with regard to outcome following resection of colorectal liver metastases. Between 20–25% of patients are cured and the operative mortality rate is less than 5%. Clearly careful selection is important and several prognostic factors are now recognized.

The actual size of a liver tumour does not necessarily preclude resection. Baer et al (1989) have suggested a simple classification of such tumours. 'Hanging' and 'pushing' tumours can be resected but infiltrating 'invasive' tumours usually cannot because of involvement of major vascular structures. Some authors also believe that several metastases should not be regarded as a contraindication to surgery (Minton et al 1989) although this is more controversial. Another poor prognostic group is patients with hepatocellular carcinoma and severe cirrhosis of the liver. Fujio et al (1989), however, have carried out resections in these patients preceeded by portal vein embolization, with possible survival benefit.

Other new techniques for patients with unresectable liver tumours which are showing some promise but require further evaluation include cryotherapy (Charnley et al 1989), repeated transient hepatic ischaemia for carcinoid tumours and pre-operative hepatic chemoembolization for hepatocelluar carcinoma (Nagasue et al 1989).

Variceal bleeding continues to pose major management problems. Factors predicting outcome both in surgical and non-surgical patients have been studied by Jacobs et al (1989). The initial prothrombin time ratio is very important. When greater than 2.2 it had a predictive power for death of 94% in 87 patients.

In an attempt to improve survival the role of prophylactic endoscopic sclerotherapy has been addressed by several groups. Most recently Potzi et al (1989) in a series of 87 patients demonstrated a tendency towards longer survival in patients with prophylactic sclerotherapy, particularly in those with alcoholic cirrhosis. Another non-surgical treatment worthy of comment is the use of oral propranolol. Kiire (1989) in a study of 50 patients with non-cirrhotic portal fibrosis showed a statistically significant reduction in gastrointestinal haemorrhage in patients receiving propranolol for 1 year.

In those patients who continue to bleed despite intensive medical treatment surgical intervention is indicated. Oesophageal transection and devascularization is a popular procedure. Al-Kraida et al (1989) have described the technique of oesophageal transection with gastro-oesophageal devascularization and splenectomy in 50 consecutive patients. In this group of patients with varices usually secondary to schistosomiasis and hepatitis B infection, a low operative mortality occurred and no recurrence of bleeding was recorded in patients surviving for follow-up periods of 2–3 years.

In patients with either extra-hepatic portal hypertension or the Budd-Chiari syndrome the traditional surgical procedures of shunting are of little value. Szczepanik & Rudowski (1989) have suggested that the former condition is best treated by repeated long-term sclerotherapy and Stringer et al (1989) have described a technique of mesoatrial shunt (in five patients) for the latter condition.

The indications for transplantation in alcoholic liver disease have been reviewed by Neuberger (1989). He concludes that it is reasonable to consider for transplantation patients with alcoholic hepatitis with no serious disease of other organs and no history of alcohol dependence.

Finally the management of bleeding varices in the elderly can be a particularly difficult condition to deal with. Hosking et al (1989) have compared the outcome of bleeding varices in patients aged under 65 with those over 65. Treatment was by active sclerotherapy and mortality due to the first bleed was dependent on severity of liver disease and was unrelated to age. Survival was 65% at 1 year and 60% at 2 years for both groups of patients. Accordingly, patients should not be denied active treatment for bleeding varices on the basis of age alone.

BREAST DISEASE

Benign disease

Benign breast disease comprises over 90% of the breast pathology seen by surgeons. One of the commonest complaints is mastalgia—both cyclical and non-cyclical. Maddox et al (1989) have suggested a classification and treatment protocol for the latter. Persistent symptoms respond to drug therapy (Danazol especially); musculoskeletal pain was relieved in over 90% of patients with injections of steroid and local anaesthetic.

Wilkinson et al (1989) have reviewed the outcome in 110 women under 35 with fibroadenomas. If not excised, these lesions often resolve. Cytology is absolutely essential to exclude malignancy if a conservative policy is followed. A period of greater than 12 months may be required for resolution and so it is simpler to remove the lump as a day case.

Breast cancer

With the introduction of a National Breast Screening Programme in the UK during 1989 there has been a significant proliferation of articles related to this aspect. Controversy still exists regarding the benefit of breast screening and recent views have been expressed from the experience in the USA (Shapiro 1989), Sweden (Holmberg et al 1989) and the UK (Forrest 1989). All these studies tend to suggest a benefit in reducing breast cancer mortality by up to 30%. However, other views would lend less support to cost/benefit analysis.

Surgeons should be involved in all aspects of screening assessment and particularly treatment. Localization biopsy of screen-detected impalpable lesions is a difficult technical exercise but is most important if in-situ lesions are to be adequately excised. Techniques for performing this have been described (Tate & Umpleby 1989) and the role of stereotactic fine needle biopsy in making accurate diagnoses has been assessed and shown to be effective (Azavedo et al 1989). Frisell et al (1989) have demonstrated from the Swedish experience that fine needle aspiration biopsy can reduce the rate of negative surgical biopsies by 90% in patients with uncertain mammograms without considerably impairing the reliability of the results.

The management of ductal carcinoma in-situ (DCIS) is still extremely controversial. Whether wide excision is sufficient for localizing DCIS is not entirely clear from a review of the literature and clinical trials assessing radiotherapy are required. Sector mastectomy or total mastectomy for multifocal DCIS is currently the treatment of choice, but again randomized trials are important in this regard. The management of residual tumour after biopsy can be a major problem (Wobbes et al 1989) and it is not certain that radiotherapy is an adequate treatment. Such patients frequently require either wider excision or mastectomy.

The primary treatment of breast cancer has always been uncertain. Conservative surgery can be safely offered to a high proportion of patients with localized breast cancer. This should be combined with breast irradiation to reduce the incidence of local recurrence. Reed & Morrison (1989) advocate wide local excision alone in the elderly with no significant effect of recurrence on survival because of the relatively high mortality rate from unrelated conditions. Others would suggest tamoxifen alone in this group or tamoxifen combined with local therapy (Leading article 1989).

Radiotherapy following surgery can be associated with problems which should be considered in patient management. Aitken et al (1989) have demonstrated reduced shoulder mobility in women receiving adjuvant radiology and Haybittle et al (1989) noted from the Cancer Research Campaign trial in Stage I and II disease that adjuvant radiotherapy after simple mastectomy for early breast cancer produces a small excess late mortality from other cancers and cardiac disease. It should be noted that survival from breast cancer was not initially improved by post-operative radiotherapy.

Recent overviews on the role of adjuvant therapy have been published (Early Breast Cancer Trialists Collaborative Group 1988) and indicate that tamoxifen is associated with a highly significant improvement in survival in women over 50 years of age whereas combination cytotoxic chemotherapy gave a reduction in the odds of death of 22% corresponding to a 9.3% higher survival at 5 years in younger women. These effects are not large but given the high prevalence of the disease, they are important. It should be noted, however, that a recent paper has suggested that in patients receiving tamoxifen a second breast cancer occurred less often but that endometrial cancer occurred more often than in controls (Fornander et al 1989).

Finally, several recent publications have addressed themselves to the question of stress (Ramirez et al 1989) in the overall management of patients with breast cancer. This aspect should be taken into account in the overall management of patients with breast cancer.

REFERENCES

Aitken R J, Gaze M N, Rodger A et al 1989 Arm morbidity within a trial of mastectomy and either nodal sample with selective radiotherapy or axillary clearance. Br J Surg 76: 568–571

Al-Kraida The late A, Qazi S A, Shaikh M U et al 1989 Transabdominal gastro-oesophageal devascularization and oesophageal transection for bleeding oesophageal varices. Br J Surg 76: 943–945

Allum W H, Powell D J, McConkey C C et al 1989a Gastric cancer: a 25 year review. Br J Surg 76: 535–540

Allum W H, Hallissey M T, Kelly Krystyna A 1989b Adjuvant chemotherapy in operable gastric cancer. 5 year follow-up of first British Stomach Cancer Group Trial. Lancet i: 571–574

Arnaud J-P, Buyse M, Nordlinger B et al 1989 Adjuvant therapy of poor prognosis colon cancer with levamisole: results of an EORTC double-blind randomised clinical trial. Br J Surg 76: 284–289

Aston N O, Owen W J, Irving J D 1989 Endoscopic balloon dilatation of colonic anastomotic strictures. Br J Surg 76: 780–782

Azavedo I, Svane G, Auer G 1989 Stereotactic fine-needle biopsy in 2594 mammographically detected non-palpable lesions. Lancet i: 1033–1036

Bade P G, Thomson S R, Hirshberg A et al 1989 Surgical options in traumatic injury to the extrahepatic biliary tract. Br J Surg 76: 256–258

Baer H U, Gertsch Ph, Matthews J B et al 1989 Resectability of large focal liver lesions. Br J Surg 76: 1042–1045

Ball A B S, Thomas P A, Evans S J 1989 Operative mortality after perforated peptic ulcer. Br J Surg 76: 521

Barillari P, de Angelis R, Valabrega S et al 1989 Relationship of symptom duration and survival in patients with colorectal carcinoma. Eur J Surg Oncol 15: 441–445

Barr H, Bown S G, Krasner N et al 1989 Photodynamic therapy for colorectal disease. Int J Colorect Dis 4: 15–19

Berne T V, Donovan A J 1989 Nonoperative treatment of perforated duodenal ulcer. Arch Surg 124: 830–832

Beynon J 1989 An evaluation of the role of rectal endosonography in rectal cancer. Ann R Coll Surg Engl 71: 131–139

Beynon J, Mortensen J J McC, Foy D M A et al 1989 Preoperative assessment of mesorectal lymph node involvement in rectal cancer. Br J Surg 76: 276–279

Bird N C, Goodman A J, Johnson A G 1989 Serum phospholipase A2 activity in acute pancreatitis: an early guide to severity. Br J Surg 76: 731–732

Brough W A, Schofield P F 1989 An improved technique of J pouch construction and ileoanal anastomosis. Br J Surg 76: 350–351

Brough W, Tweedle D 1989 An improved technique for oesophagojejunal anastomosis using the EEA Premium stapling gun. Ann R Coll Surg Engl 71: 322–323

Brower S T, Dumitrescu O, Rubinoff S et al 1989 Operative ultrasound establishes resectability of metastases by major hepatic resection. World J Surg 13: 649–657

Brunetaud J M, Maunoury V, Cochelard D et al 1989 Laser palliation for rectosigmoid cancers. Int J Colorect Dis 4: 6–8

Buyse M, Zeleniuch-Jacquotte Anne, Chalmers T C 1988 Adjuvant therapy of colorectal cancer. Why we still don't know. JAMA 259: 3571–3578

Canivet J-L, Damas P, Desaive C et al 1989 Operative mortality following surgery for colorectal cancer. Br J Surg 76: 745–747

Carty N J, Loizidou M, Taylor I 1989 The effect of syngeneic blood transfusion of chemically induced colon cancer in the rat. Surg Res Comm 7: 79–83

Charnley R M, Doran J, Morris D L 1989 Cryotherapy for liver metastases: a new approach. Br J Surg 76: 1040–1041

Choi T K, Mok F, Zhan W H et al 1989 Somatostatin in the treatment of acute pancreatitis: a prospective randomised controlled trial. Gut 30: 223–227

Cola B 1989 Inflammatory bowel disease and cancer. Int J Colorect Dis 4: 128–133

Csendes A, Braghetto I, Henriquez A et al 1989 Late results of a prospective randomised study comparing forceful dilatation and oesophagomyotomy in patients with achalasia. Gut 30: 299–304

Darzi A, Monson J R T, O'Morain C et al 1989 Extension of selection criteria for extracorporeal shock wave lightotripsy for gall stones. Br Med J 299: 302–303

Deakin M, Mayer D, Temple J G 1989 Surgery for gastro-oesophageal reflux: the Angelchik prosthesis compared to the floppy Nissen fundoplication. Two-year follow-up study and a five-year evaluation of the Angelchik prosthesis. Ann R Coll Surg Engl 71: 249–252

Dehn T C B, Kettlewell M G W, Mortensen N J McC et al 1989 Ten-year experience of strictureplasty for obstructive Crohn's disease. Br J Surg 76: 339–341

Domergue J, Rouanet P, Daures J B et al 1989 Multivariate analysis of prognostic factors for curative resectable rectal cancer. Eur J Surg Oncol 15: 93–98

Early Breast Cancer Trialists Collaborative Group 1988 Effects of adjuvant tamoxifen and of cytotoxic therapy on mortality in early breast cancer: an overview of 61 randomized trials amongst 28,896 women. New Engl J Med 319: 1681–1692

Ede R J, Williams S J, Hatfield A R W et al 1989 Endoscopic management of inoperable cholangiocarcinoma using iridium-192. Br J Surg 76: 867–869

Fornander T, Cedermark B, Mattsson A et al 1989 Adjuvant tamoxifen in early breast cancer: occurrence of new primary cancers. Lancet i: 117–120

Forrest A P M 1989 The surgeon's role in breast screening. World J Surg 13: 19–24

Fozard J B J, Dixon M F 1989 Colonoscopic surveillance in ulcerative colitis—dysplasia through the looking glass. Gut 30: 285–292

Frisell J, Eklund G, Nilsson et al 1989 Additional value of fine-needle aspiration in a mammographic screening trial. Br J Surg 76: 840–843

Fujio N, Sakai, Konoshita H et al 1989 Results of treatment of patients with hepatocellular carcinoma with severe cirrhosis of the liver. World J Surg 13: 211–218

George S M, Fabian T C, Voeller G R et al 1989 Primary repair of colon wounds. Ann Surg 209: 728–734

Gerard A, Buyse M, Nordlinger B et al 1988 Preoperative radiotherapy as adjuvant treatment in rectal cancer. Ann Surg 208: 606–614

Gerecht W B, Henry N K, Hoffman W W et al 1989 Prospective randomised comparison of mezlocillin therapy alone with combined ampicillin and gentamicin therapy for patients with cholangitis. Arch Intern Med 149: 1279–1284

Gouma D J 1989 Preoperative total parenteral nutrition in severe Crohn's disease. Surgery 103: 648–652

Granowska M, Jass J R, Britton K E et al 1989 A prospective study of the use of [III]In-labelled monoclonal antibody against carcinoembryonic antigen in colorectal cancer and of some biological factors affecting its uptake. Int J Colorect Dis 4: 97–108

Greenstein A J 1988 Perforating and nonperforating indications for repeated operations in Crohn's disease: evidence for two clinical forms. Gut 29: 588–592

Grundy A, Belli A 1988 Balloon dilatation of upper gastrointestinal tract strictures. Clin Radiol 39: 229–236

Gutman H, Kott I, Haddad M et al 1988 Changing trends in surgery for benign gallbladder disease. Am J Gastroenterol 83: 408–410

Hands L J, Papavramidis S, Bishop H et al 1989 The natural history of peptic oesophageal strictures treated by dilatation and antireflux therapy alone. Ann R Coll Surg Engl 71: 306–309

Hardcastle J D, Chamberlain J, Sheffield J et al 1989 Randomised controlled trial of faecal occult blood screening for colorectal cancer. Lancet i: 1160–1164

Haybittle J L, Brinkley D, Houghton J et al 1989 Postoperative radiotherapy and late mortality: evidence from the Cancer Research Campaign Trial for early breast cancer. Br Med J 298: 1611–1614

Heyen F, Ambrose N S, Allan R N et al 1989 Enterovesical fistulas in Crohn's disease. Ann R Coll Surg Engl 7: 101–104

Hoffman J, Rasmussen O O 1989 Aids in the diagnosis of acute appendicitis. Br J Surg 76: 774–779

Holm A, Bradley E, Aldrete J S 1989 Hepatic resection of metastasis from colorectal carcinoma. Ann Surg 209: 428–434

Holmberg L, Ponten J, Adami H-O 1989 The biology and natural history of breast cancer from the screening perspective. World J Surg 13: 25–30

Hosking S W, Bird N C, Johnson A G et al 1989 Management of bleeding varices in the elderly. Br Med J 298: 152–153

Hughes L E 1988 Local depot methylprednisolone injection for painful anal Crohn's disease. Gastroenterology 94: 709–711

Hunt T M, Taylor I 1989 The role of chemotherapy in the treatment and prophylaxis of colorectal liver metastases. Cancer Surveys 8: 72–90

Hunter J G, Becker J M, Lee R G et al 1989 Anterior lesser curvature laser seromyotomy with posterior truncal vagotomy: a potential treatment of peptic ulcer disease. Br J Surg 76: 949–952

Jacobs S, Chang R W S, Lee B et al 1989 Prediction of outcome in patients with acute variceal haemorrhage. Br J Surg 76: 123–126

Kiire C F 1989 Controlled trial of propranolol to prevent recurrent variceal bleeding in patients with non-cirrhotic portal fibrosis. Br Med J 298: 1363–1365

Kmiot W A, Keighley M R B 1989 Totally stapled abdominal restorative proctocolectomy. Br J Surg 76: 961–964

Krasner N 1989 Laser therapy in the management of benign and malignant tumours in the colon and rectum. Int J Colorect Dis 4: 2–5

Kune G A, Brough W 1989 Surgical intervention in severe acute pancreatitis: 476 cases in 20 years. Ann R Coll Surg Engl 71: 23–27

Larvin M, McMahon M J 1989 Apache II score for assessment and monitoring of acute pancreatitis. Lancet ii: 201–204

Leading article 1989 Colon Cancer: Molecular analysis marches on. Lancet i: 1236–1237

Leung J W C, Sung J J Y, Shunt S C S et al 1989 Urgent endoscopic drainage for acute suppurative cholangitis. Lancet i: 1307–1309

Lin H J et al 1988 Prospectively randomised trial of heat probe thermocoagulation v. pure alcohol injection in non-variceal peptic ulcer haemorrhage. Am J Gastroenterol 83: 283–286

London N J M, Neoptolemos J P, Lavelle J et al 1989a Serial computed tomography scanning in acute pancreatitis: a prospective study. Gut 30: 397–403

London N J M, Neoptolemos J P, Lavelle J et al 1989b Contrast-enhanced abdominal computed tomography scanning and prediction of severity of acute pancreatitis: a prospective study. Br J Surg 76: 268–272

Lorentz M, Herrman G, Kirkowa-Reimann M et al 1989 Temporary chemoembolization of colorectal liver metastases with degradable starch microspheres. Eur J Surg Oncol 15: 453–462

Lorentz T, Fok M, Wong J 1989 Anastomotic leakage after resection and bypass for oesophageal cancer: lessons learned from the past. World J Surg 13: 472–477

Maddox P R, Harrison B J, Mansel R E et al 1989 Non-cyclical mastalgia: an improved classification and treatment. Br J Surg 76: 901–904

Martin F M, Robinson A M, Thompson W R 1988 Therapeutic colonoscopy in the treatment of colonic pseudo-obstruction. Postgrad Med J 54: 519–523

Mathus-Vleigen E M H 1989 Laser treatment of intestinal vascular abnormalities. Int J Colorect Dis 4: 20–25

Mayberry J P, Ballantyne K C, Hardcastle J D et al 1989 Epidemiological study of asymptomatic inflammatory bowel disease: the identification of cases during a screening programme for colorectal cancer. Gut 30: 481–483

Mellow M H 1989 Endoscopic laser therapy in colorectal cancer. Int J Colorect Dis 4: 12–14

Milewski P, Schofield P F 1989 Massive colonic haemorrhage—the case for right hemicolectomy. Ann R Coll Surg Engl 71: 253–259

Minton J P, Hamilton W B, Sardi A et al 1989 Results of surgical excision of one to 13 hepatic metastases in 98 consecutive patients. Arch Surg 124: 46–49

Moertel L G, Fleming T R, McDonald J S et al 1990 Levamisole and flurouracil for adjuvant therapy of resected colon carcinoma. New Engl J Med 322: 352–358

Moore M, Jones D J, Schofield P F et al 1989 Current status of tumour markers in large bowel cancer. World J Surg 13: 52–59

Nagasue N, Galizia G, Kohno H et al 1989 Adverse effects of preoperative hepatic artery chemoembolization for resectable hepatocellular carcinoma: a retrospective comparison of 138 liver resections. Surgery 106: 81–86

Nakagawa K, Asaki S, Sato T 1989 Endoscopic treatment of bleeding peptic ulcers. World J Surg 13: 154–157

Neuberger J M 1989 Transplantation for alcoholic liver disease. Br Med J 299: 693–694

Nicolson M L, Neoptolemos J P, Charp J F et al 1989 Localization of lower gastrointestinal bleeding using in vivo technetium 99m-labelled red blood cell scintigraphy. Br J Surg 76: 358–361

Okuda K, Ohto M, Tsuchiya Y 1988 Role of ultrasound, percutaneous transhepatic cholangiography, CT and MRI in preoperative assessment of bile duct cancer. World J Surg 12: 18–26

Oresland T, Fasth S, Nordgren S et al 1989 The clinical and functional outcome after restorative proctocolectomy. A prospective study in 100 patients. Int J Colorect Dis 4: 50–56

Orsay C P, Merlotti G, Abcarian H et al 1989 Colorectal trauma. Dis Colon Rectum 32: 188–191

Palmer C A, Reece-Smith H, Taylor I 1989 Major abdominal surgery in the over-eighties. J R Soc Med 82: 391–393

Paterson I M, Wong J 1989 Anastomotic leakage: an avoidable complication of Lewis-Tanner oesophagectomy. Br J Surg 76: 127–129

Percivale P, Bertoglio S, Maggianu et al 1989 Long-term postoperative results in 54 cases of early gastric cancer: the choice of surgical procedure. Eur J Surg Oncol 15: 436–440

Pinna Pintor M, Northover J M A, Nicholls R J 1989 Squamous cell carcinoma of the anus at one hospital from 1948–1984. Br J Surg 76: 806–810

Potzi R, Bauer P, Reichel W et al 1989 Prophylactic endoscopic sclerotherapy of oesophageal varices in liver cirrhosis. A multicentre prospective controlled randomised trial in Vienna. Gut 30: 873–879

Pye G, Marks C G, Martin S et al 1989 An evaluation of Fecatwin/Feca EIA; a faecal occult blood test for detecting colonic neoplasia. Eur J Surg Oncol 15: 446–448

Ramirez Amanda J, Craig T K J, Watson J P et al 1989 Stress and relapse of breast cancer. Br Med J 298: 291–293

Reed M W R, Morrison J M 1989 Wide local excision as the sole primary treatment in elderly patients with carcinoma of the breast. Br J Surg 76: 898–900

Rossini F P, Ferrari A, Spandre M et al 1989 Emergency colonoscopy. World J Surg 71: 97–100

Rutgeerts P, Broeckaert L, Janssens J et al 1989 Comparison of endoscopic polidocanol injection and yag laser therapy for bleeding peptic ulcers. Lancet i: 1164–1166

Sackmann M, Delius M, Sauerbruch T et al 1988 Shock wave lithotripsy of gallbladder stones: the first 175 patients. New Engl J Med 318: 393–397

Sayfan J, Wilson D A L, Allan A et al 1989 Recurrence after strictureplasty or resection for Crohn's disease. Br J Surg 76: 335–338

Schein M, Gecelter G 1989 Apache II score in massive upper gastrointestinal haemorrhage from peptic ulcer: prognostic value and potential clinical applications. Br J Surg 76: 733–736

Serpell J W, McDermott F T, Katrivessis H et al 1989 Obstructing carcinomas of the colon. Br J Surg 76: 965–969

Shapiro S 1989 The status of breast cancer screening: a quarter of a century of research. World J Surg 13: 9–18

Shivananda A, Hordijk M I, Pena A S et al 1989 Crohn's disease: risk of recurrence and reoperation in a defined population. Gut 30: 990–995

Skipper D, Jeffrey M J, Cooper A J et al 1989 Enhanced growth of tumour cells in healing colonic anastomoses and laparotomy wounds. Int J Colorect Dis 4: 172–177

Steele G, Ravikumar T S 1989 Resection of hepatic metastases from colorectal cancer. Ann Surg 210: 127–138

Stephenson K R, Steinberg S M, Hughes D S et al 1988 Perioperative blood transfusions are associated with decreased time to recurrence and decreased survival after resection of colorectal liver metastases. Ann Surg 208: 679–687

Stringer M D, Howard E R, Green D W et al 1989 Mesoatrial shunt: a surgical option in the management of the Budd-Chiari syndrome. Br J Surg 76: 474–478

Svendsen L B, Sorensen C, Kjersgaard, Meisner S et al 1989 The influence of age upon the survival after curative operation for colorectal cancer. Int J Colorect Dis 4: 123–127

Szczepanik A B, Rudowski W J 1989 Extrahepatic portal hypertension: long-term results of surgical treatment. Ann R Coll Surg Engl 71: 222–225

Tate J J T, Umpleby H C 1989 Localization biopsy of the breast. Hospital Update 15: 69–72

Tate J J T, Rawlinson T, Royle G T et al 1988 Preoperative or postoperative colonic examination for synchronous lesions in colorectal cancer. Br J Surg 75: 1016–1019

Tate J J, Northway J, Royle G T, Taylor I 1989 Evaluation of a 'DIY' test for the detection of colorectal cancer. J R Soc Med 82: 388–390

Taylor T V 1989 Current indications for elective peptic ulcer surgery. Br J Surg 76: 427–428

Taylor T V, Knox R A, Pullan B 1989 Vertical gastric plication: an operation for gastro-oesophageal reflux. Ann R Coll Surg Engl 71: 31–36

Trudel J L, Fazio V W, Sivak M V 1988 Colonoscopic diagnosis and treatment of arteriovenous malformations in chronic lower gastrointestinal bleeding. Dis Colon Rectum 31: 107–110

Van Cutsem E, Boonen A, Geboes G et al 1989 Risk factors which determine the long term outcome of Neodymium-YAG laser palliation of colorectal carcinoma. Int J Colorect Dis 4: 9–11

Vente J P, Wiggers T H, Weidema W F et al 1989 Peri-operative blood transfusions in colorectal cancer. Eur J Surg Oncol 15: 371–374

Walther B S, Zilling T, Johnsson F et al 1989 Total gastrectomy and oesophagojejunostomy with linear stapling devices. Br J Surg 76: 909–912

Wells G R, Taylor E W, Lindsay G et al 1989 Relationship between bile colonization, high risk factors and postoperative sepsis in patients undergoing biliary tract operations while receiving a prophylactic antibiotic. Br J Surg 76: 374–377

Wilkinson S, Anderson T J, Rifkind E et al 1989 Fibroadenoma of the breast: a follow-up of conservative management. Br J Surg 76: 390–391

Williams N S 1989 Stapling technique for pouch anal anastomosis without the need for purse-string sutures. Br J Surg 76: 348–349

Williams J G, Hughes L E 1989 Effect of perioperative blood transfusion on recurrence of Crohn's disease. Lancet ii: 131–133

Wilson C, Heads A, Shenkin A et al 1989 C-reactive protein, antiproteases and complement factors as objective markers of severity in acute pancreatitis. Br J Surg 76: 177–181

Wobbes Th, Tinnemans J G M, van der Sluis R F 1989 Residual tumour after biopsy for non-palpable ductal carcinoma in situ of the breast. Br J Surg 76: 185–186

Index

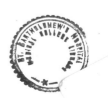